T0213844

Lecture Notes in Computer Science   **9638**

Commenced Publication in 1973
Founding and Former Series Editors:
Gerhard Goos, Juris Hartmanis, and Jan van Leeuwen

More information about this series at http://www.springer.com/series/7409

Alexander Meschtscherjakov
Boris De Ruyter · Verena Fuchsberger
Martin Murer · Manfred Tscheligi (Eds.)

Persuasive Technology

11th International Conference, PERSUASIVE 2016
Salzburg, Austria, April 5–7, 2016
Proceedings

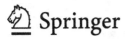 Springer

Editors

Alexander Meschtscherjakov
University of Salzburg
Salzburg
Austria

Boris De Ruyter
Philips Research Europe
Eindhoven
The Netherlands

Verena Fuchsberger
University of Salzburg
Salzburg
Austria

Martin Murer
University of Salzburg
Salzburg
Austria

Manfred Tscheligi
University of Salzburg
Salzburg
Austria

and

Austrian Institute of Technology
Vienna
Austria

ISSN 0302-9743   ISSN 1611-3349   (electronic)
Lecture Notes in Computer Science
ISBN 978-3-319-31509-6   ISBN 978-3-319-31510-2   (eBook)
DOI 10.1007/978-3-319-31510-2

Library of Congress Control Number: 2016933467

LNCS Sublibrary: SL3 – Information Systems and Applications, incl. Internet/Web, and HCI

Printed on acid-free paper

This Springer imprint is published by Springer Nature
The registered company is Springer International Publishing AG Switzerland

Preface

Persuasive Technology is a vibrant and highly interdisciplinary research field that focuses on the design, development, and evaluation of interactive technologies with the aim of changing users' attitudes and behaviors. Attitude and behavior change is achieved by means of persuasive strategies, such as social influences embodied in the design of interactive technologies, without any coercion or deception. Persuasive technologies are used to change people's behavior in various domains such as healthcare, sustainability, education, or marketing.

PERSUASIVE, the International Conference on Persuasive Technology, is the leading venue for ground-breaking research and novel designs of persuasive technologies. It is the annual conference in which to discuss the latest persuasive theories, strategies, applications, and artifacts with academics and practitioners from all over the world. Over the past decade the conference was held at exciting places such as Chicago, Padua, Sydney, Linköping, Columbus, Copenhagen, Claremont, Oulu, Palo Alto, and Eindhoven.

PERSUASIVE 2016 was the 11th edition of the conference and took place in April 2016 in Salzburg, Austria. The conference theme was "Contextual Persuasion: Supporting Life Situations and Challenges by Persuasive Design." With this conference theme, the ubiquity and situatedness of persuasive interactions was emphasized: How are interactions with persuasive technologies influenced and facilitated by spatial, temporal, social, or individual conditions and characteristics? How can we analyze, design, and evaluate for specific contexts or conditions?

On April 4, a Doctoral Consortium, a tutorial on "Mobile Persuasion Design," and a Persuasive Game Jam were held as part of the pre-conference program. On April 5, seven half-day workshops were held. On April 6 and 7, the main conference was held in seven single-track sessions, including oral presentations of accepted short and long papers, as well as a poster and demo session during which accepted work-in-progress and demonstrations were presented. It also included an opening keynote by Mark Aloia, Global Lead for Behavior Change at Philips HealthTech, and a closing keynote by Cees Midden, Professor of Human–Technology Interaction at Eindhoven University of Technology.

This volume contains the accepted short and long papers presented during the main track. Overall, 73 papers were submitted (59 long papers with a maximum length of 12 pages and 14 short papers with a maximum length of 6 pages) with 197 authors from more than 20 countries from Asia, Australia, Europe, North and South America.

Papers were selected for presentation at the conference after a thorough peer-review process. The submitted papers were reviewed by experts in the field of persuasive technologies in a double-blinded review process. Overall, 63 reviewers were randomly (excluding any conflict of interest) assigned to the papers. They provided a detailed textual review of the assigned paper and rated each paper, leading to a ranking of the papers. The Program Committee chairs examined the papers and their reviews and compiled the final list of papers to be presented at the conference.

From the 73 submitted papers, 30 were accepted, yielding an acceptance rate of 41.1 %. From the 59 long papers submitted, 27 were accepted (i.e., acceptance rate of 45.8 %). From the 14 submitted, three were accepted (i.e., acceptance rate of 21.4 %).

In addition to the papers presented in this volume, the conference also published adjunct proceedings, which included the accepted work-in-progress submissions to the posters track, the accepted demo submissions to the demos track, the accepted position papers to the doctoral consortium, as well as a description of the seven workshops:

- User Experience Design for Persuasion and Behavior Change
- Empowering Cities for Sustainable Well-Being
- The Challenge of Device Overload: Using the Persuasive Framework to Effectively Use Modern Technologies to Encourage Health-Promoting Behaviors
- Where Are We Bound for? Persuasion in Transport Applications
- Persuasive Designs for Learning – Learning in Persuasive Design
- Behavior Change Support Systems (BCSS 2016): Epic for Change, the Pillars for Persuasive Technology for Smart Societies
- Personalization in Persuasive Technology Workshop

To make this conference a success, a great number of people supported in various ways. We would like to thank the authors for their high-quality contributions, and the reviewers for their valuable feedback. Furthermore, we would like to express our appreciation to the organizational and scientific committees, who took care of the workshops, tutorials, doctoral consortium, posters, demos and showcases, the game jam, and the main conference.

April 2016

Alexander Meschtscherjakov
Boris De Ruyter
Verena Fuchsberger
Martin Murer
Manfred Tscheligi

Organization

General Chair

Manfred Tscheligi   University of Salzburg and Austrian Institute
of Technology, Austria

Program Chairs

Boris De Ruyter   Philips Research, The Netherlands
Alexander   University of Salzburg, Austria
  Meschtscherjakov

Organizational Chairs

Verena Fuchsberger   University of Salzburg, Austria
Martin Murer   University of Salzburg, Austria
Alexander   University of Salzburg, Austria
  Meschtscherjakov

Poster Chairs

Alexandra Millonig   Austrian Institute of Technology, Austria
Rita Orji   McGill University, Canada

Demo and Showcase Chairs

Marc Busch   Austrian Institute of Technology, Austria
Margaret Morris   Intel, USA

Doctoral Consortium Chairs

Jaap Ham   Eindhoven University of Technology, The Netherlands
Cees Midden   Eindhoven University of Technology, The Netherlands
Luciano Gamberini   University of Padua, Italy

Workshop Chairs

Maurits Kaptein   Tilburg University, The Netherlands
Peter Fröhlich   Austrian Institute of Technology, Austria

Persuasive [Game] Design Jam Chairs

Bernhard Maurer   University of Salzburg, Austria
Agnis Stibe   MIT Media Lab, USA

Tutorial Chair

Harri Oinas-Kukkonen   University of Oulu, Finland

Social Media Chair

Agnis Stibe   MIT Media Lab, USA

Local Arrangements

Carina Bachinger   University of Salzburg, Austria
Kristina Karl   University of Salzburg, Austria
Alexandra Leitner   University of Salzburg, Austria

Scientific Committee

Magnus Bang   Linkoping University, Sweden
Shlomo Berkovsky   CSIRO, Australia
Robert Biddle   Carleton University, Canada
Marc Busch   Austrian Institute of Technology, Austria
Cheryl Campanella Bracken   Cleveland State University, USA
Samir Chatterjee   Claremont Graduate University, USA
Luca Chittaro   HCI Lab, University of Udine, Italy
Janet Davis   Whitman College, USA
Berardina De Carolis   University of Bari, Italy
Boris De Ruyter   Philips Research, The Netherlands
Peter De Vries   University of Twente, The Netherlands
Sebastian Egger   Austrian Institute of Technology, Austria
Alexander Felfernig   Graz University of Technology, Austria
BJ Fogg   Stanford University, USA
Jill Freyne   CSIRO, Australia
Peter Fröhlich   Austrian Institute of Technology, Austria
Verena Fuchsberger   University of Salzburg, Austria
Luciano Gamberini   University of Padua, Italy
Mark Gilzenrat   CNN Digital, USA
Manuel Giuliani   University of Salzburg, Austria
Thomas Grah   University of Salzburg, Austria
Ulrike Gretzel   University of Queensland, Australia
Marco Guerini   FBK_Irst, Italy
Magdalena Gärtner   University of Salzburg, Austria
Jaap Ham   Eindhoven University of Technology, The Netherlands

Steering Committee

Harri Oinas-Kukkonen	University of Oulu, Finland
Magnus Bang	Linkoping University, Sweden
Shlomo Berkovsky	CSIRO, Australia
Samir Chatterjee	Claremont Graduate University, USA
BJ Fogg	Stanford University, USA
Peter Hasle	Aalborg University, Denmark
Cees Midden	Eindhoven University of Technology, The Netherlands

Sponsors

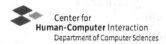

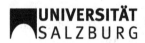

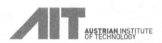

Contents

Methods and Models

Games and Gamification

Interventions for Behavior Change

Design Strategies and Techniques

Individual Differences

Tailoring Web Pages for Persuasion on Prevention Topics: Message Framing, Color Priming, and Gender

Luca Chittaro[✉]

Human-Computer Interaction Lab, University of Udine, via delle Scienze 206, 33100 Udine, Italy
luca.chittaro@uniud.it
http://hcilab.uniud.it

Abstract. On the Web, as in more traditional influence contexts, the most effective persuasive strategies often depend on the individual characteristics of the message recipient. Unfortunately, most persuasive technology applications currently employ a one-size-fits-all approach to interventions. The study we illustrate investigates two different techniques (message framing and color priming) that can be used in tailoring a persuasive Web page about a prevention topic. The findings of our study highlight interactive effects between message framing and color priming, and advance the results in the literature by showing that red enhances the effects of framing in a gender-based fashion. The obtained results also provide practical guidance for automatic tailoring of persuasive Web pages about prevention topics, suggesting a strategy based on gender, an information about the user that is typically readily available in social network profiles, and other Web sites to which people register.

Keywords: Tailoring · Web pages · Color priming · Message framing · Gender differences · Prevention · Health · Safety · Persuasive technology

1 Introduction

Individual characteristics of the message recipient often affect the effectiveness of persuasive strategies on the Web as well as in other influence contexts. Unfortunately, most persuasive technology applications currently employ a one-size-fits-all approach to interventions, failing to deliver tailored persuasion that leverages user's characteristics [1]. In particular, Web audiences are large and heterogeneous, and influencing them with a one-size-fits-all intervention is difficult.

Software systems that are able to tailor content and presentation of Web pages based on a user's profile exist–see [2] for a review – and could be used for tailoring Web-based persuasive interventions. However, these tailoring systems need to be programmed with proper rules to deliver the most effective content and presentation based on user's characteristics. In persuasive interventions, the definition of such rules should be guided by theoretical frameworks of persuasion, and needs to be supported by studies of how different people are affected by different versions of a Web page.

© Springer International Publishing Switzerland 2016
A. Meschtscherjakov et al. (Eds.): PERSUASIVE 2016, LNCS 9638, pp. 3–14, 2016.
DOI: 10.1007/978-3-319-31510-2_1

Two important features of Web pages that could affect their effectiveness are the framing of the message contained in the page (for example, a message about health can be framed in terms of gain or loss associated with following or not the recommended behavior [28]), and the colors used by the page (for example, different background colors of a Web page can prime different attributes related to its content, influencing viewers [22]). The study in this paper focuses on both persuasion techniques (message framing and color priming), exploring how they could be exploited in tailoring a persuasive Web page. More specifically, the purpose of the paper is to (i) investigate message framing and color priming in Web pages that deal with prevention topics, (ii) study possible gender differences in users' susceptibility to the considered techniques, which could be very important for automatically tailoring Web pages based on gender as an individual user's characteristic, (iii) derive possible design guidance for tailoring Web interventions on prevention topics.

2   Related Work

A persuasive message can be framed in terms of the benefit (gain) or cost (loss) associated with adopting or not its recommendation. Several studies have shown that loss and gain frames affect people's attitudes and behavior in a different way even when they describe objectively equivalent situations, see [19, 27, 28] for reviews. In particular, the effects of framing can change with the addressed type of behavior, with gain framing being more effective when the message is a prevention recommendation (e.g., sun screen use, physical exercise, vaccinations,...), and loss framing more effective when it is a detection recommendation (e.g., checkups, breast self-exam, HIV testing,...).

However, most studies did not consider gender as a possible individual difference that may affect the influence of loss or gain framing on message recipients, see [19]. The few studies which considered gender in health communication (e.g., about sunscreen [27] and condoms [18] to prevent health risks) or in other domains (e.g., filling honestly the tax return to prevent risks such as fines, penalties and jail sentences [16]) suggest that gain framing could be more effective with women, while men could be more sensitive to loss framing. It is also worth noting that Fagley and Miller [10, 11], who studied gender differences in risky decision problems, go as far as saying that framing experiments which do not address possible gender effects may simply reflect the gender that predominates in the sample and be uninterpretable.

Another important feature of Web pages that can affect users is color. Research on color priming has investigated effects of color on different aspects of cognition and behavior, e.g. [7–9, 14, 23]. A study about Web persuasion was proposed by [22], who considered simple Web pages containing a product description and showed how background color can influence consumers. Participants who examined a car description on a Web page with a red and orange flame-like background were later more likely to mention safety as an important attribute for buying a car than participants who were exposed to a different (green) background, showing that red can help in priming safety. One of the color priming studies conducted by [23] focused specifically on prevention aspects. Participants read descriptions of three pairs of brands on a computer screen and then reported their brand preferences. Within each pair, one brand highlighted a negative outcome people try to avoid, whereas the other brand highlighted a positive outcome people try to approach. For example, one of the pairs concerned toothpaste, with brand A particularly good for cavity prevention and brand B particularly good for tooth whitening. Across the three pairs, a red background increased preference for the brand that emphasized prevention. After ruling out mood as an alternative explanation with a post-hoc study, the study concluded that a red background contributes to activating avoidance motivation.

Gerend and Sias [13] investigated color priming together with message framing in persuasion about preventive behavior. In particular, the study concerned printed materials (a red or grey leaflet recommending a vaccination), in which the message was presented as either loss-framed or gain-framed. The results showed an interaction between color priming and message framing: loss framing was more effective but only when primed with red. Participants in this study were all male (a limitation that is acknowledged by its authors), and this could explain why the sample was more sensitive to the loss frame. The fact that red enhanced the effect of loss framing is consistent with the increase in risk avoidance motivation pointed out by [23] and with the role of red as a safety prime found by [22]. Moreover, Gerend and Sias [13] suggest that the enhancing interactive effect of color red could originate from the fact that red primes threat via associations with blood and danger, and acts as a peripheral threat cue that affects processing of persuasive health messages. More generally, other authors point out that red, as the single color most commonly associated with danger [34], has been shown to make people more vigilant [23], and the amount of attention directed to the message is an important aspect for the success of a persuasive intervention. Both perspectives would be consistent with the activation of a recently postulated "human alarm system" [6], a psychological system that people use to detect and handle threatening cues and, when activated, prompts people to process more alertly what is going on (for a discussion of the human alarm system, and some of its effects on judgment see [32]).

3   Method

The goal of our study was to advance the investigation of message framing and color priming in Web pages for prevention topics, aiming at deriving possible guidance for tailored persuasion based on gender.

We considered fires as a prevention domain of interest for their social relevance, e.g. in 2014, in the US alone, 19'050 civilians were hurt (3,275 dead, 15,775 injured) as the result of fires [17], with home fires accounting for 84 % of the death toll, and a fire occurring every 86 s in the country. Adjusting for population, the fire death rate of some former USSR countries such as Russia, Latvia, and Estonia, is about ten times higher than the fire death rate of the US [5]. Fire risks are thus an important worldwide safety issue, and also a public health issue because they lead to hospitalizations of survivors, who can suffer long-term or even lifelong health consequences.

Current approaches to foster awareness of personal fire safety on the Web have explored the creation of different pages based on a two-groups age segmentation, producing a version of the Web site devoted to children, e.g. [24, 30], and one to adults, e.g. [25, 31]. Web pages targeted at adults currently follow a one-size fits all approach that uses the same messages for all visitors.

The study in this paper explores if tailoring message framing and color in this kind of Web pages could increase their effectiveness. Among the topics dealt with by fire prevention campaigns, the described experiment focuses on domestic smoke alarms, a preventive measure that significantly increases occupants' chances of surviving a deadly home fire [25, 31].

3.1   Design, Participants, and Hypotheses

We followed a between-groups design in which participants read a Web page about fire prevention that stressed the importance of having smoke alarms in houses. The textual message of the Web page was either gain- or loss-framed. More specifically, the message in the loss-framed (respectively, gain-framed) version of the Web page pertained how many people die (could be saved) every year if fires were prevented, the negative effects of noticing late a fire in the house (the positive effects of noticing early a fire in the house), the negative effects of the lack of smoke alarms in the house (the positive effects of the presence of smoke alarms in the house). Table 1 compares the two versions of the message, highlighting the parts that differ.

The study was conducted on a sample of 126 (65 male, 61 female) non-colorblind participants, recruited at the university library or through personal contact. They were volunteer undergraduate, graduate and doctoral students enrolled in different programs (Agricultural Science, Business Administration, Computer Science, Foreign Languages, Engineering, Literature,…), and people from other occupations who received no compensation. Age ranged from 19 to 38 (M = 25.3, SD = 4.0).

Participants were told that the purpose of the study was to evaluate a Web page. They first filled a short demographic questionnaire. Then, they read the Web page assigned to them on a computer screen. No interaction with the computer keyboard or mouse was required to read the page. Color priming was manipulated by making the background and the two uppercase section titles in the Web page either red or grey, equated on value (the relative lightness versus darkness of a color). As a result, four versions of the Web page were created (gain-framed with red or grey, loss-framed with red or grey), and each participant read one of the four pages. In all versions of the Web page, the text paragraphs were contained in a rectangular white area and were displayed in black lettering over the white area to maximize readability. The rectangular white area was placed over the red or grey background that filled the page, and its size and position did not change. The only factors that changed were message frame (gain, loss) and color prime (red, grey) as already described above. The Web page did not contain any other text (e.g., menus, links, copyright,…). After examining it, participants were asked about their:

Table 1. Gain- and loss-framed message. For reader's convenience, the section titles and the text paragraphs in the message are an English translation of the original (non-English) ones, and we have highlighted differences between the gain- and loss-framed versions in italic.

Gain-Framed Version	Loss-Framed Version
HOME FIRES	HOME FIRES
Fire has always been a leading cause of accidental death. Just think that *if there were no* fires in buildings, more than 5000 people a year *would be saved* in Europe alone.	Fire has always been a leading cause of accidental death. Just think that *because of* fires in buildings, more than 5000 people a year *die* in Europe alone.
Homes are particularly exposed to the possibility of fire, due to a relevant concentration of electrical devices, sources of heat and flammable materials.	Homes are particularly exposed to the possibility of fire, due to a relevant concentration of electrical devices, sources of heat and flammable materials.
Several studies show that in common home environments, *detecting early* the presence of a fire *can help prevent reaching* conditions of non-sustainability (that is, the death of people).	Several studies show that in common home environments, *detecting late* the presence of a fire *can put at risk of reaching* conditions of non-sustainability (that is, the death of people).
Fortunately, many families *saved their lives* because they *did install* an important safety feature in their homes: smoke alarms.	*Unfortunately*, many families *lost their lives* because they *did not install* an important safety feature in their homes: smoke alarms.
With smoke alarms, you *are warned* that smoke is entering your bedroom while you are sleeping: in this way, you wake up *in time*, when *it is still possible* to escape from the building.	*Without* smoke alarms, you *are not warned* that smoke is entering your bedroom while you are sleeping: in this way, you wake up *too late*, when *it is not anymore possible* to escape from the building.
The causes of a fire can be very common and trivial: a short circuit in an electrical appliance, a cigarette left burning on an ashtray, a cloth over a lit lamp,... *The presence* of a smoke alarm *allows* us to detect these events early and *frees us from* a deadly trap.	The causes of a fire can be very common and trivial: a short circuit in an electrical appliance, a cigarette left burning on an ashtray, a cloth over a lit lamp,... *The absence* of a smoke alarm *does not allow* us to detect these events early and *imprisons us in* a deadly trap.
THE SOLUTION IS SIMPLE	THE SOLUTION IS SIMPLE
Fire alarms are cheap and easy to install. It is advisable to install a smoke alarm outside each bedroom or sleeping area of the house. If you live in a multi-story home, you need to install a smoke alarm on each floor.	Fire alarms are cheap and easy to install. It is advisable to install a smoke alarm outside each bedroom or sleeping area of the house. If you live in a multi-story home, you need to install a smoke alarm on each floor.

- Perceived level of attention and alertness to the Web page. We were interested in assessing this aspect because, in general, when a persuasive attempt employs textual messages, it is fundamental that the user attentively reads the information contained in them. Moreover, in this study, it is important to assess if and when the threatening cue (color red) is actually able to increase the level of attention and alertness as the color priming literature would suggest it is able to.

• Attitudes towards the specific prevention solution (smoke alarms) recommended by the page. We particularly focused on beliefs concerning the effectiveness of the recommended solution (response efficacy), because a broad array of theoretical perspectives – see [12, 26, 28, 33] for thorough discussions - suggests that perceived response efficacy is an important predictor of the likelihood of the recommended behavior being carried out by the message recipient.

Based on the previously surveyed literature on color priming, which has shown the general role of red in increasing vigilance and priming safety, and the specific study [13] which has shown (on a male sample) that the enhancing effect of red on persuasion shows itself with the loss frame (to which men are likely more sensitive), we hypothesized that we were going to obtain a similar result with men in our study. However, since our study extends the investigation to women, who are likely more sensitive to the gain frame, we hypothesized that we were going to obtain the best results in terms of attention and persuasion with women through the gain frame, enhanced by the general role of red mentioned above.

3.2   Measures

To measure the level of attention and alertness, we employed the items used in [32]. We asked participants whether the Web page led them to be alert *(1 = very weakly, 7 = very strongly)* and to be attentive *(1 = very weakly, 7 = very strongly)*, and their answers to the two items were averaged to form a reliable scale of participants' alertness (Cronbach's alpha = .78).

   To measure participants' attitudes towards the recommended prevention solution, we used three questions that respectively asked how useful, important, and effective is to have smoke alarms in houses. Answers were given on a 7-point Likert scale *(1 = not at all, 7 = a lot)*, and were averaged to form a reliable scale of perceived response efficacy (Cronbach's alpha = .92).

4   Results

We conducted a three-way ANOVA with framing (loss, gain), color priming (red, gray), and gender (male, female) as factors. The results of the analysis yielded:

• for attention, a main effect of gender, $F(1,118) = 10.17$, $p < .01$, $\eta_p^2 = .079$, and an interaction among all three factors, $F(1,118) = 10.53$, $p < .01$, $\eta_p^2 = .082$;
• for response efficacy, a main effect of gender, $F(1,118) = 5.24$, $p = .024$, $\eta_p^2 = .042$, and an interaction among all three factors, $F(1,118) = 5.94$, $p = .016$, $\eta_p^2 = .048$.

Since a triple interaction among the independent variables characterized attention as well as perceived response efficacy, we followed a standard unfolding procedure to determine its meaning, by computing separately subsidiary two-way ANOVAs. Unfolding of the triple interaction for attention (see Fig. 1) showed that, in men, color red generated more attention with loss (M = 4.97, SD = 1.66) rather than gain framing (M = 3.35, SD = 1.14), $F(1,28) = 9.08$, $p < .01$, $\eta_p^2 = .25$, and the gain frame generated less attention when coupled with red (M = 3.35, SD = 1.14) rather than grey (M = 4.22, SD = 1.15), $F(1,29) = 4.39$, $p = .045$, $\eta_p^2 = .13$. On the contrary, in women, it was the gain frame that generated more attention when coupled with red (M = 5.33, SD = 1.05) rather than grey (M = 4.37, SD = 1.33), $F(1,28) = 4.90$, $p = .035$, $\eta_p^2 = .15$. Finally, the difference in attention between women and men was statistically significant only for the gain frame enhanced with red, with higher attention elicited in women (M = 5.33, SD = 1.05) rather than men (M = 3.35, SD = 1.14), $F(1,26) = 23.95$, $p < .001$, $\eta_p^2 = .47$.

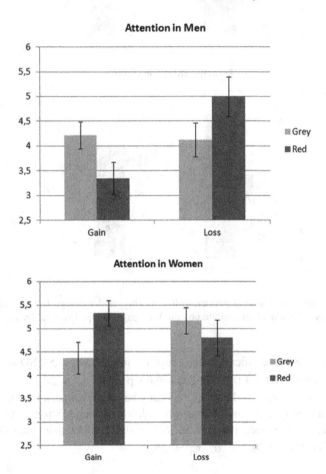

Fig. 1. Triple interaction among gender, color priming, and message framing on attention elicited by the Web page. Capped vertical bars denote ± 1 SE (Color figure online).

Unfolding of the triple interaction for response efficacy (see Fig. 2) revealed no statistically significant differences in men, while in women the gain frame produced

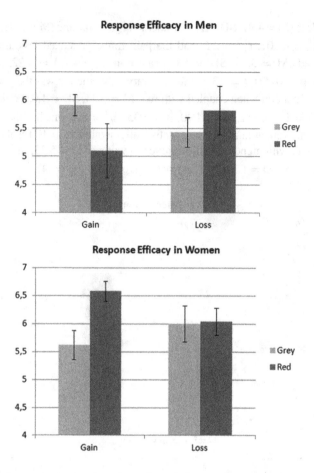

Fig. 2. Triple interaction among gender, color priming, and message framing on perceived response efficacy of smoke alarms elicited by the Web page. Capped vertical bars ± 1 SE (Color figure online).

higher perceived response efficacy when coupled with red (M = 6.58, SD = 0.71) rather than grey (M = 5.62, SD = 1.01), F(1,28) = 9.05, p < .01, η_p^2 = .24.

The difference in perceived response efficacy between women and men was statistically significant only in the gain frame with red, which elicited stronger perception of response efficacy in women (M = 6.58, SD = 0.71) rather than men (M = 5.10, SD = 1.73), F(1,26) = 9.20, p < .01, η_p^2 = .26.

5   Discussion

The results for attention and response efficacy confirmed our expectation that the effects on women and men were going to differ, and better results were in general going to be obtained by employing a gain frame strategy with women and a loss frame strategy with men, enhancing it with red color priming in both cases.

The finding that, for male participants, loss framing was more effective in eliciting attention but only when primed with red is consistent with and reinforces the results of the previously mentioned study by Gerend and Sias [13] of a male-only sample that read printed materials about a vaccination. In particular, the pattern suggested by the charts concerning men in Fig. 1 (and also in Fig. 2) is remarkably similar to the one found in that study when they measured the effectiveness of their persuasive message. However, to the best of our knowledge, our study is the first to extend the investigation of the interactive effects of message framing and color priming to women, showing that a different pattern characterizes women, with gain framing (instead of loss framing) primed with red as the possible strategy of choice.

Our results contribute evidence to what has been suggested (but not extensively studied in different conditions and domains) by some authors in the literature (see Sect. 2), i.e. that in communication about prevention topics a gain framing strategy could be more effective with women, while men could be more sensitive to loss framing. However, our study suggests that for this difference to become significant, the persuasive intervention may have to enhance the framing of the textual message with further stimuli. In our case, the additional stimulus was a peripheral threat cue (red color in the page). An interesting consideration concerns how a subtle cue (such as page color) peripheral to the information being processed can actually have considerable effects. Previous research on Web pages had shown that different choices of background color can change the perception of Web page loading time [15], can influence final scores on general knowledge tests conducted through Web pages [14] or influence users into considering some features of a product description more important than others [22]. In our study, color priming was instead effective in amplifying the effects of a persuasive framing strategy in terms of attention obtained by the Web page and elicited perception of efficacy of the recommendation made by the Web page. Taken together, these different studies highlight how the design of persuasive Web pages should be very careful and grounded on persuasion research, even for those peripheral page features such as background color that are typically dealt with only from the point of view of usability (e.g., readability of information) and aesthetics (e.g., pleasant and coherent color schemes).

It is worth remembering that color priming is context-dependent: while red activates avoidance motivation [23] when associated with safety topics, it can have different effects in other contexts, e.g. in interpersonal relationships it can enhance male (physical and sexual) attraction towards a woman [9] instead of avoidance motivation. One should thus be careful in trying to generalize the results of our experiment outside the context of messages about risk prevention.

On a practical level, our findings indicate that gender-based tailoring of Web pages in persuasive interventions concerning prevention topics can be effective. The versions of the Web page we tested produced different results in participants, based on their gender. For an automated system that has access to gender information, e.g. most applications in social networks, it would be very easy to present the user with the version of the Web page that maximizes the desired effects.

As a final consideration, a limitation of the study might involve cultural aspects: the meaning attributed by people to colors can be culture-dependent (e.g., in some cultures black is the color of mourning, while in others it is white) and our experiment involved only a European sample. However, our finding on color concerned red, whose impact is supposed to be universal [7].

6   Conclusions

This paper explored the effectiveness of a loss frame versus a gain frame strategy in formulating a persuasive message for a Web page that included either a grey or red color prime. We focused on possible gender differences that could provide design guidance for rules that drive automated systems for Web page tailoring.

First, the results of the study support the idea of gender-based tailoring of Web pages in persuasive attempts concerning prevention topics: the most effective conditions were different between men and women.

Second, it confirms gender differences in the effectiveness of message framing hypothesized in the literature [16, 18, 27]: gain framing was the best strategy for female users, while loss framing could be more suited to male users.

Third, it confirms the interactive effects between message framing and color priming obtained in the literature with men [13], but extends those results by showing that red enhances the effects of framing in a gender-based fashion: it is better to associate red to a gain frame for female users and to a loss frame for male users. This extended result provides practical guidance for automatic tailoring of persuasive Web pages about prevention topics.

A particular situation in which the suggested automatic tailoring could become less effective concerns users who access social networks or Web sites with a fake profile in which they misrepresent their gender. However, in the context of large-scale campaigns, the benefits of maximizing effectiveness on the large number of people who build real profiles on the social network will overshadow the suboptimal results that could be obtained with the smaller number of those who fake their identity. Moreover, it must also be noted that automatic technologies able to detect gender misrepresentation on the Web are available, e.g. Twitter claims that its gender recognition technology is 90 % accurate [29]. Gender recognition technologies based on multilingual automatic text analysis [3] allow a social network to detect user's gender also when the profile does not include gender information (as in current Twitter profiles).

We now plan to carry out further studies to extend and refine rules for tailoring persuasive Web pages based on simple information about the visitor that can be readily available, such as gender. For example, recent research on health and safety campaigns, e.g. [4, 20, 21], has suggested that men could be less sensitive than women to messages that resort to high physical threats (such as death and injuries), while they might respond better to humorous appeals, a difference that – if confirmed – could be important for Web content tailoring.

References

1. Berkovsky, S., Freyne, N.J., Oinas-Kukkonen, H.: Influencing individually: fusing personalization and persuasion. ACM Trans. Interact. Intell. Syst. **2**, 2 (2012)
2. Bunt, A., Carenini, G., Conati, C.: Adaptive content presentation for the web. In: Brusilovsky, P., Kobsa, A., Nejdl, W. (eds.) The Adaptive Web. LNCS, vol. 4321, pp. 409–432. Springer, Heidelberg (2007)
3. Burger, J.D., Henderson, J., Kim, G., Zarrella, G.: Discriminating gender on twitter. In: Proceedings of the Conference on Empirical Methods in Natural Language Processing (EMNLP 2011), pp. 1301–1309. Stroudsburg, USA: Association for Computational Linguistics (2011)
4. Conway, M., Dubé, L.: Humor in persuasion on threatening topics: Effectiveness is a function of audience sex role orientation. Pers. Soc. Psychol. Bull. **28**, 863–873 (2002)
5. CTIF - International Association of Fire and Rescue Services (2008). World Fire Statistics 13
6. Eisenberger, N.I., Lieberman, M.D.: Why rejection hurts: A common neural alarm system for physical and social pain. Trends Cogn. Sci. **8**, 294–300 (2004)
7. Elliot, A.J., Maier, M.A.: Color and psychological functioning. Curr. Dir. Psychol. Sci. **16**, 250–254 (2007)
8. Elliot, A.J., Maier, M.A., Moller, A.C., Friedman, R., Meinhard, J.: Color and psychological functioning: The effects of red on performance attainment. J. Exp. Psychol. Gen. **136**, 154–168 (2007)
9. Elliot, A.J., Niesta, D.: Romantic red: Red enhances men's attraction to women. J. Personal. Soc. Psychol. **95**, 1150–1164 (2008)
10. Fagley, N., Miller, P.M.: The effects of framing on choice: Interactions with risk-taking propensity, cognitive style, and sex. Pers. Soc. Psychol. Bull. **16**, 496–510 (1990)
11. Fagley, N., Miller, P.M.: Framing effects and arenas of choice: Your money or your life? Organ. Behav. Hum. Decis. Process. **71**, 355–373 (1997)
12. Floyd, D.L., Prentice-Dunn, S., Rogers, R.W.: A meta-analysis of research on Protection Motivation Theory. J. Appl. Soc. Psychol. **30**, 407–429 (2000)
13. Gerend, M.A., Sias, T.: Message framing and color priming: how subtle threat cues affect persuasion. J. Exp. Soc. Psychol. **45**(4), 999–1002 (2009)
14. Gnambs, T., Appel, M., Batinic, B.: Color red in web-based knowledge testing. Comput. Hum. Behav. **26**(6), 1625–1631 (2010)
15. Gorn, G.J., Chattopadhyay, A., Sengupta, J., Tripathi, S.: Waiting for the Web: How screen color affects time perception. J. Mark. Res. **41**(2), 215–225 (2004)
16. Hasseldine, J., Hite, P.A.: Framing, gender and tax compliance. J. Econo. Psychol. **24**, 517–533 (2003)
17. Haynes, M.J.: Fire Loss in the United States during 2014. National Fire Protection Association, Quincy, MA (2015)
18. Kiene, S.M., Barta, W.D., Zelenski, J.M., Cothran, D.L.: Why Are You Bringing Up Condoms Now? Eff. Message Content Framing Eff. Condom Use Message. Health Psychol. **24**, 321–326 (2005)
19. Levin, I.P., Schneider, S.L., Gaeth, G.J.: All frames are not created equal: A typology and critical analysis of framing effects. Organ. Behav. Hum. Decis. Process. **76**, 149–188 (1998)
20. Lewis, I., Watson, B., Tay, R.: Examining the effectiveness of physical threats in road safety advertising: The role of the third-person effect, gender, and age. Transp. Res. Part F **10**, 48–60 (2007)

21. Lewis, I., Watson, B., White, K.M.: An examination of message-relevant affect in road safety messages: Should road safety advertisements aim to make us feel good or bad? Transp. Res. Part F **11**, 403–417 (2008)
22. Mandel, N., Johnson, E.J.: When Web pages influence choice: Effects of visual primes on experts and novices. J. Consum. Res. **29**(2), 235–245 (2002)
23. Mehta, R., Zhu, R.J.: Blue or Red? Exploring the Effect of Color on Cognitive Task Performances. Science **323**, 1226–1229 (2009)
24. National Fire Protection Association (2013a). Safety Information for kids. http://www.nfpa.org/itemDetail.asp?categoryID=1803&itemID=42601&URL=Safety%20Information/For%20kids, Last Accessed 27 November 2015
25. National Fire Protection Association (2013b). Safety Information for Consumers. http://www.nfpa.org/safety-information/for-consumers, Last Accessed 27 November 2015
26. Rogers, R.W.: Cognitive and physiological processes in fear appeals and attitude change: A revised theory of Protection Motivation. In: Cacioppo, J.T., Petty, R.E. (eds.) Social Psychophysiology: A sourcebook, pp. 153–176. Guilford Press, New York (1983)
27. Rothman, A.J., Salovey, P., Antone, C., Keough, K., Martin, C.D.: The influence of message framing on intentions to perform health behaviors. J. Exp. Soc. Psychol. **29**, 408–433 (1993)
28. Rothman, A.J., Salovey, P.: Shaping perceptions to motivate healthy behavior: The role of message framing. Psychol. Bull. **121**, 3–19 (1997)
29. Twitter (2012). http://advertising.twitter.com/2012/10/gender-targeting-for-promoted-products.html, last accessed 27 November 2015
30. U.S. Fire Administration (2013a) Fire Safety for Kids. http://www.pct3vfd.com/news/firesafetykids/html/index.html, Last Accessed 27 November 2015
31. U.S. Fire Administration (2013b) Fire Safety for Citizens. http://www.ready.gov/home-fires, Last Accessed 27 November 2015
32. van den Bos, K., Ham, J., Lind, E.A., Simonis, M., van Essen, W.J., Rijpkema, M.: Justice and the human alarm system: The impact of exclamation points and flashing lights on the justice judgment process. J. Exp. Soc. Psychol. **44**(2), 201–219 (2008)
33. Witte, K., Allen, M.: A meta-analysis of fear appeals: Implications for effective public health campaigns. Health Educ. Behav. **27**, 591–616 (2000)
34. Wogaiter, M.S., Conzola, V.C., Smith-Jackson, T.L.: Research based guidelines for warning design and evaluation. Appl. Ergon. **33**, 219–230 (2002)

Supporting Users in Setting Effective Goals in Activity Tracking

Katja Herrmanny, Jürgen Ziegler, and Aysegül Dogangün[✉]

Personal Analytics, Interactive Systems Research Group,
University of Duisburg-Essen, Duisburg, Germany
{katja.herrmanny,juergen.ziegler,ayseguel.dogaguen}@uni-due.de

Abstract. In this paper we present the development of the pedometer app *Move My Day* which implements goal setting as its main persuasive design principle. Manual goal input as well as two strategies to support users in setting realistic goals, namely reference routes and personal goal recommendation, were implemented. The proposed algorithm for adaptive personal goal recommendation is designed in a way that it recommends short-term goals considering motivational aspects and gradually raises goals in the long term to meet physical activity recommendations. In a 12 week field study, we investigated the potentials of the two support strategies. Results indicate that about half of the users appreciate goal setting support and that especially personal goal recommendation seems to have potential to support users in setting effective physical activity goals.

Keywords: Persuasive technology · Behavior change support system · Activity tracking · Goal setting · Personalization · Pedometer · Physical activity

1 Introduction

Physical activity plays an important role for a healthy lifestyle as it can prevent and alleviate wide-spread diseases, such as diabetes, coronary heart disease, hypertension or types of cancer. Increasing physical activity is thus a goal frequently addressed in persuasive systems research. One of the core design principles used in these systems is goal setting. According to the goal setting theory [1] pursuing a goal has a motivating effect on performance. To be motivating and effective, goals should be precise, challenging and achievable. Moreover, self-set goals should be preferred over externally assigned goals as they have been shown to be more effective [1]. However, research [2] has revealed that people have problems in setting realistic goals, especially for moderate-intensity physical activity. Also our own research results of an online pre-study ($n = 194$, age: $M = 27$, range $= 14–74$) showed that participants had problems in estimating realistic goal distances. From these results and findings reported in the literature, it becomes clear that better strategies for supporting users in setting realistic activity goals are required when designing persuasive technologies to increase physical activity.

While from a motivational point of view goals should be challenging and realistic, these goals should also conform to common physical activity recommendations provided from a medical perspective. A key problem is that users start from very different

© Springer International Publishing Switzerland 2016
A. Meschtscherjakov et al. (Eds.): PERSUASIVE 2016, LNCS 9638, pp. 15–26, 2016.
DOI: 10.1007/978-3-319-31510-2_2

initial activity levels. For many users, standard activity recommendations would be too high compared to their current activity level to constitute a realistic next goal. For others, these goals are achievable but may not be challenging. Therefore, we propose an adaptive algorithm that is designed to gradually raise goals in the long term to meet standard activity recommendations, but recommends realistic and motivating short-term goals. The algorithm calculates suggestions of individual step goals for a week.

As an alternative support strategy we suggest reference routes, i.e. usually well-known or user-specific routes or distances which are transformed to the corresponding number of steps aiming at making these goals more precise.

We implemented a pedometer app integrating these strategies as well as the possibility to manually enter goals and investigated the supportive potential of these strategies in an empirical field study.

2 Related Work

Adaptivity of persuasive systems for behavior change is often addressed in research [3–5]. Based on a literature review, op den Akker et al. [6] identified adaptive goal setting, among others, as an important research topic. The authors recommend to define a user-specific, challenging and achievable goal based on the user's prior activity data. However, most activity tracking devices and applications that allow goal setting just assign fixed, non-adaptive goals or provide the opportunity to set a goal without any support. Example applications for assigned goals are the *Houston* system [7], *Fish'n'Steps* [8], and *UbiFit* [9]. An example for user-generated activity goals is an application targeting persons 50 + on a PDA [4] which enables users to set daily and weekly individual goals, but does not provide any goal setting support. Until now, only few approaches provide user-specific, adaptive goals or goal recommendations.

An early approach used a fixed threshold to select a goal level [10]. Users who achieved more than 5000 steps a day as baseline were given 10000 steps as their new goal. Those below 5000 steps were given a goal of 5000 steps a day. Burns et al. [11] also used participants' baseline activity in their application *ActivMon*, measured in the first study week, to define a goal level of 5 % more than baseline activity.

A smartphone application developed by King et al. [12] allows users to type in their weekly activity goal or choose among three suggested goals based on health recommendations. The suggested goals increase week by week, provided the previous week goal has been reached. Otherwise, a lower goal is recommended.

The persuasive system *Move2Play* offers a personalized recommendation of a training plan [13]. It bases on a user model, a domain model and the common recommendation of 10000 steps a day. The user model contains information e.g. on the user's fitness and active time slots. The domain model contains data e.g. about the current day, the user's age and sex. The author does not mention how this data is considered in the recommendation nor describe the concrete algorithm.

Also the virtual training system *MOPED* [14] implements user-specific and adaptive recommendations in terms of specific exercises. Therefore, a user model was initialized with manually entered information about sex, age, weight etc. During usage, further data are added such as fitness test results and historical training data such as exercise level or frequency as well as the user's heart rate. Based on these data, recommendations for the exercise count and speed of the concrete exercises are calculated.

3   Move My Day

We developed the pedometer App *Move My Day* to investigate our research question. Three versions with different functions were developed as described in Sect. 4.1. (Three additional versions were developed for another investigation that is not topic of this paper.) Goal setting is the predominant persuasive design principle. Permanent graphical and textual feedback indicates the progress towards the goal (see Fig. 1). In another view a list of selectable goal components is presented, i.e. distances used as goals or sub-goals. The app allows for goals consisting of more than one component. Moreover, the app contains views for recording reference routes (see Sect. 3.1), for typing in goals, and for viewing one's personal history. History includes records, average steps per day and week as well as statistics of the previous days and weeks. In another view, the app offers the opportunity to manually correct the step number counted by the system. This function was integrated to obtain valid data also in case of special situations e.g. when the smartphone's battery was exhausted or the user forgot it at home that day.

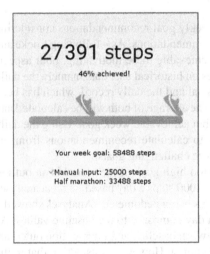
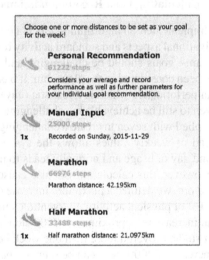

Fig. 1. Screenshots of the home view and goal selection of the pedometer app *Move My Day*

Goals are set for one week starting on Monday. They are not assigned automatically, but are set by the users themselves, however, supported by the app. The app provides three different ways to set a goal– two of them implement support strategies, one is unsupported. First, goals can be chosen from a list of pre-defined reference routes which are described in the following section. These reference routes are provided to make goals more concrete and conceivable than just numerical step counts. Second, as an alternative to reference routes, *Move My Day* provides a personal goal recommendation that is updated each Monday. Its calculation is based on historical user data, general health recommendations, as well as on motivational aspects and is described in detail in Sect. 3.2. Third, users can type in their goals manually, without any support of the app. It is possible to combine different types of goal components into one goal. However, in some study conditions not all of the three methods are available (see Sect. 4.1).

3.1 Reference Routes

Reference routes represent well-known or self-recorded distances. For instance, one pre-defined reference route is the distance of a marathon converted to an approximate number of steps. Further reference routes refer to the distance between two well-known cities, formula one race tracks, or routes popular with tourists (e.g. Avenue de Champs Élysées in Paris). Varying the area of interest ensures that each user can associate at least some reference routes with a distance. Varying length of the routes ensures that different activity levels can be considered. Moreover, it enables users to either select one single week goal or a number of smaller sub-goals. Besides pre-defined reference routes, users can record own routes, e.g. when making a walking tour. They can be labelled individually and do appear in the reference route list to be chosen as a goal.

3.2 Calculating Goal Recommendations

We implemented an algorithm to calculate weekly goal recommendations considering motivational aspects and standard activity recommendations. As – following Locke and Latham – goals should be challenging and achievable to be motivating, both aspects have been considered in the algorithm. It bases on historical user data, namely the daily mean performance which is a realistic (day) goal and the daily record, which has been proven to still be achievable but challenging. The average of both will be calculated and multiplied with seven to create a challenging but achievable week goal. Using the daily instead of weekly values allows the system to calculate recommendations from the second day of usage and normally leads to more challenging goals.

However, this calculation can also cause too high goals if the record is an outlier. Therefore, we defined a maximum increase of 2000 steps a day based on meta analyses [15, 16] of physical activity intervention studies using pedometers. Analyses showed a mean increase of approximately 2000 steps a day compared to the baseline values. As most studies covered more than one week between baseline and intervention outcome, an increase of 2000 steps can be seen as challenging. However, considering that in the described case the record is even higher, the new goal can still be seen as achievable.

Especially in the beginning of app usage, identical or very similar average and record step counts could hinder increase or lead to an increase that is considered to be too low against the background of the goal setting theory [1]. To avoid this, the algorithm includes a check whether the goal is at least 10 % higher than the average step number. If it is not, the initially calculated goal recommendation will be replaced by the average step count per day plus 10 % and again multiplied with seven to get a week goal. This is a higher increase than Burns et al. [11] suggested to keep the goal challenging.

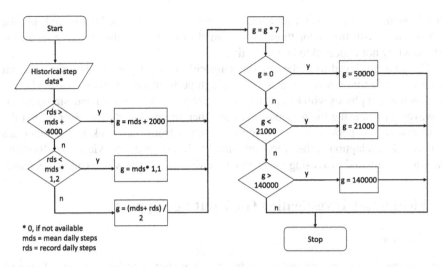

Fig. 2. Flow chart of the goal recommendation algorithm

The algorithm should also consider specific situations. These situations are:

- Historical data are not yet available (cold-start situations).
- The previous step count is unrealistically low (e.g. because usage started the day before, but not in the morning, or the person is far too little active).
- The user has already achieved a high average level that should not raise to unreachable values.

To meet these demands, thresholds are used to ensure reasonable overall minimum and maximum values (see Fig. 2). Also, a default value is used to alleviate the cold start problem which exists in the first week of usage. Modelled after the physical activity recommendations of the WHO [17], the default, minimum and maximum values are age-dependent, dividing age groups below 18 years and above. If the user has not entered his or her age, calculation for adults is used. The default goal recommendation for adults in case that no historical values are available is 50000 steps a week. This is above mean step levels former research has identified, but below health recommendations that propagate 10000 steps a day respectively 70000 steps a week [18]. Thus, it can be seen as a challenging but achievable goal for an average person. For children and adolescents, who are recommended much higher levels of physical activity, the default goal is 100000 steps. Unrealistically low goal recommendations, e.g. caused by reasons described above, are replaced by a minimum value of 21000 steps for adults and 63000 steps for children and adolescents. Referring to Tudor-Locke et al. [19] the minimum chosen for adults can be classified as "Limited Activity", which is in the lower range of physical activity but above "Basal Activity". As WHO activity recommendations for persons under 18 years are three times higher than those for adults, the minimum value for children and adolescent has been defined as the one for adults multiplied with three. As maximum values that are implemented to avoid unachievable goals we chose 140000 steps for adults (which is two times the recommendation of 10000 steps a day) and

300000 steps for children and adolescents. In this case, we decided not to multiply the 140000 steps with the factor three as it seemed to be an unrealistic high goal and is consequently not expected to be motivating.

The goals retrieved from the described algorithm are adaptive to the user's current medium-term activity level. In phases with high performance, goals increase whereas they decrease in phases with low performance due to the decreasing mean step number. However, by not using the previous week as other approaches do (see Sect. 2) but the mean and record performance, too high variations from one week to the other are avoided. Goal adaption is therefore very smooth. In the long-term view, the algorithm tends to recommend increasing goals by integrating the record which cannot decrease.

4   Field Study Investigating Goal Setting Support

4.1   Method

We performed a comparative field study to investigate users' preferences regarding goal setting strategies and the supportive potentials of the personal goal recommendation and reference routes. We published *Move My Day* at Google Play Store and promoted the app via press to generate a representative sample. Before downloading, prospective users were informed about taking part in a scientific study by using the app.

Users' app usage behavior was logged and stored on a server for data analysis. Logged data include test condition, created goal components, selected goal components, steps performed, app usage (i.e. opening the app), relevant technical data as well as gender, year of birth and former experience with activity tracking if provided by the user. Besides this information retrieved directly from the app, there were no other types of data collection. Also, there was no direct contact between the investigator and the users. Moreover, no end date of the study was communicated. Users can use the app without time limit. This study design was chosen to get real usage data without any bias evoked by the study situation. When starting the app for the first time, users were randomly assigned to one of three study conditions. The conditions contain either the adaptively calculated goal recommendation, reference routes or both. Additionally, we integrated the opportunity of setting goals manually in all conditions, in order to investigate, if users want to get supported by the app or not. This design decision results in the following conditions:

- Condition Rec + M: This condition included adaptively calculated goal recommendations as well as the possibility to manually type in a goal.
- Condition Ref + M: This condition included the opportunity to choose from reference routes or goals typed in manually.
- Condition Rec + Ref + M: This condition included all three possibilities to set a goal.

4.2   Data Processing and Analysis

The observation period covered 12 weeks. Logged data were filtered to meet our inclusion criteria for a high data quality:

- First usage week was eliminated as we supposed that users would test the functions and select different goal components just to try them.
- If users terminated using the app during the investigation period, also the last incomplete week was eliminated.
- Only weeks of active usage were included in the analysis. Our defined criterion for active usage was opening the app at least seven times a week.
- Further criteria were used to check the trustworthiness of data, especially regarding manual corrections. Criteria include negative step counts resulting from manual corrections, unrealistic high step counts (more than 70000 steps a day), and manual corrections on Sunday with nearly the amount of missing steps for reaching the goal.

Unfortunately, due to technical problems some data was not stored for some data sets resulting in further exclusions. Furthermore, we removed combined goals (i.e. goals consisting of more than one type of goal component) from statistical comparison of the support strategies as no clear allocation is possible. As there is a naturally high variation in step performance and goals, statistical methods considering such variance had to be chosen. Therefore, we focus on descriptive data, effect sizes and report confidence intervals for better interpretation of the results. As there is an ongoing debate about the informative value of significance testing, we also provide results of significance tests for the sake of completeness.

4.3 Results

Sample. After the described exclusions, a sample size of 79 participants (27 male, 34 female) and 206 weeks remained. Mean age was 47 years ($n = 62$, min $= 12$, max $= 72$). 18 participants didn't indicate their age or sex. Asked about previous experience with activity tracking (at least one month during the last year), 12 indicated to have experience, 50 were unexperienced and 17 did not indicate any experience information.

Investigation of Used Goal Components. We first investigated the number of sub-goals, a goal consisted of. Mostly, a goal included one component (142 times), followed by two (34 times), three (14 times), four (9 times), seven (6 times), and five (1 time). In condition Ref + Rec + M users could choose between all three types of goal components. 48 % of set goals were entered manually whereas for 44 % a support strategy was used (ref. route: 24 %, personal rec.: 20 %). 8 % were combined goals. Also in condition Rec + M most goals were manual inputs (64 %), followed by recommendation (31 %) and combined goals (5 %). In condition Ref + M most goals were supported by reference routes (65 %), 39 % were unsupported inputs and 6 % combined goals. Notably, all reference routes in all conditions were predefined ones. Even though users recorded own routes, they were not set as goals.

Investigation of Steps Per Week. We compared the steps users took per week between the three conditions as well as between the types of goal. Results are presented in Tables 1 and 2. Participants in condition Rec + Ref + M achieved higher performance than those in condition Rec + M and Ref + M, however with high standard deviation. Calculation of effect size showed a small effect

($\eta^2_{part} = .024$). Difference is statistically not significant ($F(2, 75) = 0.699, p = .500$). Comparing the number of steps taken between the different types of set goals, highest performance was found for goals based on recommendation followed by reference routes and manual input. Analysis shows a small effect and no statistical significance ($F(2, 100) = 1.486, p = .230, \eta^2_{part} = .018$).

Table 1. Descriptive results of achieved steps per week, grouped by condition

Condition	n	min	max	M	SD	95 % CI
Rec + M	50	2730	98424	36954.08	27346.47	29182.30 - 44725.86
Ref + M	39	913	70288	34378.62	18216.04	28473.66 - 40283.57
Rec + Ref + M	36	591	95428	44361.81	30877.15	33914.48 - 54809.13

Table 2. Descriptive results of achieved steps per week, grouped by used type of goal

Type of goal	n	min	max	M	SD	95 % CI
Recommend.	9	4145	80133	42195.67	26702.71	21670.15 - 62721.19
Ref. Route	28	591	70288	35462.86	22439.32	26761.80 - 44163.92
Man. Input	41	913	92783	31774.44	25923.79	23591.88 – 39957.00

Investigation of Set Step Goals. Set goals were also compared between the conditions and the types of chosen goals. Mean goals were very similar for all study conditions (see Table 3). For all conditions they comply on average with common physical activity recommendations. Regarding the type of goal the targeted steps also comply with physical activity recommendations for personal recommendation and reference routes. For manual input they are slightly below (see Table 4).

Table 3. Descriptive results of set goals, grouped by condition

Condition	n	min	max	M	SD	95 % CI
Rec + M	55	3500	200000	56159.27	38062.04	45869.66 - 66448.88
Ref + M	85	8	220789	55659.46	42905.84	46404.88 - 64914.03
Rec + Ref + M	66	1770	345456	53745.38	55145.24	40188.99 - 67301.77

Table 4. Descriptive results of set goals, grouped by used type of goal

Type of goal	n	min	max	M	SD	95 % CI
Recommend.	30	21000	97398	52412.87	21658.91	44325.30 - 60500.44
Ref. Route	71	3031	220789	58959.63	46988.02	47837.75 - 70081.52
Man. Input	92	8	200000	45589.48	33199.60	38714.04 - 52464.92

As mean goals are of limited informative value when investigating if realistic goal setting can be supported, further analysis focused on the difference between actually set goals and a reasonable goal. Based on goal setting theory [1], a reasonable goal should be challenging and achievable. However, there are large inter-personal performance differences. Goals that seem high or even not achievable for one person might not even be challenging for another. Thus, we investigated deviation of set goals from an individually realistic level. This level was estimated by the steps actually reached.

Comparing the mean deviation values between the different types of goals shows that performance was overestimated in all groups (see Table 5). Highest deviations are revealed for combined goals, lowest for goals based on the personal recommendation. This is a small effect (η^2_{part} = .018). A Kruskal-Wallis test shows that differences are statistically not significant ($\chi^2(2)$ = 2.27, p = .322).

Table 5. Descriptive results of deviations (pos. and neg.) between estimated realistic performance and set goals, grouped by used type of goal

Type of goal	n	min	max	M	SD	95 % CI	Mean rank
Rec.	9	-32089	30083	-5396.56	20201.27	-20924.63 - 10131.51	47.89
Ref. Route	28	-85527	41399	-12180.25	28826.70	-23358.08 - -1002.42	47.64
Man. Input	41	-172566	27783	-17361.44	32306.63	-27558.67 - -7164.21	39.88

Comparing the step count deviations ensures a uniform level of deviation. However, additionally we compared the percentage deviations from the realistic goal level in order to consider highly varying goals and performances. Therefore, we calculated the absolute value of mean percentage differences between the estimated realistic performance and set goals (see Table 6) and compared them between the types of goal. Again, we found a small effect (η^2_{part} = .046) and no significance ($F(2, 75)$ = 1.807, p = .171).

Table 6. Descriptive results of the absolute value of percentage deviations between estimated realistic performance and set goals, grouped by used type of goal

Type of goal	n	min	max	M	SD	95 % CI	Mean rank
Rec.	9	10.21	406.63	75.17	125.80	22.77 – 176.94	40.22
Ref. Route	28	0.06	10105.92	764.54	2267.26	52.33 – 1752.71	36.39
Man. Input	41	0.91	1093,32	162.79	228.81	80.48 – 254.19	41.46

Realistic goal setting might not only be supported when participants make use of a type of goal component. Also just offering these types of goal component could have a supportive effect on manually entered goals. Therefore, we compared the deviations for the manually entered goals of all conditions. As Table 7 shows, differences between goals and estimated realistic level as well as standard deviations are obviously lower in condition Rec + Ref + M than in the other conditions. For condition Ref + M descriptive analysis shows a slightly lower negative mean value and lower standard deviation than for Rec + M. For this comparison between the study conditions a Kruskal Wallis test revealed a significant effect ($\chi^2(2)$ = 9.40, p = .009). Effect size is medium-ranged (η^2_{part} = .104). Post hoc testing indicates a significant difference between Rec + M and Rec + Ref + M (p = .041) as well as Ref + M and Rec + Ref + M (p = .012).

Table 7. Descriptive results of deviations (pos. and neg.) between estimated realistic perform-ance and manually entered goals, grouped by condition

Condition	n	min	max	M	SD	95 % CI	Mean rank
Rec + M	20	-172566	27783	-21018.15	39976.46	-39727.71 - -2308.59	19.00
Ref + M	10	-60739	10274	-28474.50	25241.67	-46531.30 - -10417.70	15.00
Rec + Ref + M	11	-19803	23069	-610.09	10301.07	-7530.44 - 6310.26	30.09

4.4 Discussion

When having all three opportunities of goal setting, participants used supported and unsup-ported goal setting equally. When just one support strategy was provided, users preferred manual goal input or reference routes, depending on the study condition. Personal goal recommendation was used less than the other opportunities, but still in 20-31 % of set goals. Obviously it is a matter of individual preference whether users want goal setting support or not and which strategy they like. Regarding reference routes only predefined ones were selected although participants had used the recording function. Taking a deeper look at the recorded routes showed that step numbers were very low and thus not suitable for week or day goals. Labeling of these routes, e.g. "Home to work", indicates, that people used the recording function to evaluate the step number of their everyday routes. Consid-ering that the observation period did not cover holiday time, it seems plausible to assume that there was not yet much opportunity to record suitable routes (e.g. a longer walk, or a hiking trip). Thus, investigating the use of personal reference routes remains an interesting research aspect for long-term evaluation.

The absolute goal levels did not differ substantially between the study conditions, whereas deviations between personally realistic and actually chosen manually entered goals did. The significant medium-sized effect indicates that adding both supportive strategies, reference routes as well as personal recommendation, to the manual goal provides larger support in goal setting than just one of these opportunities even when these components are not selected.

When comparing absolute goal levels between the types of set goals, those based on reference routes were apparently the highest, those on manual input the lowest. However, evaluating how realistic these goals were, shows a unified picture: Goals based on personal recommendation obviously had lowest mean deviation between goals and estimated realistic goal level as well as lowest standard deviation for all calculations (absolute difference and percentage difference), indicating that the personal recommen-dation has most potential in supporting users in setting realistic activity goals. Goals based on reference routes do not seem superior to manually entered goals regarding user support. Although there is no statistically significant effect, at least descriptive differ-ences between the achieved steps are in accordance with this tendency as highest performance was achieved when using the personal recommendation. In general, natu-rally high inter-personal variation regarding goals as well as step performance makes valuation of statistical significance difficult. However, descriptive data, found small effects and a unified picture regarding the different calculations indicate, that the found differences might not be random effects.

5   Conclusion and Limitations

We presented the app *Move My Day* which implements goal setting as its core persuasive design principle. Two strategies to support users in setting realistic goals, namely reference routes and personal recommendation calculation, as well as manual goal input were implemented. In a 12 week field study, we investigated the potentials of these supportive strategies. Results show that users set goals with and without support equally, if all types of goal setting are provided. Reference routes were the preferred support strategy, but also the personal recommendation was used. However, on average the chosen goals that based on personal recommendation tended to be more realistic than goals from other sources and might have led to descriptively higher performance.

Even though the found effects are not strong, results indicate that many users appreciate being supported in goal setting and that personal recommendation based on the described algorithm might have a supportive influence in realistic goal setting. When defining goals by manual input, providing reference routes and personal recommendation as additional supportive information seems to be most effective. However, in order to investigate users' acceptance and preferences regarding the type of goal setting and the influence of just offering support on manual goal input, in our study design all conditions additionally contained the possibility of unsupported goal setting. For further investigation it would be interesting to only provide one opportunity of goal setting per condition and have a larger sample size, to alleviate comparison of the strategies. However, for the design of activity tracking technologies we recommend integrating manual input as well as goal setting support, ideally user-adaptive.

Regarding self-recorded reference routes, long-term data will reveal if people use them for their goals and if they are effective in supporting realistic goal setting.

Although the developed algorithm for personal goal recommendation shows promising results, there might be limitations for long-term use. In long-term use, the algorithm will get more and more insensitive to new records or variations in the mean performance. Possibly it will be necessary to neglect older information units in order to remain the flexibility of the algorithm, which is topic of our further evaluation. We also plan to differentiate days of work, holiday and illness to improve the recommendation. We will investigate these aspects in a long-term analysis of the ongoing study.

References

1. Locke, E.A., Latham, G.P.: Building a practically useful theory of goal setting and task motivation: A 35-year odyssey. Am. Psychol. **57**(9), 705–717 (2002)
2. Saini, P., Lacroix, J.: Self-setting of physical activity goals and effects on perceived difficulty, importance and competence. In: 4th International Conference on Persuasive Technology (Persuasive), pp. 33–39. ACM Press, New York (2009)
3. Hawkins, R.P., Kreuter, M., Resnicow, K., Fishbein, M., Dijkstra, A.: Understanding tailoring in communicating about health. Health Educ. Res. **23**(3), 454–466 (2008)
4. King, A.C., Ahn, D.K., Oliveira, B.M., Atienza, A.A., Castro, C.M., Gardner, C.D.: Promoting physical activity through hand-held computer technology. Am. J. Prev. Med. **34**(2), 138–142 (2008)

5. op den Akker, H., Jones, V.M., Hermens, H.J.: Tailoring real-time physical activity coaching systems: a literature survey and model. User Model. User-Adap. Inter. **24**(5), 351–392 (2014)
6. op den Akker, H., Klaassen, R., op den Akker, R., Jones, V.M.; Hermens, H.J.: Opportunities for smart & tailored activity coaching. In: 26th IEEE International Symposium on Computer-Based Medical Systems (CBMS), pp. 546–547. IEEE Press (2013)
7. Consolvo, S., Everitt, K., Smith, I., Landay, J.A.: Design requirements for technologies that encourage physical activity. In: SIGCHI Conference on Human Factors in Computing Systems (CHI), pp. 457–466. ACM Press, New York (2006)
8. Lin, J.J., Mamykina, L., Lindtner, S., Delajoux, G., Strub, H.B.: Fish'n'Steps: Encouraging physical activity with an interactive computer game. In: Dourish, P., Friday, A. (eds.) UbiComp 2006. LNCS, vol. 4206, pp. 261–278. Springer, Heidelberg (2006)
9. Consolvo, S., Klasnja, P., McDonald, D.W., Avrahami, D., Froehlich, J., LeGrand, L., Libby, R., Mosher, K., Landay, J.A.: Flowers or a robot army? In: 10th International Conference on Ubiquitous Computing (UbiComp), pp. 54–63. ACM Press, New York (2008)
10. Bickmore, T.W., Caruso, L., Clough-Gorr, K.: Acceptance and usability of a relational agent interface by urban older adults. In: CHI 2005 Extended Abstracts, pp. 1212–1215. ACM Press, New York (2005)
11. Burns, P., Lueg, C., Berkovsky, S.: Activmon: Encouraging physical activity through ambient social awareness. In: CHI 2012 Extended Abstracts, pp. 2363–2368. ACM Press, New York (2012)
12. King, A.C., Hekler, E.B., Grieco, L.A., Winter, S.J., Sheats, J.L., Buman, M.P., et al.: Harnessing different motivational frames via mobile phones to promote daily physical activity and reduce sedentary behavior in aging adults. PLoS ONE **8**(4), e62613 (2013)
13. Bielik, P.: Personalized training plan recommendation and activity tracking for a healthier lifestyle. Bull. ACM Slovakia **3**(4), 39–40 (2011)
14. Buttussi, F., Chittaro, L.: MOPET: A context-aware and user-adaptive wearable system for fitness training. Wearable Comput. Artif. Intell. Healthc. Appl. **42**(2), 153–163 (2008)
15. Bravata, D.M., Smith-Spangler, C., Sundaram, V., Gienger, A.L., Lin, N., Lewis, R., Stave, C.D., Olkin, I., Sirard, J.R.: Using pedometers to increase physical activity and improve health: a systematic review. JAMA **298**(19), 2296–2304 (2007)
16. Kang, M., Marshall, S.J., Barreira, T.V., Lee, J.O.: Effect of pedometer-based physical activity interventions: A meta-analysis. Res. Q. Exerc. Sport **80**(3), 648–655 (2009)
17. World Health Organization: Global recommendations on physical activity for health (2010). http://whqlibdoc.who.int/publications/2010/9789241599979_eng.pdf?ua=1
18. Choi, B.C.K., Pak, A.W.P., Choi, J.C.L.: Daily step goal of 10,000 steps: A literature review. Clin. Invest. Med. **30**(3), 6 (2007)
19. Tudor-Locke, C., Johnson, W.D., Katzmarzyk, P.T.: Accelerometer-determined steps per day in US adults. Med. Sci. Sports Exerc. **41**(7), 1384–1391 (2009)

Persuasive and Culture-Aware Feedback Acquisition

Malik Almaliki[1]([✉]) and Raian Ali[2]

[1] Taibah University, Medina, Kingdom of Saudi Arabia
mrmalki@taibahu.edu.sa
[2] Bournemouth University, Bournemouth, UK
rali@bournemouth.ac.uk

Abstract. User feedback is an important factor to improve software quality. For example, it can provide information on missing features and clarify user trends and preferences for future improvement. However, gathering user's feedback is not an easy process since the majority of users lack motivation and interest in providing feedback, especially in a constant and frequent style. In addition, studies have noted that the cultural differences among users also play a role in affecting their motivations to feedback acquisition. In this paper, we empirically investigate the role of culture in affecting users' perception and motivations to give feedback. Our study identifies some key differences between Western and Middle Eastern users on what motivate them to provide feedback and what could have an influence on the quality of the feedback they give. This also makes the case for the need to design a persuasive and culture-aware feedback acquisition.

Keywords: User's feedback · Persuasive technology · Software engineering

1 Introduction

In the context of software system, the software's ability to adapt to different cultures in users' space is important for improving its success in wider contexts and constructs a key requirement for professional and ethical reasons [1]. Generally speaking, most software designs follow a western cultural cues. This has caused a design gap when users coming from different cultures (i.e. eastern cultures) use the software within their cultural context. An example is clearly seen in the different ways people from all over the world use social networks. This is perhaps due to the fact that software industry is largely led by western management and developers [2]. Therefore, software systems that are marketed worldwide need to be tailored to fit the different cultures [3] as designs that are successful in one culture may fail dramatically in others [4, 5].

User's feedback constructs an important source for information needed for planning software evolution and adaptation [6]. This means that users need to be persuaded to provide feedback frequently. However, persuading users is not an easy task as the majority of users have little motivation and interests in providing such feedback in an on-going style [7]. Moreover, motivating users would highly depend on their culture and values. This sheds the lights on the potential use of persuasive technology in order to empower users' willingness to give feedback thus their experience and software's success.

© Springer International Publishing Switzerland 2016
A. Meschtscherjakov et al. (Eds.): PERSUASIVE 2016, LNCS 9638, pp. 27–38, 2016.
DOI: 10.1007/978-3-319-31510-2_3

Persuasive technology refers to the technology that is designed to change the attitudes or behaviors of users through persuasion and social influence, but not through coercion [8]. It has been used as an effective approach to increase users' engagement in many areas including the area of human-computer interaction. Recent research indicates that persuasive technology is more effective when it is tailored to the culture of its intended target audience [9]. However, little research has explicitly investigated the relationship between persuasive technology and culture [10].

In this paper, the authors qualitatively (using a focus group approach) study the effect and impact of cultural backgrounds on users' social motives to give feedback. The study's focus is on two different cultural backgrounds: Middle Eastern users and European users. The paper also advocates the need to design the acquisition process taking into account the persuasion goal of feedback acquisition in different cultures. The results of this study are meant to help devising a persuasive and systematic method for conducting a socially aware feedback acquisition that can adapt to different types of users in terms of their cultural backgrounds (Middle Eastern and European users). This will ultimately maximize feedback quality, users' satisfactions and motivations to give feedback.

The paper is structured as follows. In Sect. 2 we briefly discuss feedback acquisition and its relation to cultural backgrounds. In Sect. 3 we describe the research method adopted. In Sect. 4 we present and discuss the results of our study and in Sect. 5 we present our conclusion.

2 Feedback Acquisition and Cultural Differences

In [7] the authors conducted an empirical study to investigate users' behaviour to feedback requests and discover what motivates them to provide feedback. The study consisted of two phases: a qualitative and a quantitative phase. In the qualitative phase 7 interviews were conducted whereas in the quantitative phase, a survey was used and 100 responses were collected. The results of their study showed a preliminary indication that the variant cultural backgrounds of users has a noticeable impact on their behaviour and how they are socially motivated to give feedback. The preliminary results and survey questions related this aspect are provided in [22].

While a number of researchers have already investigated cultural differences in relation to software such as how graphics, language, object formatting, colours, and layout of web sites and other user preferences is perceived in different cultures [11–14], to the our best knowledge no studies have yet investigated how users with different backgrounds behave in response to feedback acquisition and how their culture frame affect their motivations to feedback requests. This paper aims at qualitatively investigating this aspect to help improving the design of a persuasive and culture-aware feedback acquisition.

3 Research Method

In empirical research, researchers might need to qualitatively follow up or build upon quantitative results for the purpose of explaining or further investigating the quantitative results [15]. This design is suitable for researchers who need qualitative data to explain significant, non-significant or surprising quantitative results [16, 17]. The results discussed in [7] indicated that the variant cultural backgrounds of users have a noticeable impact on users' behaviour and how they are socially motivated to give feedback. This was only an indicator which would need confirmation and clarification. To achieve that, this study follows up the quantitative results in [7] with a qualitative phase through focus groups which is a powerful tool to get insights and stimulate discussions in a small group of participants.

A focus group is a qualitative research method in which a group of people are gathered to be asked about their opinions, beliefs, or attitudes regarding an issue, phenomena, service, etc. The questions are asked in an interactive setting which allows participants to talk freely about their thoughts to other group members. Due to the nature of the study where social/group interaction is needed and the type of the asked questions which mainly relate to the culture impact (Middle Eastern and European cultures) on social perception of feedback acquisition of both the feedback provider and those who watch it, this paper adopted Focus Group as a data collection method in this investigatory study.

3.1 Focus Group Design

Four Semi-structured focus groups were conducted in two countries (Saudi Arabia and the UK) with 27 participants to further explore how Middle Eastern and European users behave in response to feedback acquisition and how their culture frame affect their motivations to feedback requests. Participants were carefully selected in order to guarantee a high level of diversity and to avoid bias (e.g. various age groups, backgrounds and gender). The first two focus groups took place on June-2014 in the UK and were conducted with European participants to investigate how their culture impacts their perception to feedback acquisition. Whereas the other two focus groups were held on July-2014 and conducted with Saudi participants to investigate the Middle Eastern culture's impact to feedback acquisition. Each focus group session lasted for about an hour which makes an amount of four hours in total.

The focus groups protocol was developed in the light of the results discussed in [7] in which an indication to cultural differences between European and Middle Eastern users on what motivate them to provide feedback was discovered. In particular, the four social factors (*Feedback acquisition as a social activity, Social recognition, Volume of already given feedback and Visibility and similarity of others feedback*) that influence how Middle Eastern and European users are socially motivated to give feedback served as a foundation to develop the protocol of the focus group. The focus group protocol is available in [22].

The protocol was iteratively reviewed and revised by 3 researchers to ensure clarity and understandability. Participants were briefed to the session and the discussed topic through a 10 min presentation in which some example of feedback acquisition in software application were also given to more familiarise the participants with the discussed topic. Each participant received £15 amazon vouchers as an appreciation for taking part in the study.

3.2 Sampling

Purposeful sampling is a common technique in qualitative research [18]. In this study, purposeful sampling was used to recruit the participants. The inclusion criteria of this study allowed for participants who are European or were born and raised in Europe to take part in the first two focus groups dedicated to study European people (7 participants for the first focus group and 6 for the second). On the other hand, participants who are Saudis or were born and raised in Saudi Arabia were recruited to take part in the other two focus groups dedicated to study Middle Eastern people in which 7 participants took part in each focus group.

In addition, the inclusion criteria allowed for participants within an age range of 18 to 71 and average computer users who use typical and diverse set of popular software applications rather than domain specific software for everyday life activities. This sampling criterion were developed to allow for more variety in selecting participants and reflecting users' experience with popularly used software applications. This can maximize the generalizability of the results. For more details about the participants' characteristics (e.g. age, gender, home country, etc.) please refer to [22].

The authors assumed that Saudi users could be a good fit to represent the Middle Eastern culture. It is due to the fact that Saudi Arabia is one of the largest countries in the Middle East and could fairly represent users' cultures in the region when it comes to the use of software. Statistics indicate that Saudi Arabia has over 6 million active Facebook users which is the highest Facebook user rate in the region. With more than 3 million active Twitter users, Saudi Arabia takes the lead not only in the Middle East, but in the world in its Twitter users' growth rate. In addition, More than 90,000,000 videos are watched daily on YouTube in Saudi Arabian which is more than any daily YouTube video views number in the world [19]. Based on this statistics, the available resources to the authors and time, the authors assumes that Saudi Arabia is a reasonable fit to be adopted in this study to represent Middle Eastern culture to feedback acquisition.

3.3 Analysis

Focus groups were audio taped and transcribed verbatim analysis was performed in several steps which included: (1) initial exploration of the gathered data by reading the transcripts; (2) coding data by labelling and segmenting the text; (3) using codes to generate themes by gathering similar codes together; (4) connecting, comparing and interrelating themes. Credibility of the findings was maximized by using an inter-coder agreement check and academic advisor's auditing [18, 20].

4 Findings

As previously stated, the focus group design covered how a number of social factors influence Middle Eastern and European users with regard to feedback acquisition. In this section, these social factors are used to structure, represent and discuss the main themes of the findings. The themes and codes that highlight the encountered behavioural differences between the two studied groups (Middle Eastern and European users) to feedback acquisition are shown in Table 1.

Table 1. A breakdown of the themes and codes of the analysis.

Theme1: Visibility and similarity of others feedback
Anonymity of feedback providers.
Cross conversation
Feedback objectivity and relevancy
Language used among given feedback.
Gender,
social position or a personal relationship with a feedback provider
Theme2: Volume of already given feedback
Feedback objectivity and relevancy.
Theme3: Social recognition
Feedback objectivity and relevancy.
Suitable and unsuitable uses of social recognition
More beneficial with close friends and small community.
Social recognition can result in ignoring unrecognized users' feedback
Social recognition might result in addiction especially for young users.
Theme4: Feedback acquisition as a social activity
Feedback objectivity and relevancy.

4.1 Visibility and Similarity of Others Feedback

Generally speaking, the responses from Middle Eastern participants and European participants are noticeably different when they were asked whether the visibility of others feedback (the ability to others feedback before giving feedback) and the similarity of their feedback to others feedback would have effect on their willingness to give feedback. Although feedback visibility plays a role in motivating both Middle Eastern and European participants to give feedback, Middle Eastern participants seemed to be more concerned and socially motivated by this factor than European participants. This trend became more obvious when they were asked whether knowing the similarity of their feedback to others would affect their willingness to give feedback. One the participants mentioned in this regard *"I'm normally interested in replying to reviews that I do not agree with"*. Figure 1 gives a general view of how the different cultures' impact on this social factor could affect the quality of given feedback. In addition, the following dimensions of this theme were extracted from the participants' responses:

Anonymity of Feedback Providers. Users ability to give feedback anonymously (i.e. using nicknames instead of the real names) is shown to play a role in motivating both parties (Middle Eastern and European users) to give feedback especially when the given feedback is publicly open and seen by other users. This is perhaps due to several factors (i.e. dissociative anonymity, invisibility, solipsistic introjection, dissociative imagination, and minimization of authority) as discussed in [7] which allow users to enjoy more freedom in expressing their opinion about a product or a software service. One of the participants said "I would be more interested in truly engaging when no one knows me. It feels like you are free to say whatever you like and you will still be unknown". However, anonymity does not seem to be a motivating factor when a feedback provider is part of an online closed community such as a Facebook group. In general, users prefer to know the identity of the feedback provider in their closed social network/community since it makes them more comfortable participating and discussing a software service or a product.

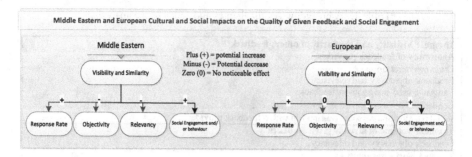

Fig. 1. The effect of feedback visibility and similarity in Middle Eastern and European culture.

On the downside, anonymity seems to affect the objectivity and relevancy of provided feedbacks by both parties but it is more prominent with the Middle Eastern than European users. Their overall responses indicated that anonymity could results in the so-called *online disinhibition effect* [21] which gives users space to escape from their social constrains. However, this feeling of freedom can result in an overexpression and less objectivity and relevancy of their opinion about a service or a product. One of the participants commented *"The problem is that some people think they can say anything or be unfair or even harm others because nobody knows them. That's not the point of being anonymous"*. Figure 2 gives a clearer view of how the different cultures' impact on this social factor could affect the quality of given feedback.

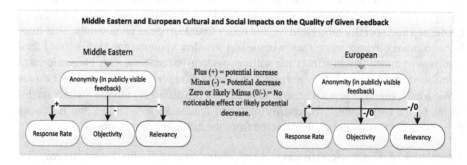

Fig. 2. The effect of anonymity on feedback in Middle Eastern and European culture.

Cross Conversation, Feedback Objictivety and Relevancy and Language Used. In the context of cross conversation (irrelevant feedback) and how it affects the provided feedback, users' responses indicated that feedback given by European users might enjoy a slightly higher degree of relevancy and objectivity than the feedback given by Middle Eastern users. This is perhaps due to the fact that Middle Eastern users are more socially engaged which could put some constrains on the relevancy and objectivity of their given feedback However, in all cases cross conversation (irrelevant feedback), subjectivity and the harshness degree in the language used among already given feedback can results in a low response rate by both parties (Middle Eastern and European users). It can also result in a harm to the software product or the provided service.

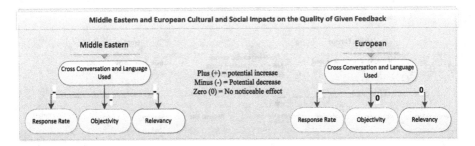

Fig. 3. The effect of cross conversation and language used on feedback in Middle Eastern and European culture.

An example of this was given by one of the participants "if *the cross conversations or the harshness of the used language leverage among users feedback such as two large groups of users fighting around irrelevant specific religious or political party, this can highly result in users from either group degrading and disliking the service or the product just to cause a harm to the service provider who they think he might be from the opposite party*". Figure 3 gives a clearer view of how the different cultures' impact on this social factor could affect the quality of given feedback.

Gender, Social Position or a Personal Relationship with a Feedback Provider.
Being able to know/see the gender, social position or your personal relationship with a feedback provider gives a clear view about how users from the different two cultures (Middle Eastern and European cultures) are socially motivated to give feedback. In the European culture, users do not seem to be influenced by these factors to give feedback at all. This is perhaps due to the fact that they feel more socially- free-wheeling than Middle Eastern users as described by some of the participants. A participant commented *"I believe living in this community (European community) makes you less socially-dependent and do not easily accept to accomplish things with the help of your parents or friends for example. You always want to do things by yourself. This is how we grew up"*.

On the other hand, users coming from Middle Eastern culture are significantly different to the European users in their perception of these factors. They feel highly motivated by these factors to give feedback especially with people/users they know (i.e. having a personal relationship with the person asking for feedback or the users giving feedback). Interestingly, the gender of a feedback provider is considered to be source of curiosity that motivates Middle Eastern users to give feedback which is not the case with the European users. Males/females would find it interesting to see how females/males think of a particular software service or product. One of the participants said *"I would really love to see how males' feedback would be on a certain aspect of a software such as the interface colours. You know we love girly colours and this will always make my feedback clashes with males which is fun"*.

On the down side, motivating Middle Eastern users by these factors can result in a questionable quality of their given feedback in terms of its objectivity and relevancy to the discussed software service or product. Some of the Middle Eastern participants mentioned

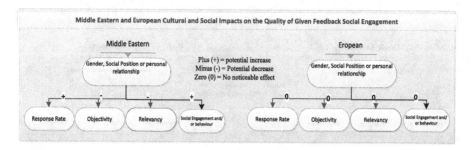

Fig. 4. The effect of gender, position or relationship on feedback in Middle Eastern and European culture.

that they always tend to be supportive and on the side of their friends (i.e. software service provider who is asking for their feedback) regardless of the discussed product and their real opinion about it. Although this can be harmful to the quality of the feedback, it gives a nice example of a caring relationship among users. Figure 4 gives a clearer view of how the different cultures' impact on this social factor could affect the quality of given feedback.

4.2   Volume of Already Given Feedback

When participants were asked whether the number of feedback already provided on a software service or a product would affect their willingness to give feedback, Middle Eastern users showed a consensus on that they would like to provide feedback if there were only few feedback given rather than a large number of already given feedback. One of the participants commented *"it makes me feel sorry when only few reviews are given especially when the app or service is good. I would certainly find a time to write my own review and help"*. In comparison, European users had a similar attitude but they perceive this as a less important factor when compared to Middle Eastern users.

Feedback Objectivity and Relevancy. The degree of feedback relevancy and objectivity given by both parties (Middle Eastern and European users) does not seem to be influenced by the volume of already given feedback. However, the low number of already given feedback can sometimes impose potential risk to the software service or product. Several users from both parties indicated that when a low number of feedback/ reviews is already given it makes them lose interest in the provided service since it does not seem to be popular among users otherwise it would be highly reviewed by a large number of users. One of the participants commented *"The first thing I do before down-loading an app is to look at the number of reviews. A low number means to me less popular and useful"*. Figure 5 gives a clearer view of how the different cultures' impact on this social factor could affect the quality of given feedback.

4.3   Social Recognition

Participants were asked whether being recognized by the community as feedback providers would affect their willingness to give feedback. The responses from the two groups were noticeably different. Users from Middle Eastern backgrounds indicated that being socially recognized as a feedback provider is an influential factor that could positively maximize their willingness to give feedback. There could be still some constraints on this, e.g., some participants commented that *"it is nice to be visible only when others can see their feedback which led to some changes on the system"*.

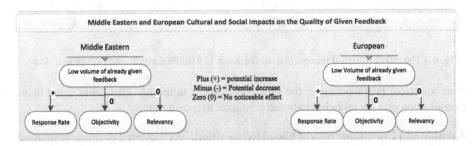

Fig. 5. The effect of feedback volume on feedback in Middle Eastern and European culture.

On the other hand, European users seemed to be far less motivated by the same aspect as few participants would have thought in a similar way. In fact, some of the European participants mentioned that some of the socially recognized feedback providers might have been selected and sponsored by the software/service provider for marketing reasons (e.g. being a celebrity). One of the participants commented *"You know nowadays in advertisements they use popular names and faces to attract people. It can be the same case for feedback too"*. Although Middle Eastern users are also aware of this threat but they would still be more interested in the social aspect (social recognition) regardless of the potential threats it might cause. Generally, these potential threats could result in users having negative attitudes towards the provided software service or the product. Figure 6 gives a general view of how the different cultures' impact on this social factor could affect the quality of given feedback. In addition, the following dimensions of this theme were extracted from the participants' responses:

Feedback Objectivity and Relevancy. Social recognition as a motivating factor to feedback acquisition does not seem to play a role in affecting the objectivity and relevancy of feedback given by European users. In contrast to, the degree of relevancy and objectivity of feedback given by Middle Eastern users to the provided service might be slightly harmed. This is due to the fact that Middle Eastern users are more socially involved with their community and this can push them sometimes to act differently when they are being socially recognized as feedback providers. One of the participants commented *"You know lots of people could be watching me. I will always try my best to be ideal in their eyes"*. This indeed could have negative impact on their given feedback such as imposing favouritism in their opinions regarding the provided software service which made them socially recognized at the first place. However, this social aspect could have a positive impact on the social behaviour within the online society of Middle Eastern users since socially recognized users would feel more socially constrained and

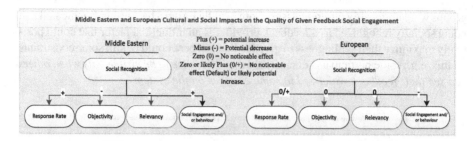

Fig. 6. The effect of social recognition on feedback in Middle Eastern and European culture.

their behaviour is always under the spot light of the community. This could result in an overall improved social behaviour and an online user community.

Suitable and Unsuitable uses of Social Recognition. As indicated by users' responses from both parties (Middle Eastern and European users) social recognition could be more beneficial and motivating if it is used in a small and closed community of users where all of the users somehow know each other (i.e. Facebook groups). This makes users more interested in being socially recognized to people who they know and more motivating for users to follow up a socially recognized person who they know and trust. One of the participants commented *"It would be nice if we are all friends and know each other. I will trust and follow who I know and I will be happy to be recognized in front of people who care about me, right?"*

On the other hand, users indicated that social recognition can lead to users following socially recognized users only and ignoring the feedback of unrecognized users even if their feedback is far better in quality. This of course could harm the provided software service and its reputation since vital information and knowledge about the provided service could be overlooked. In addition, some users mentioned that social recognition could lead to users' addiction to the used software especially young users who are eager to be socially recognized and more socially active. It is a trade-off between using this factor to benefit users or harm them and the provided service.

4.4 Feedback Acquisition as a Social Activity

Similar to the above dimension, Middle Eastern users showed a much higher interest in conducting feedback acquisition as a social activity (i.e. social games) and emphasized that it would increase their willingness to give feedback. This was true especially for young users. Example of such an activity could be the users' ability to visualize how their direct and indirect social contacts are rating a certain service and how their feedback influenced the trend in their community. Compared to this, the majority of interviewed European showed a negative trend towards this factor. In fact, they believe feedback requests should be straightforward and simple by default and conducting it as a social activity could make the process of feedback acquisition more discouraging, complex and distracting from the main purpose which is evaluating a provided software service. One of the participants said in this regard *"I think it should not look more than what it is supposed to do. It is to get your feedback and not a game to play with"*.

Feedback Objectivity and Relevancy. Conducting the feedback acquisition as a social activity could have a harmful effect on the objectivity and relevancy of the given feedback by Middle Eastern users. It is perhaps due to users' engagement with the activity more than the provided service as well as the burden of social constraints. One of the participants commented *"I imagine I would be nicer about my opinion to people I know more than others"*. Although this might result in given feedback that does not reflect users' true opinion about the provided software service, it could also result in a more socially active users which could be a positive sign to the software and the users' community. Users' satisfaction with the social activity should not affect their view about the software service. This highlights the need to carefully design and apply this factor. Figure 7 gives a clearer view of how the different cultures' impact on this social factor could affect the quality of given feedback.

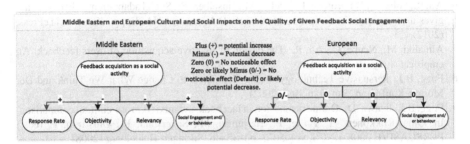

Fig. 7. Eeffect of feedback acquisition as a social activity in Middle Eastern and European culture.

In general, this paper advocated that culture variations has a noticeable impact on how Middle Eastern and European users' behaviour in response to feedback acquisition and how they are socially motivated to give feedback. The results suggest that having carfully tailopred persuasive method for the design of an adaptive and cultural-aware feedback acquisition could highly improve the quality of the collected feedback as well as users' satisfactions and response rate to feedback acquisition.

5 Conclusion

In this paper reported on an empirical study that investigated qualitatively the culture impact on users' behaviour and motivations to feedback acquisition. The result highlighted key differences between Middle Eastern and Western users with regard to their social motives to give feedback. Generally, European users found to be more socially-independent and showed less interest in being socially motivated to give feedback than Middle Eastern users. The paper also advocates the need to have a persuasive and culture-aware feedback acquisition which opens the gate for further research in this area.

Acknowledgment. We would like to acknowledge that this research was supported by an FP7 Marie Curie CIG grant (the SOCIAD Project). We would also like to thank the participants who took part in our study for their valuable input.

References

1. Yunker, J.: Beyond borders: Web globalization strategies. New Riders, Boston (2002)
2. Reinecke, K., Bernstein, A.: Culturally adaptive software: moving beyond internationalization. In: Aykin, N. (ed.) HCII 2007. LNCS, vol. 4560, pp. 201–210. Springer, Heidelberg (2007)
3. Nielsen, J., Pfeil, U., Zaphiris, P., Ang, C.S.: International user interfaces Cultural differences in collaborative authoring of Wikipedia. J. Comput. Mediated Commun. 12(1), 88–113 (1996)
4. Honold, P.: Culture and context: An empirical study for the development of a framework for the elicitation of cultural influence in product usage. Int. J. Hum.-Comput. Interact. 12(3–4), 327–345 (2000)
5. Abdelnour-Nocera, J., Clemmensen, T., Kurosu, M.: Reframing HCI through local and indigenous perspectives. Int. J. Hum. Comput. Interact. 29, 201–204 (2013)
6. Ali, R., Solís, C., Omoronyia, I., Salehie, M., Nuseibeh, B.: Social adaptation - when software gives users a voice. In: Filipe, J., Maciaszek, L.A. (eds.), ENASE, pp. 75–84. SciTePress, (2012)
7. Almaliki, M., Ncube, C., Ali, R.: The design of adaptive acquisition of users feedback: An empirical study, RCIS (2014)
8. Fogg, B.J.: Persuasive Technology: Using Computers to Change What We Think and Do. Morgan Kaufmann, San Francisco (2002)
9. Fogg, B.J., Iizawa, D.: Online persuasion in facebook and mixi: A cross-cultural comparison. In: Oinas-Kukkonen, H., Hasle, P., Harjumaa, M., Segerståhl, K., Øhrstrøm, P. (eds.) PERSUASIVE 2008. LNCS, vol. 5033, pp. 35–46. Springer, Heidelberg (2008)
10. Khaled, R.: Culturally-relevant persuasive technology (2008)
11. Marcus, A.: Global/intercultural user interface design. Hum. Comput. Interact. Des. Issues, Solutions, Appl. 107, 355–381 (2003)
12. Callahan, E.: Interface design and culture. Ann. Rev. Inf. Sci. Technol. 39(1), 255–310 (2005)
13. Aykin, N., Quaet-Faslem, P.H., Milewski, A.E.: Cultural ergonomics. Handbook of Human Factors and Ergonomics, Third Edition, 177–190 (2006)
14. Frandsen-Thorlacius, O., Hornbæk, K., Hertzum, M., Clemmensen, T.: Non-universal usability?: a survey of how usability is understood by Chinese and Danish users. In: SIGCHI Conference on Human Factors in Computing Systems, ACM (2009)
15. Creswell, J.W., Plano Clark, V.L., Gutmann, M.L., Hanson, W.E.: Advanced mixed methods research designs. Sage, Thousand Oaks, CA (2003)
16. Morse, J.M.: Approaches to qualitative-quantitative methodological triangulation. Nurs. Res. 40(2), 120–123 (1991)
17. Tashakkori, A., Teddlie, C.: Mixed methodology: Combining qualitative and quantitative approaches. Sage Publications, Thousand Oaks (1998)
18. Creswell, J.W.: Qualitative Inquiry And Research Design: Choosing Among Five Approaches, 3rd edn. Sage Publications Inc., Thousand Oaks (2013)
19. Socialclinic: The State of Social Media in Saudi Arabia. The Social Clinic (2013). http://www.thesocialclinic.com/the-state-of-social-media-in-saudi-arabia-2012-2/
20. Miles, M.B., Huberman, A.M.: Qualitative data analysis: An expanded sourcebook, 2nd edn. Sage, Thousand Oaks (1994)
21. Suler, J.: The online disinhibition effect. Cyber Psychol. Behav. 7(3), 321–326 (2004)
22. Almaliki, M.: Engineering an Adaptive and Socially-aware Feedback Acquisition. Ph.D. thesis, Bournemouth University, 88–102 (2015)

Theoretical Reflections

Crowd-Designed Motivation: Combining Personality and the Transtheoretical Model

Roelof A.J. de Vries[✉], Khiet P. Truong, and Vanessa Evers

University of Twente, Enschede, The Netherlands
{r.a.j.devries,k.p.truong,v.evers}@utwente.nl

Abstract. Current approaches to design motivational technology for behavior change focus on *either* tailoring motivational strategies to individual preferences *or* on implementing strategies from behavior change theory. Our goal is to combine these two approaches and translate behavior change theory to text messages, tailored to personality. To this end, we conducted an online survey with 481 participants exploring the relationship between behavior change theory (the Transtheoretical Model) and personality in the context of physical activity. Our results show that (1) people's personalities correlate with their stage of change and (2) people's personalities and their stages of change correlate to preferences for certain processes of change. We discuss the implications of the results for designing motivational technology.

Keywords: Behavior change · Persuasion strategies · Personality · Processes of change · Stages of change · Transtheoretical model

1 Introduction

Over the past few years, human-computer interaction (HCI) research, in particular persuasive technology research, has focused on designing motivational technology, assisting or encouraging people to change their behavior [1]. To increase the effectiveness of the strategies used in these technologies, researchers aim for personalization [2]. This can be done by, for example, tailoring the strategies to certain user characteristics, like personality [3]. Additionally, authors have been advocating the use of behavior change theory [4] aiming to increase the effectiveness of the strategies used in these technologies. However, using theory or models when designing motivational technology for behavior change comes with a challenge: there is no well-established method to translate theoretical constructs and insights to persuasive or motivational interaction designs to be used in practice.

We aim to combine these two approaches to increase the effectiveness of persuasive and motivational strategies. For our long-term goal, the objective is to design a smartphone application that motivates users through text messages

© Springer International Publishing Switzerland 2016
A. Meschtscherjakov et al. (Eds.): PERSUASIVE 2016, LNCS 9638, pp. 41–52, 2016.
DOI: 10.1007/978-3-319-31510-2_4

to become regular runners by implementing strategies from behavior change theory or models and tailoring these text messages to personality.

The strategies that we aim to translate and personalize come from the Transtheoretical Model (TTM) of behavior change [5]. According to the TTM, behavioral change consists of five stages of change. When moving through these stages, people encounter processes of change, i.e., experiences and actions that influence the progression through the stages [6]. Different processes are associated with different stages of change [7]. For example, rewarding desirable behavior (i.e., Reinforcement Management) is expected to be most useful in stages where desirable behavior is performed (i.e., in the Action or Maintenance stage), whereas making someone aware of the risks of undesirable behavior (i.e., Consciousness Raising) is expected to be most useful in stages where the undesirable behavior is still performed (i.e., in the Precontemplation, Contemplation or Preparation stage). We expect that when designing messages that capture a process of change that fits with the stage of change a person is in, the effectiveness of the messages will increase. To increase the effectiveness even further, we could account for the individual preferences people have for persuasive strategies [8,9], for example based on their personality [10], which is similar to a persuasion profile [11].

In this paper we report on the first step in a novel approach to translate and personalize strategies from behavior change theory to inform the design of motivational technology. Using a crowdsourcing platform, we measured the participants' stage of change, personalities and preference for a certain process of change. We show that (1) personality is correlated to the stage of change a person is in, and (2) personality and stage of change are related to the preference for a certain process of change.

In the following sections we report on theoretical background, related work, our expectations, the design and results of the crowdsourcing study with questionnaires, and we end with a discussion and conclusion.

2   Theoretical Background: TTM and Personality

The Transtheoretical Model (TTM) from Prochaska et al. [5] is a dynamic, integrative behavior change model focused on the individual. The stages of change associated with the TTM can be practically applied [12] and classify people into (not necessarily linearly) progressing stages for changing behaviors, i.e., Precontemplation, Contemplation, Preparation, Action, and Maintenance. While the stages of change are useful in explaining when changes in cognition, emotion, and behavior take place, the processes of change help to explain how and why the progression through these stages occur. Ten covert and overt processes will usually be experienced when successfully progressing through the stages of change and attaining the desired behavioral change. The ten processes can be divided into two groups: Experiential processes and Behavioral processes. Experiential processes are focused on changing people's ideas and Behavioral processes are focused on changing people's actions, see Table 1 for an overview. The effectiveness of the processes of change depends on their associated stages of change.

Table 1. The processes of change divided in experiential and behavioral processes with a short description.

Experiential processes
Consciousness raising (CR): The individual seeks increased knowledge about the causes, consequences and cures for their problem behavior
Dramatic relief (DR): The individual's emotions about the problem behavior and possible solutions are evoked
Environmental reeval. (ER): The impact that the individual's problem behavior has on their environment is reevaluated
Social liberation (SOL): Attempts are made to increase alternatives for the individual's former problem behavior
Self-reevaluation (SR): Cognitions and emotions regarding the individual with respect to their problem behavior are reevaluated
Behavioral processes
Self-liberation (SEL): The individual has the belief that he can change and commits to it by choosing a course of action
Helping relationships (HR): The individual seeks trust and open discussion about the problem behavior as well as support for the healthy behavior change
Counterconditioning (CC): The individual substitutes positive behaviors for the individual's problem behavior
Reinforcement manag. (RM): Steps or changes made by the individual are rewarded when in a positive direction or punished when in a negative direction
Stimulus control (SC): Stimuli that may cue a lapse back to the problem behavior are avoided and prompts for more healthier alternatives are inserted

If we could also account for individual preferences, for example those caused by differences in personality [10], we could increase the effectiveness even further.

Personality is a way to describe long-lasting individual characteristics (similarities and differences) between people. In the psychology literature, a lot of different personality classifications can be found. The most important one is the Big Five [13] model, also known by its acronym for the personality traits; OCEAN. This framework classifies people in five dimensions: Openness to experience, (**O**), Conscientiousness (**C**), Extraversion (**E**), Agreeableness (**A**) and Neuroticism (**N**). A well-known measure for this five-factor model is the NEO-PI-R [14]. Although there are other personality theories, we chose to work with this model: it is practical in use, it is temporally stable [15], and measurement tools (i.e., questionnaires) for the model are widely available and well validated [16].

3   Related Work

The use of theory or models, such as the TTM, has been advocated in designing strategies to change behavior (e.g., [17,18]) because this will help evaluate this theory or model and the use of this theory or model then offers an explanation when the designed intervention strategy does or does not work. Hence, a theoretical foundation will help in understanding and targeting determinants of behavior, like the stages of change or personality. However, there is little guidance on how to apply theory to the design of intervention strategies [18].

In the context of changing or determining physical activity behavior, some direct relations have been found between physical activity and certain personality traits. Overall, Extraversion and Conscientiousness seem to be positively correlated with physical activity and exercise behavior [19–21] while Neuroticism appears to be negatively correlated to physical activity [21].

Research on personality as a factor for tailoring messages to encourage physical activity has been rather limited. The most closely related works can be found in [22,23]. In a study by Courneya et al. [22], exercise behavior, motives, barriers, and preferences were correlated to the Big Five. Among other things, it was found that: the personality trait Openness was related to the motive of fun and enjoyment; Conscientiousness was related to the motive of fitness and health; Extraversion was related to the motive of socializing and meeting people, Agreeableness was negatively related to preference for competitive exercises; and Neuroticism was related to the barriers of lack of energy, lack of motivation and embarrassment. From these correlations, one could derive guidelines on how (not) to tailor motivational messages to each personality type. Another study [24] also addressed the relation between personality and motives in exercise participation. It was found that different personalities have different motives for change in exercise participation, indicating that people with different personalities should be motivated in different ways to participate in exercise. Halko et al. [23] explores the relationship between personality (Big Five) and persuasion in the context of health-promotion with mobile applications. Their results showed that all personality types had different preferences for (mobile) persuasive messages (for healthy living). Finally, there have been some studies that suggest that the stages of change can benefit from personalization [25], that future research should tailor messages that promote physical activity to people's personalities [26], and that "Individuals with certain personality traits are more likely to be perceptive toward the idea of physical activities" [3, p. 8]. All these studies indicate that personality is a decisive factor in explaining the individual nature of people and their motivations and barriers for physical activity participation.

There has been some recent research into the role of personality when designing tailored persuasive strategies [9,27,28]. For example, Kaptein et al. [9] developed six persuasive strategies and a questionnaire to measure the user's susceptibility to those six persuasive strategies. They tested a setup where they tailored to the user's susceptibility versus a contra-tailored setup in the context of snacking and found a greater decrease in the tailored version. In a study about tailored persuasive messages for advertisement (advertising mobile phones), Hirsh et al. [27] let participants rate the level of persuasiveness of the messages that were tailored to each personality type. For example, people with the Extraversion personality type would receive messages like "With XPhone, you'll always be where the excitement is" [27, p. 579] because extraverts are especially sensitive to rewards and social attention. The results show a clear benefit in tailoring messages to personality type features. Similar results were obtained in a study [28] where an application was developed to persuade users to study more using persuasion strategies that were tailored to users' personalities: different personalities indeed preferred different (persuasive) study behaviors. All these studies show promising results and are good examples of how persuasive strategies and personality targeted design can influence participants and increase their participation in a HCI context.

4   Expectations

Our long-term goal is to develop technology that motivates people to exercise and adhere to exercising for a longer period of time such that long-term behavior change can be accomplished. We argue that motivational text messages tailored to personality, as a stable, distinctive factor, and framed in behavior change theory, will contribute to longer-term exercise adherence.

In the current work, we explored the relation between personality and the stages, and between personality and the stages, and the processes of change. For the first relation, we expected to find that personality correlates to the stages of change. More specifically, given that Extraversion and Conscientiousness have been found to correlate positively to fitness and health [19–22], and Neuroticism was found to correlate negatively to physical activity [21], we expected to find a positive correlation for Conscientiousness and Extraversion and a negative correlation for Neuroticism in relation to stage of change. For the second relation, we expected to find that different personality traits together with the stages of change related to different processes of change, but we had no expectation specifically, about how traits, stages and processes related.

5   Study

Our study was framed as an online crowdsourcing (language-elicitation) task with questionnaires. The same study was also described in [29] but reports on different results. In the current paper, we focused on the results of the questionnaires. The participants were gathered through Amazon Mechanical Turk (AMT), with a link to SurveyMonkey where the study was hosted. In the questionnaires, we measured the participants' personalities, their self-assessed stage of change and the processes of change.

5.1   Sample

The sample size consisted of 500 people. The data of 19 respondents was excluded because their questionnaires were incomplete. The final sample included 481 respondents (250 male and 231 female). The minimum age was 18 and the maximum was 68. The average age was 31.09 (SD = 9.22) and the median 29.

With respect to education, 201 respondents received some college education, 183 obtained a college degree, 46 obtained a masters degree, 42 completed their high school, 5 obtained a PhD and 4 received other types of education.

The AMT requirements for the respondents were that they had already completed >1000 tasks on AMT, >98 % of them were approved successfully and the respondents were located in the United States. These requirements ensured that respondents were already familiar with surveys, that they were serious about filling in the survey (only 19 were not, which is low for online anonymous surveys) and that they had some proficiency in English.

5.2 Questionnaire Measures

To measure participants' personality we used the 50-item IPIP representation of the revised version of Costa and McCrae's [14] NEO Personality Inventory[1] which posed 50 statements (for example, "Make plans and stick to them."). Participants were asked to answer how self-descriptive they found these statements (on a 5-point Likert scale, 1 being "very inaccurate" and 5 being "very accurate"). We used a 1-item stage of change measure for exercise [30] where participants were given a description of regular exercise and of the five stages and rated their stage based on that description. Additionally, we used a 30-item processes of change measure[2] for exercise [31] which asked how often certain experiences or habits (for example, "I feel more confident when I exercise regularly.") occurred in the last month (each measured by three items, ratings from 1 (never) to 5 (always)).

The reliability of the measures was overall very good (see Table 2 for personality and Table 3 for processes). The only disputable measure was that of Social liberation, with a Cronbach's alpha of .63 which we found still acceptable (and also comparable to other relevant work [7]). Otherwise the reliability scores were between .75 and .90.

5.3 Procedure

Participants were recruited through AMT. They were informed of their compensation, the goal of the survey experiment and the estimated completion time. On SurveyMonkey, the goal of this survey was summarized and participants were asked to complete a consent form. Our study was framed as an online crowdsourcing (language-elicitation) task with questionnaires. First, the participants were given a crowdsourcing language-elicitation task: the description and analysis of this task fall outside the scope of this paper. Second, participants were asked to fill out questionnaires for personality, stage of change and processes of change. We address the results of these questionnaires in the current paper.

---

[1] adopted from http://ipip.ori.org/.

[2] adopted from http://www.uri.edu/research/cprc/measures.htm.

Table 2. Averages (M), standard deviations (SD), and Cronbach's alpha's (α) for all the construed scales. Scales are added, instead of averaged to keep origin clear. Personality scales are 10 items with scoring from 1 to 5 added up (possible scores from 10 to 50). Ordinal regression with stage of change as dependent variable and the personality traits (OCEAN) as independent variables. (N = 481)

Trait	M	SD	α	ratio	sig	CI
Openness to exp.	38.94	6.65	.77	1.015	.252	[0.989 − 1.042]
Conscientiousness	37.75	7.43	.89	1.025	.074	[0.998 − 1.055]
Extraversion	31.02	8.91	.90	1.050	**.000**	[1.028 − 1.075]
Agreeableness	38.24	6.14	.80	0.969	.057	[0.939 − 1.001]
Neuroticism	24.61	8.91	.90	0.971	**.024**	[0.946 − 0.996]

The participants were debriefed about the detailed goals of this survey and given a completion code to fill in on AMT to receive payment. The survey took about 45 min to complete. Participants were compensated 3 US dollars for their participation.

6   Results

Data from 481 participants was analyzed. Important to note is that the self-assessed stages of change measure was not equally distributed: 175 participants rated themselves to be in the *Maintenance stage* (M), 114 in the *Preparation stage* (P), 91 in the *Action stage* (A), 68 in the *Contemplation stage* (C), and 33 participants rated themselves in the *Precontemplation stage* (PC).

6.1   Relation Between Personality and Stages of Change

Based on literature we expected that certain personality traits scores significantly relate to self-assessed stage of change. An ordinal logistic regression was run to determine the effect of the traits (OCEAN) on the self-assessed (ordinal) stages of change. The general model (OCEAN) statistically significantly predicted the stages of change over and above the intercept-only model, $\chi^2(5) = 66.526$, $p < .001$. Concerning the contributing factors, an increase in Extraversion was associated with an increase in stage of change, with an odds ratio of 1.051 (95 % CI, 1.028 to 1.075), $\chi^2(1) = 18.578$, $p < .001$. However, a decrease in Neuroticism was associated with an increase in stage of change, with an odds ratio of 0.971 (95 % CI, 0.946 to 0.996), $\chi^2(1) = 5.091$, $p < .024$. The other personality traits were not significantly ($p < 0.05$) related to stage of change (see Table 2). Overall, the influence of the relations (as expressed in the odds ratio) is small.

Table 3. Averages (M), standard deviations (SD), and Cronbach's alpha's (α) for all the construed scales. Scales are added, instead of averaged to keep origin clear. processes of change are 3 items with scoring from 1 to 5 added up (possible scores from 3 to 15). Standardized regression coefficients of personality traits, stages of change and the processes of change are reported. (N = 481) $^1p < 0.05$, $^2p < 0.01$, $^3p < 0.001$.

PoC	M	SD	α	R^2	SoC β	O β	C β	E β	A β	N β
CR	8.81	3.38	.89	.246	**0.398**^{3}	**0.102**^{1}	0.014	**0.151**^{2}	0.005	0.018
DR	9.10	3.10	.75	.112	**0.278**^{3}	0.080	**0.127**^{1}	0.072	-0.068	0.115
ER	10.65	2.88	.75	.071	0.087	**0.160**^{2}	**0.114**^{1}	0.072	0.011	0.047
SOL	10.64	2.57	.63	.121	0.087	0.064	**0.147**^{2}	**0.171**^{2}	**0.171**^{2}	**0.143**^{1}
SR	12.34	2.75	.86	.260	**0.389**^{3}	**0.225**^{3}	0.014	-0.010	**0.119**^{1}	0.007
SEL	10.98	3.07	.82	.476	**0.619**^{3}	**0.083**^{1}	**0.112**^{2}	0.045	0.006	-0.001
HR	7.81	3.75	.90	.194	**0.297**^{3}	-0.077	0.035	**0.203**^{3}	0.027	-0.046
CC	8.08	3.29	.85	.462	**0.578**^{3}	-0.005	**0.146**^{2}	**0.111**^{2}	0.008	-0.011
RM	11.21	3.11	.84	.310	**0.441**^{3}	**0.164**^{3}	0.062	0.058	0.074	0.001
SC	8.30	3.45	.77	.335	**0.471**^{3}	0.053	**0.115**^{1}	**0.126**^{2}	-0.033	-0.015

6.2   Relation Between Personality and Stages and Processes

We expected that the stages of change and different personalities would relate to different self-assessed processes of change in relation to exercise, but we had no expectation specifically, about how traits, stages and processes related. We were interested in understanding the relations between the continuous personality trait variables (O, C, E, A and N) of the compound variable personality and the continuous variables of the processes of change, which we can assess with regression coefficients. Hence we carried out multiple regression analyses. In Table 3 the standardized regression coefficient (β) scores are reported for the predictor variables stages of change and personality traits (OCEAN) and the outcome variables of the processes of change (10 times). The regression coefficient results suggest that different personality traits scores relate differently to processes of change. All processes are significantly correlated to at least one personality trait, and all personality traits are significantly related to at least one process. It should be noted that although there are significant personality-trait-to-process relations, the stages of change are usually a much larger predictor (this can be seen from the standardized β reported in Table 3). The personality trait results could be considered 'nuances' to the already existing relation between stages and processes.

7   Discussion

Using theory in practice is not always easy and effective. Although there is a general consensus on the value of most behavior change theories and more specifically the Transtheoretical Model, there is also still plenty of room to increase the effectiveness and salience of such theories by identifying more determinants (e.g., personality) for specific situations (e.g., the exercise domain) and by revealing new dependencies between them. As a first step towards combining personality and behavior change theory to motivate people to exercise, we assessed the possibility of personality-based tailoring of the processes of change through crowdsourcing and self-assessment measures. We conclude that (1) personality traits (E and N) relate to the stages of change and (2) personality traits and the stages of change relate to preferences for certain processes of change. In this section we discuss the implications of the results separately for each expectation.

7.1   Relation Between Personality and Stages of Change

The results of the study show that people's personalities are related to their progression through the different stages of change for exercise behavior, specifically that the Extraversion trait was positively correlated with people progressing through the stages, while the Neuroticism trait was negatively correlated with progressing through the stages. In other words, people scoring higher on Extraversion are more likely to be in higher stages of change, while people scoring higher on Neuroticism are more likely to be in the lower stages of change. No significant relation was found between Conscientiousness and the stages of change. Although the correlations of personality traits to the stages of change are relatively small, this is similar to other research on personality and physical activity [21] and considered still important for the health context. For Extraversion and Neuroticism, which are significantly correlated to the stages, one tentative explanation could be that people change their personality when changing their behavior. But, because it is believed that personality is temporally stable [15], a more likely explanation is that people with low Extraversion and high Neuroticism scores need different motivations and see different barriers when trying to change their behavior (compared to high Extraversion, low Neuroticism scoring people) then those addressed in current motivational technology and programs and therefore these people have more difficulties in changing their behavior.

7.2   Relation Between Personality and Stages and Processes

Our study also shows that there are relations between different personality traits and different processes of change they find important in relation to exercise. Conscientiousness is related to six processes, Openness to Experience and Extraversion are related to five, Agreeableness to two, and Neuroticism to one. Interesting to see is that Neuroticism, which correlated negatively to the stages of change, does not (significantly) relate to many processes. This could support our previous interpretation that the processes believed to help people through the stages are not very appealing to people scoring high on Neuroticism and therefore they also do not progress through the stages. Similar results with health-promoting strategies for people scoring high on Neuroticism were found in previous work [23]. Conscientiousness, which we expected to relate to the stages of change did not, but in turn correlated to the most processes. Previous work also suggested a relation between Conscientiousness and the stages of change, but found that this was fully mediated by the relation between Conscientiousness and certain processes [32]. In any case, the results show a relation between different processes of change and personality traits, which serves as an indication that the tailoring of processes to personality trait preferences could be very helpful in making the messages more salient for behavior change.

7.3   Limitations of the Current Study

There were some limitations to the present study. Firstly, we used a cross-sectional design which does not provide strong evidence for causation, only correlation. A second limitation is that we ran our study on AMT. This could misrepresent the 'general' population, although some studies have reported that AMT can give very good representation of general society, especially for online survey standards [33]. A third limitation is the self-assessment nature of the measures, which asks people to *think* about what strategies influence them. This does not necessarily mean these strategies *will* influence them, or that they will be influenced by textual representations of these strategies.

8   Conclusion

As part of a larger study, we sought to leverage certain HCI practices, like crowd-sourcing, to explore theory on behavior change from psychological research to come to useful and practical insights about how to further adapt the processes of change to (robust) user characteristics (e.g., personality traits). We identified new dependencies between the different processes, stages and personality traits in the context of the exercise domain. And we made a first step in translating theoretical constructs and principles of behavior change theories to information structures and interaction designs. These findings can help inform developers of motivational and persuasive technology who want to use the TTM as a foundation for long-term behavior change and who want to use personality to tailor to individuals. Concretely, we argue that: (1) when designing for behavior change, one should take into account the relation between someone's personality and the stages of behavior change; (2) when designing for more than one-size-fits-all, one should take into account the relation between someone's personality and the preference for different processes of change.

In future research, we will address the limitations of the current study (see Sect. 7.3), and carry out a long-term in-the-wild study to look into the effectiveness of personality-tailored behavior change messages.

Acknowledgments. This research was funded by COMMIT/ and is part of the P3 project SenseI: Sensor-Based Engagement for Improved Health. We would like to thank Maartje de Graaf for her input.

References

1. Hekler, E.B., Klasnja, P., Froehlich, J.E., Buman, M.P.: Mind the theoretical gap: interpreting, using, and developing behavioral theory in HCI research. In: Proceedings of the SIGCHI Conference on Human Factors in Computing Systems, PP. 3307–3316. ACM (2013)
2. Noar, S.M., Benac, C.N., Harris, M.S.: Does tailoring matter? meta-analytic review of tailored print health behavior change interventions. Psychol. Bull. **133**(4), 673–693 (2007)
3. Arteaga, S.M., Kudeki, M., Woodworth, A., Kurniawan, S.: Mobile system to motivate teenagers' physical activity. In: Proceedings of the 9th International Conference on Interaction Design and Children, pp. 1–10. ACM (2010)
4. Chatterjee, S., Price, A.: Healthy living with persuasive technologies: framework, issues, and challenges. J. Am. Med. Inform. Assoc. **16**(2), 171–178 (2009)
5. Prochaska, J.O., DiClemente, C.C.: Stages and processes of self-change of smoking: toward an integrative model of change. J. Consult. Clin. Psychol. **51**(3), 390 (1983)
6. Spencer, L., Adams, T.B., Malone, S., Roy, L., Yost, E.: Applying the transtheoretical model to exercise: a systematic and comprehensive review of the literature. Health Promot. Pract. **7**(4), 428–443 (2006)
7. Marcus, B.H., Rossi, J.S., Selby, V.C., Niaura, R.S., Abrams, D.B.: The stages and processes of exercise adoption and maintenance in a worksite sample. Health Psychol. **11**(6), 386 (1992)
8. Lacroix, J., Saini, P., Goris, A.: Understanding user cognitions to guide the tailoring of persuasive technology-based physical activity interventions. In: Proceedings of the 4th International Conference on Persuasive Technology, p. 9. ACM (2009)
9. Kaptein, M., De Ruyter, B., Markopoulos, P., Aarts, E.: Adaptive persuasive systems: a study of tailored persuasive text messages to reduce snacking. ACM Trans. Interact. Intell. Syst. (TIIS) **2**(2), 10 (2012)
10. Alkış, N., Temizel, T.T.: The impact of individual differences on influence strategies. Personality Individ. Differ. **87**, 147–152 (2015)
11. Kaptein, M., Markopoulos, P., de Ruyter, B., Aarts, E.: Personalizing persuasive technologies: Explicit and implicit personalization using persuasion profiles. Int. J. Hum. Comput. Stud. **77**, 38–51 (2015)
12. Nigg, C.R., Geller, K.S., Motl, R.W., Horwath, C.C., Wertin, K.K., Dishman, R.K.: A research agenda to examine the efficacy and relevance of the transtheoretical model for physical activity behavior. Psychol. Sport Exercise **12**(1), 7–12 (2011)
13. Goldberg, L.R.: The development of markers for the big-five factor structure. Psychol. Assess. **4**(1), 26 (1992)
14. Costa, P.T., McCrae, R.R.: Normal personality assessment in clinical practice: The NEO personality inventory. Psychol. Assess. **4**(1), 5 (1992)
15. Rhodes, R.E., Courneya, K.S., Jones, L.W.: Personality and social cognitive influences on exercise behavior: adding the activity trait to the theory of planned behavior. Psychol. Sport Exerc. **5**(3), 243–254 (2004)
16. McCrae, R.R., Costa Jr., P.T.: A five-factor theory of personality. Handbook of personality: Theory and research **2**, 139–153 (1999)
17. Cole-Lewis, H., Kershaw, T.: Text messaging as a tool for behavior change in disease prevention and management. Epidemiol. Rev. **32**(1), 56–69 (2010)
18. Michie, S., Johnston, M., Francis, J., Hardeman, W., Eccles, M.: From theory to intervention: mapping theoretically derived behavioural determinants to behaviour change techniques. Appl. psychol. **57**(4), 660–680 (2008)

19. Gallagher, P., Yancy, W.S., Denissen, J.J.A., Kühnel, A., Voils, C.I.: Correlates of daily leisure-time physical activity in a community sample: Narrow personality traits and practical barriers. Health Psychol. Official J. Div. Health Psychol. Am. Psychol. Assoc. **32**(12), 1227–1235 (2013)
20. Hoyt, A.L., Rhodes, R.E., Hausenblas, H.A., Giacobbi, P.R.: Integrating five-factor model facet-level traits with the theory of planned behavior and exercise. Psychol. Sport Exerc. **10**(5), 565–572 (2009)
21. Rhodes, R.E., Smith, N.E.I.: Personality correlates of physical activity: a review and meta-analysis. Br. J. Sports Med. **40**(12), 958–965 (2006)
22. Courneya, K.S., Hellsten, L.A.M.: Personality correlates of exercise behavior, motives, barriers and preferences: An application of the five-factor model. Personality Indiv. Differ. **24**(5), 625–633 (1998)
23. Halko, S., Kientz, J.: Personality and persuasive technology: an exploratory study on health-promoting mobile applications. In: Persuasive technology, pp. 150–161 (2010)
24. Ingledew, D.K., Markland, D.: The role of motives in exercise participation. Psychol. Health **23**(7), 807–828 (2008)
25. Ferron, M., Massa, P.: Transtheoretical model for designing technologies supporting an active lifestyle. In: Proceedings of the Biannual Conference of the Italian Chapter of SIGCHI, p. 7. ACM (2013)
26. Latimer, A.E., Brawley, L.R., Bassett, R.L.: A systematic review of three approaches for constructing physical activity messages: what messages work and what improvements are needed? Int. J. Behav. Nutr. Phys. Act. **7**, 36–53 (2010)
27. Hirsh, J.B., Kang, S.K., Bodenhausen, G.V.: Personalized persuasion: tailoring persuasive appeals to recipients' personality traits. Psychol. Sci. **23**(6), 578–581 (2012)
28. Adnan, M., Mukhtar, H., Naveed, M.: Persuading students for behavior change by determining their personality type. In: 2012 15th International Multitopic Conference (INMIC), pp. 439–449 (2012)
29. De Vries, R.A.J., Truong, K.P., Kwint, S., Drossaert, C.H.C., Evers, V.: Crowd-designed motivation: Motivational messages for exercise adherence based on behavior change theory. In: Proceedings of the SIGCHI Conference on Human Factors in Computing Systems. ACM (in press, 2016)
30. Norman, G., Benisovich, S., Nigg, C., Rossi, J.: Examining three exercise staging algorithms in two samples. In: 19th Annual Meeting of the Society of Behavioral Medicine (1998)
31. Nigg, C., Norman, G., Rossi, J., Benisovich, S.: Processes of exercise behavior change: Redeveloping the scale. Ann. Behav. Med. **21**, S79 (1999)
32. Bogg, T.: Conscientiousness, the transtheoretical model of change, and exercise: a neo-socioanalytic integration of trait and social-cognitive frameworks in the prediction of behavior. J. Pers. **76**(4), 775–802 (2008)
33. Mason, W., Suri, S.: Conducting behavioral research on amazon's mechanical turk. Behav. Res. Methods **44**(1), 1–23 (2012)

The EDIE Method – Towards an Approach to Collaboration-Based Persuasive Design

Sandra Burri Gram-Hansen[✉]

Department of Communication and Psychology, Aalborg University, Aalborg, Denmark
burri@hum.aau.dk

Abstract. This paper presents the initial steps towards a collaboration-based method for persuasive design – the EDIE method (*Explore, Design, Implement, Evaluate*). The method is inspired by Design-Based Research, but developed to combine different design approaches that have dominated the persuasive technology field over the past decade. The rhetorical notion of Kairos is considered a key element in the EDIE method, resulting in a distinct focus on participatory design and constructive ethics. The method is explained through a practical example of developing persuasive learning designs in collaboration with the Danish Ministry of Defence and the Installation Management Command.

Keywords: Persuasive design · Energy and environmental behaviour · Sustainability · Design-Based research · Participatory design · Constructive ethics · Persuasive design framework

1   Introduction

In this paper, the initial steps towards a collaboration-based method for persuasive design is presented and discussed. The framework is based upon the Design-Based Research Methodology (DBR) [1], but distinguishes itself by combining different context- and system-oriented approaches from the persuasive technology field, and by enabling ethics to be applied constructively throughout the design process. The method constitutes some of the results found by applying DBR when exploring the potential of persuasive learning designs in the Danish army.

Over the past decade, different methods to persuasive design have been discussed and exemplified, as researchers have taken either a primarily system-oriented [2] or primarily user-centred approach to the design process [3, 4]. Simultaneously, the theoretical underpinning of the notion of persuasive technologies has been explored and developed through both practical exemplifications and thorough literary investigations [5, 6]. Across these different approaches the rhetorical notion of Kairos [7] continuously establishes itself as a key concept to persuasion, both from a narrow system-oriented angle and a wider more contextual perspective. From the foundation of this classical rhetorical understanding of timing and appropriateness, it has been argued that persuasive initiatives are only successful when applied within the intended use context,

© Springer International Publishing Switzerland 2016
A. Meschtscherjakov et al. (Eds.): PERSUASIVE 2016, LNCS 9638, pp. 53–64, 2016.
DOI: 10.1007/978-3-319-31510-2_5

that the notion of persuasion and subsequently persuasive technologies hold a strong ethical demand, and that a user-centred approach to design is a requisite to successful persuasive designs [6].

Within the persuasive technology research field, several researchers have argued that Value Sensitive Design and Participatory design are particular relevant to the development of persuasive designs [10–12], partly due to the ethical implications related to designing for behaviour change, and partly in respect to the rhetorical notion of Kairos. Kairos sums up the concept of the opportune moment, in consideration of time, place and manner in which a persuasive initiative is taken. Kairos constitutes both a narrow understanding of the appropriate time for something to take place, and a wider more philosophical understanding of appropriateness within an intended use context. In order for designers to grasp this opportune moment, they must strive to create an appropriate balance between the persuasive initiative and the intended use context. [7]. Whilst both the temporal and location-based perspectives of Kairos may possibly be defined and formalised without user involvement, detecting the appropriate manner is dependent on user participation [6]. As designers we may share our ideas regarding new approaches to digital learning, but only those who understand the practice of the intended use context can determine whether or not our ideas may be both applicable and persuasive.

This paper presents the argument that the system-oriented and user-centred approaches, which have been developed and/or discussed in relation to persuasive technology, may be constructively combined in the development process. Considering Kairos throughout the design process facilitates this bridge between design approaches, leading to the initial version of the EDIE method - a collaboration-based persuasive design approach.

2   The EDIE Method

As previously stated the Edie method is inspired by and developed in accordance with the DBR methodology - an iterative process for developing, testing, evaluating, and refining design solutions. As a research methodology it is most often applied in the context of learning and education, but the applicability of the approach is not restricted to this domain. By design based, it is understood that research is conducted as designs are developed and implemented in practice and that the research is oriented towards exploring best practices or generating directions for future design processes [1]. Particular attention is directed towards DBR's consistent focus on stakeholder collaboration and the mentioned focus on the intended use context. By maintaining yet adjusting this constituent, both the wider notions of Kairos and the ethical demand related to persuasion, may be taken into consideration.

The EDIE method is a collaboration-based persuasive design methodology, constituted by the four phases *Explore, Design, Implement, Evaluate* (EDIE) visualised in Fig. 1. The method aims to facilitate a bridge between the human-centred and the system-centred approaches, which have dominated the persuasive technology field. Rather than focusing solely on either the user-centred or the system-oriented aspects of persuasive design, the method provides directions for designers to include both perspectives in the design process, and to let the different perspectives constructively influence each other.

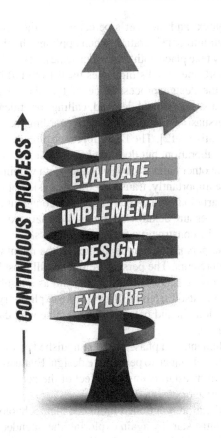

Fig. 1. The EDIE method - a collaboration-based persuasive design method

The different steps in the process, enable designers to consider and apply aspects of e.g. persuasive system design [13] and ambient persuasion [14], while consistently considering the intended use context and applying ethics constructively throughout the design process. Thereby, both the wider and the narrow perspectives of Kairos are acknowledged and considered.

2.1 Basic Distinctions

Whilst DBR and similar approaches are iterative both in the understanding that all four steps can be repeated several times, and internally within the test and refinement phase, it is predominantly a research methodology, and iterations will expectedly come to an end once the research questions have been answered. Persuasion on the other hand can be understood as a continuous process of shaping, reinforcing or changing the behaviour of users [2, 15], as users are constantly influenced not only by the persuasive system with which they are interacting, but also by changes to their use context and their community of practice. From a persuasive design perspective, it is important to acknowlededge that when a technology is added to a context, whether this be within the physical or digital realm, the context and the user's perception of the context is altered [6]. In order for this to be taken into consideration when applying the the EDIE method, iterations must continuously take place both on a wider scale and within the different phases.

Furthermore, the EDIE method distinguishes itself from DBR by including ethical reflections throughout the design process. One of the distinct claims of persuasive design, may be seen as a strong ethical demand, calling for ethical reflections not only regarding the overall persuasive intention, but also regarding the appropriateness of the different persuasive initiatives [12]. The DBR approach already emphasises the importance of stakeholder collaboration, but does not have a distinct focus on applied ethics. The EDIE method on the other hand, considers ethics both within the individual phases of the process, and more importantly, transfers ethical considerations from one phase to another. Furthermore, participatory design is applied throughout the four phases of the EDIE method, in order to ensure acknowledgment of domain experts, and to enable the ethical considerations to be constructive for design process.

As mentioned above, persuasion can be defined as the intent to shape, reinforce or change attitudes and behaviours. The persuasive intent will most likely spring from an already established need for behavioural influence, and as a result, the first step of the EDIE method distinguishes itself from DBR by a more exploratory approach to gaining an understanding of the domain and potentially determine why the intended behaviour does not already take place.

The design and implementation phases are distinguished by the inclusion of theories and methods with specific relevance to persuasive design. Evaluation in the fourth phase however, is directed towards establishing the effect of the persuasive initiatives, rather than determine best practice or design directions.

In consideration of the aforementioned influence that technologies can have on the context, new iterations must start by again exploring the intended use context in order to identify significant changes. This particular distinction is visualised by the on-going spiral in Fig. 1.

3   Applying the EDIE Method in Practice

The Danish Military is a highly complex organisation with a combination of armed forces, technical staff and civilian employees. As such, employee tasks and work facilities differ greatly as 33% of the military employees are office workers, whilst others rarely work indoors.

In order to optimise and standardise learning material across Danish Military Establishments, an increasing amount of learning material is digitalised and distributed centrally. One of the topics, which have been developed as a digital resource, is material regarding environmental legislation and appropriate environment behaviour in the Danish military. To ensure that the information is fully disseminated, all employees are required to complete the e-learning course *"The Environmental Driver's License"* (EDL) with a minimum of 80% correct answers to the included questions.

Whilst EDL does ensure standardised dissemination of environment material, this traditional e-learning course is nonetheless faced with several fundamental challenges:

- Far from all Danish military establishments are equipped with sufficient digital resources to enable the majority of their employees to attend an e-learning course
- The learning material presented in EDL does not differentiate between the different segments of employees in the Danish Military

Whilst the practical issue regarding insufficient digital resources may easily be solved, the problems related to lack of differentiation in the learning material constitutes a greater challenge. When all employees are required to relate to all the learning material, the topic may be perceived as less relevant to the individual employee, thus they may be lead to believe that the EDL is generally meant for someone else in the organisation. The lack of relevance to individual employees may potentially have negative consequences both in relation to transferability of the knowledge acquired (it may be difficult to transfer the content of EDL to practical tasks at the military establishments), and also to the long-term effect of the e-learning course.

The aforementioned problems related to EDL formed the basis of a new approach to environment education, initiated by the Installation Management Command (IMC) in 2014. In order to not just inform employees about environmental requirements in the Danish Military, but to also motivate a more environment friendly attitude and behaviour in the organization, IMC initiated the development of a prototype for environmental education which distinctively draws upon motivational elements, and which reforms the notion of digital learning within the organization.

The persuasive learning design discussed in this paper aims to educate the drafted recruits in appropriate waste management and action in case of accidents. The central element in this persuasive learning design is the prototype of a location- and situation-based game *Acttention*, which has been designed and developed specifically to meet the requirements of the Danish Military. As such, the content is targeted directly towards the drafted recruits, whilst the game is designed to be flexible and easily adjusted to fit the needs of other employee groups. In the following sections, the individual steps of the EDIE method are elaborated and exemplified in practice.

3.1 Phase 1 - Explore

In order to gain a better understanding of the intended use context, and to define any particular requirements, that needed to be taken into consideration, Phase 1 constituted a thorough analysis of intended use context and the existing solutions.

The intended use context was explored through a combination of field visits and observation studies at the different army bases and supported by wider segmentation and target group analysis.

The segmentation analysis was based on a quantitative evaluation of the army employees' attitude towards environmental education in the organization [16]. From the analysis it was clear that whilst a majority of the respondents find energy and environmental considerations important, they do not consider the subject a primary concern to their function in the army. Moreover, the analysis concluded that 20% of the respondents were hesitant or even reluctant towards the subject of energy and environmental education within the organization. As such, the analysis underpinned the relevance of persuasive design in the case due to the understanding learning takes place in the learner, and is dependent on his or her motivation towards the subject. Consequently, traditional learning designs would likely prove to be insufficient.

In order to accommodate the requirement that the learning design should be applicable across different army bases, two very different army establishments were selected as test locations for the pilot project, and field visits and in-situ interviews were conducted at both locations. Observation studies and similar ethnographic methods are often applied in relation to participatory design, and also exemplified by Davis when she argued towards the potential of participatory design in relation to persuasive technologies [4]. However, ethnography and similar approaches to understanding the intended use context may hold even more potential, if considering the rhetorical notion of Kairos a key concept to persuasion. Ethnography may facilitate the understanding of the contextual perspective, which also sums up the three dimensions of Kairos. Additionally, as the field research was done in collaboration with all primary project participants, the experiences shared formed the initial basis of a constructive ethical approach throughout the design process [12].

The field research was followed up by a series of creative workshops attended by representatives from the army, the navy and the air force, as well as from the IMC and the Danish Ministry of Defence. Apart from providing valuable insights regarding the basis of the mentioned reluctance towards the energy and environmental learning designs, the workshop also aimed to establish a mutual understanding between the participants. Thereby, the workshop also served as an initial step towards facilitating the collaboration between stakeholders throughout the design process – an outcome that was considered particularly important when working in a context with strong and evident hierarchical structures. Moreover, the workshops were planned and executed in consideration of ontological ethics, thus strengthening the constructive influence of ethics [12].

The workshop participants applied LEGO and Play-Dough as they created prototypes of future green army barracks, leading to a number of specific requirements for the architects to take into consideration. As the workshop progressed, it furthermore constituted a significant contribution to the context exploration, as they provided a number of rich explanations to practice within the intended use context. Amongst the specific requirements uncovered during the workshop was the need for environmental education to be included in other activities. Part of the reluctance towards the subject is related to a well-known challenge in educational systems – that there is much to teach and very little time to do it.

In order to also include evaluations of the existing technical solution, the PSD model [13] was applied to analyse and evaluate the EDL. The PSD framework facilitated a deeper understanding of the existing learning design, and helped initiate the discussion of the potential of persuasive principles in learning technologies. The system analysis led to the conclusion that the EDL failed to reduce and tailor the complex learning material. The analysis clarified that one of the primary challenges of the EDL was the intent to educate and motivate all employees through the same system. As mentioned, this not only constituted a practical problem, it also imposed an educational challenge as people are rarely motivated by material that they do not find relevant. For instance, smokers who do not wish to stop smoking are seldom influenced by the many campaigns regarding the subject, whereas smokers who have an endogenous wish to quit smoking may be able to find help and support through the different initiatives. As a result, it was decided that the prototype should focus on a specific group of employees (drafted recruits in the Danish Army), but that the design should be scalable in way that would enable it to be transferred to other groups of employees a later time.

3.2 Phase 2 - Design

Based on the information gathered from the analysis of practical problems, steps were taken towards the development of a learning design that would both provide information regarding appropriate environmental behaviour and motivate the learners to change both their attitude and their behaviour. As was the case in the first phase, the design phase was also conducted as a participatory design process. At this stage, the design group was narrowed in and consisted of representatives from the IMC, researchers, and technical developers with a background in experience design. All participants had been involved in the first phase of the process, ensuring that not only practical but also ethical considerations were brought along into this second phase.

In the acknowledgement that the employees do not see energy and environmental issues as core focus areas, the persuasive learning design was developed with an intent to influence the community of practice in the Danish Military. By doing so, the design distinguished itself from traditional approaches to environmental education within the army, by recognising that the learners do not consider the learning content important.

With a specific focus on army recruits, it was determined that traditional e-Learning solutions such as the EDL would not be suitable, partly due to the age group (18–20 year olds), and partly due to the daily practice of this particular segment. Recruits spend most of their working hours outdoors, and the segment consists of a highly diverse group of learners, where some may be on their way to university, whilst others will have struggled all through school. Physical training is a high priority for the recruits, as many of them are in poor physical condition when they enlist. Competition is high within the segment, and training often includes an element of behaviourism, where good results are rewarded. As a result, the design moved towards a location-based game, which could be implemented as part of the physical training.

The initial design proposal presented by the technical developers consisted solely of the *Acttention* game. It was designed as a location-based game where the recruits would interact with touch screens, be presented with waste management related questions, and then sent to a relevant location on the Military base in order to link the content of the question to a specific location. However, very early in the design process, this solution was found inadequate both from a learning perspective and from a persuasive perspective. As a learning technology, the game lacked information regarding the appropriate action in different situations; information which was a necessity if the game was to facilitate learning, rather than merely be a quiz game with a 33% chance of giving a correct answer. From a persuasive design perspective, the game lacked transparent persuasive intentions both with regards to the in-game situation and with regards to the long-term effect. There was no apparent link between the individual components of the game, and an overall persuasive intention.

In order to address this issue, an instructional film based on the existing content from EDL, was created to ensure that all recruits were presented with knowledge regarding appropriate waste management. Consequently, the game was transferred from being a learning game to becoming a tool for motivating reflections regarding appropriate behaviour. A series of different scenarios with different solutions were implemented, designed to simulate situations the recruits might find themselves in when needing to recall their knowledge about appropriate waste management.

Persuasive design was considered both in the wider and more contextual aspect of implementing a new technology within a context, and in the specific design of the game. From a contextual perspective, the combination of specifically tailored learning material and the distinct respect towards the general attitude that environmental education is regarded as low priority, both became motivational elements in the learning design. Also, the instruction film included examples from both the army bases and civilian life, in order to highlight that the information provided by the film was relevant not only in relation to personnel working on Danish army bases. By doing so, the instruction film aimed to address one of the long-term goals of the Danish drafting procedure – educating valuable members of society.

System specifically, persuasive design was taken into consideration with regards to the user interaction with the touch screens and more specifically the feedback offered by the system. In order to ensure that the Acttention game facilitated learning without requiring too much attention, user feedback was provided as a combination of brief test messages (e.g. right answer, wrong code), and supported by brightly coloured icons. Furthermore, the correct answer was highlighted in green while wrong answers were highlighted in red. Research conducted by Ham and Midden has shown that whilst users have no relation to other colour codes such as blue/yellow, the combination of red/green is subconsciously understood as positive and negative [14].

3.3   Phase 3 - Implement

Prior to testing the design with recruits, a pre-test was conducted at one of the designated army bases, by a group of university students from a Masters program in Information Architecture. None of the students had any knowledge about practice in the army, but their feedback was considered significant as their education enables them to provide very specific system-oriented evaluations. As such, this test enabled us to test the functionality of the game within the intended use context, and at the same time incorporate some final adjustments to the design. For instance, the students found that the red/green colour-based feedback should be extended, and that the possibility to skip the feedback should be removed if the learner had solved a scenario incorrectly.

The first iteration of tests with recruits took place in November 2014 at Almegaard army base on the small Danish island Bornholm, and involved 62 recruits representing three platoons. This particular army base distinguishes itself by being one of the bases, in which the physical facilities are preserved as listed buildings although the buildings are still at use.

Almegaard is also one of the smaller army bases in Denmark, which means that most locations, such as recruit quarters, garage area and environment area are less than 1 km apart and can be reached on foot. Other army bases are much larger and the different game related locations might be located so far apart that they cannot all be included. As such, Almegaard served well as a location for the first test iteration, as it enabled a test of the full range of the game.

The test took place over three days, thus enabling the design team to iteratively evaluate and adjust from day to day. Adjustments to the setup were done in careful consideration of data comparability, but whilst the overall learning design remained the same, some changes were made in order to ensure higher stability in the game. Time wise, it would have been possible to conduct all three tests during one day. However to also exemplify the design's ability to adapt to the practice within the intended use context, the trial was included as an element within a three day course which besides from waste management also included *first aid* and *fire and rescue*.

For each individual test of the learning design, the participating recruits met in the army base auditorium, where they were informed about the overall plan for the event as well as the evaluation activities that would take place during their participation in the Acttention learning design.

The recruits then watched the short 15-minute instruction film before heading out to the Acttention game base. Here they were given further information about how to play the Acttention game, and divided in to smaller teams of 5–6 members. The Acttention game is run via three touch screens and one administration screen, and these were set up in a sheltered location with easy access to the surrounding perimeters. The recruits were provided with individual chip bracelets, which enabled them to register their individual interaction with the system, thereby ensuring that all recruits were presented with all the learning scenarios in the game.

Whilst a member of the design team gave the introduction to the course and evaluation, the commissioned officers were present and engaged throughout the process. Their involvement both served as a way of introducing them to the learning design in practice, thereby ensuring that they can handle future use of the system themselves, but it also served as a way to ensure credibility of the learning design in the eyes of the participating recruits and as an empowerment of the commissioned officers.

As the terms of the game and the team competition was explained, the recruits' seriousness was replaced with a more playful and relaxed attitude – still without losing focus on what was being required of them. The team spirit and the more relaxed and collaborative attitude was facilitated further by elements such as selecting a team name and enabling the system to *tailor* the touch screens to the different teams.

3.4   Phase 4 - Evaluate

The evaluation phase was specifically designed to evaluate both the learning outcome and the persuasive potential of the design. From a design perspective there was a high interest in evaluating if the persuasive learning design had motivated a more positive attitude towards environmental education amongst the participants, however, as the design had been developed within a learning context, it was also vital to ensure that the recruits had not only enjoyed themselves but also acquired the necessary knowledge. The evaluation methods combined qualitative and quantitative methods, in order to ensure that both the learning potential and the persuasiveness of the design were assessed through the same evaluation process. In practice, this included questionnaires, observation studies and in situ interviews

Preliminary findings indicated that the combination of instructional film and location-based learning facilitated a transition from individual learning to collaborate learning. This blended learning approach and in particular the collaborative activities in the team-based learning game, ensured that all members of the platoon were able to engage in the learning experience and reflect upon the learning material.

Results from the first test showed that more than 71% of the recruits completed with results that meet or exceed the expectations of the Defence Academy. From a persuasive perspective, the learning design was well received by the recruits, who found it particularly positive to be physically active while learning, and who found the competitive element to be highly motivating. After completing the game, 78% of the recruits indicated that they found the learning material relevant and useful, and 81% indicated that learning about appropriate waste management had been fun. In light of the previously mentioned negativity towards the subject, the feedback regarding the learning experience was perceived as highly positive.

Moreover, the design enabled persuasion to take place at different user levels. Whilst the recruits may have been persuaded by engaging in the Acttention learning design, the commissioned officers and instructors were motivated and persuaded by a combination of experiencing Acttention in practice during the test iterations and more importantly having some sense of ownership of the learning design. To a great extent, this can be credited to the participatory design activities that have facilitated the entire development process. Feedback from the involved instructors and officers stated that it was a welcomed change to traditional communication within the organisation to see that their domain knowledge and input was distinctively taken into consideration in this new approach to digital learning. Both identified in the overall design decision to implement environmental education into a physical training session, and also specifically within the different scenarios.

4   Final Reflections - Future Research

Through the practical application of the EDIE method, it has been possible to combine context- and system-oriented approaches to persuasive design, whilst including ethical considerations throughout the design process. The consistent focus on participatory design facilitates both a deeper understanding of the intended use context, and the inclusion of ethical reflections in relation to persuasive designs.

By ensuring a continuous engagement by both designers and instructors, the methodology distinguishes itself from other similar design approaches, where participatory design most often takes place with a group of domain experts and only few representatives of the design team. In the acknowledgement that persuasive design is highly context dependent, the methodology presented in this paper suggests that all members of the design team must share experiences within the intended use context in order to partake in the design process. Not only to ensure that all members of the team acquire sufficient knowledge about the intended use context, but also to ensure that crucial information is transferred from one phase of the methodology to another. In consideration of Kairos, it may be argued that only users, who are already a part of the intended use context, fully understand what may be appropriate within that context. Consequently, the individual members of the design team's different interpretations of the intended context, all become equally important pieces of a puzzle, which they must participate in putting together.

Furthermore, the consistent attendance of all designers ensured that a mutual understanding was established between them, based on the interactions that took place and the experiences that were shared. Several researchers have argued that ethics is a distinctive aspect of persuasive design. When taking ontological ethics into consideration, this persuasive design methodology facilitates that ethics becomes constructive for the entire design process.

Future research will involve a thorough clarification of the different phases of the EDIE method, so that they more precisely incorporate the different aspects of persuasive design. In 2016 the framework is to be applied in two individual cases equally complex to the one presented in this paper. From this it is expected that the individual phases of the approach will be more distinctly described, as will the specific considerations related to applying ethics constructively in the design process.

Acknowledgements. The practical exemplification presented in this paper was arranged and conducted in collaboration with Thilde Møller Larsen from The Defence Installation Management Command, Denmark

References

1. Reeves, T.C.: Design research from a technology perspective. Educ. Des. Res. **1**(3), 52–66 (2006)
2. Oinas-Kukkonen, H., Harjumaa, M.: A systematic framework for designing and evaluating persuasive systems. In: Oinas-Kukkonen, H., Hasle, P., Harjumaa, M., Segerståhl, K., Øhrstrøm, P. (eds.) PERSUASIVE 2008. LNCS, vol. 5033, pp. 164–176. Springer, Heidelberg (2008)
3. Lockton, D., Harrison, D., Stanton, N.A.: The design with intent method: a design tool for influencing user behaviour. Appl. Ergonomics **41**(3), 382–392 (2010)
4. Davis, J.: Generating directions for persuasive technology design with the inspiration card workshop. In: Ploug, T., Hasle, P., Oinas-Kukkonen, H. (eds.) PERSUASIVE 2010. LNCS, vol. 6137, pp. 262–273. Springer, Heidelberg (2010)
5. Torning, K., Oinas-Kukkonen, H.: Persuasive system design: state of the art and future directions. In: Proceedings of the 4th International Conference on Persuasive Technology. ACM, Claremont (2009)
6. Gram-Hansen, S.B., Ryberg, T.: Persuasion, learning and context adaptation. Special Issue Int. J. Conceptual Struct. Smart Appl. **1**(2), 28–37 (2013)
7. Kinneavy, J.L.: Kairos in classical and modern rhetorical theory. In: Sipiora, P., Baumlin, J.S. (eds.) Rhetoric and Kairos, Essays in History, Theory and Practice. State University of New York Press, Albany (2002)

8. Amiel, T., Reeves, T.C.: Design based research and educational technology: rethinking technology and the research agenda. Educ. Technol. Soc. **11**, 29–40 (2008)
9. Gram-Hansen, S.B., Ryberg, T.: Acttention – influencing communities of practice with persuasive learning designs. In: MacTavish, T., Basapur, S. (eds.) PERSUASIVE 2015. LNCS, vol. 9072, pp. 184–195. Springer, Heidelberg (2015)
10. Davis, J.: Design methods for ethical persuasive computing. In: Proceedings of the 4th International Conference on Persuasive Technology. ACM, Claremont (2009)
11. Davis, J.: Towards participatory design of ambient persuasive technology. In: Proceedings of Pervasive 2008 Workshop, Australia, Sydney (2008)
12. Gram-Hansen, S.B., Ryberg, T.: From participatory design and ontological ethics, towards an approach to constructive ethics. In: Ethicomp 2015, ACM SIGCAS, Leicester (2015)
13. Oinas-Kukkoen, H., Harjumaa, M.: Persuasive systems design: key issues, process model, and system features. Commun. Assoc. Inf. Syst. **24**, 28 (2009)
14. Ham, J., Midden, C.: Ambient persuasive technology needs little cognitive effort: the differential effects of cognitive load on lighting feedback versus factual feedback. In: Ploug, T., Hasle, P., Oinas-Kukkonen, H. (eds.) PERSUASIVE 2010. LNCS, vol. 6137, pp. 132–142. Springer, Heidelberg (2010)
15. Miller, G.R.: On being persuaded, some basic distinctions. In: Dillard, J.P., Pfau, M. (eds.) The Persuasion Handbook, Developments in Theory and Practice. Saga Publications, London (2002)
16. Operate, Målgruppeanalyse og Segmentering (2012)

Persuasive Backfiring: When Behavior Change Interventions Trigger Unintended Negative Outcomes

Agnis Stibe[1(✉)] and Brian Cugelman[2,3]

[1] MIT Media Lab, Cambridge, MA, USA
agnis@mit.edu
[2] Statistical Cybermetrics Research Group,
University of Wolverhampton, Wolverhampton, UK
brian@alterspark.com
[3] AlterSpark, Toronto, ON, Canada

Abstract. Numerous scholars study how to design evidence-based interventions that can improve the lives of individuals, in a way that also brings social benefits. However, within the behavioral sciences in general, and the persuasive technology field specifically, scholars rarely focus-on, or report the negative outcomes of behavior change interventions, and possibly fewer report a special type of negative outcome, a backfire. This paper has been authored to start a wider discussion within the scientific community on intervention backfiring. Within this paper, we provide tools to aid academics in the study of persuasive backfiring, present a taxonomy of backfiring causes, and provide an analytical framework containing the intention-outcome and likelihood-severity matrices. To increase knowledge on how to mitigate the negative impact of intervention backfiring, we discuss research and practitioner implications.

Keywords: Backfire · Taxonomy · Behavior change · Intention-outcome matrix · Likelihood-severity matrix · Persuasive technology · Intervention design

1 Introduction

Scholars have focused on the ways in which technology can produce positive outcomes, such as increasing users' physical activity [29], reducing binge drinking [10], quitting smoking [26], or managing mood and anxiety disorders [14]. There is considerable research on this topic, with several systematic reviews and meta-analyses that focus on a wide variety of positive outcomes [9, 38].

However, few papers report negative outcomes, and possibly fewer report a special class of negative outcomes, called a *backfire*, which we define as an intervention that triggers audiences to adopt the opposite target behavior, rendering the intervention partially responsible for causing the behavior it was designed to reduce or eliminate.

Examples of backfiring interventions include drug use reduction programs that trigger drug use by accidently creating a social norm that triggers some youth to feel like everyone else is trying drugs except for them; traffic safety campaigns that use

© Springer International Publishing Switzerland 2016
A. Meschtscherjakov et al. (Eds.): PERSUASIVE 2016, LNCS 9638, pp. 65–77, 2016.
DOI: 10.1007/978-3-319-31510-2_6

shame which accidently triggers denial and resentment which leads to increased dangerous driving; binge drinking screeners that trigger some youth who drink less than average to feel pressured to catch up to their peers; or a tobacco industry sponsored anti-smoking campaign that encouraged parents to lecture their children on not smoking which triggered more youth to smoke [20].

In this paper, we aim to start a wider scientific discussion on intervention backfiring, to provide analytical frameworks to help structure this discussion, to support academic research on the topic, and to raising practitioners' awareness of the potential risks of intervention backfires so they can better manage the potential risks.

2   Background

Numerous fields provide recommendations on how to design behavior change interventions, including social marketing [1, 25], evidence-based behavioral medicine [12, 13], several health behavior change approaches [2, 7, 33], socially influencing systems [36, 37], persuasive technology [15], and classic persuasion literature [32].

However, the application of evidence-based intervention design frameworks does not guarantee that intervention designers will achieve positive outcomes. In practice, scientific models are more likely to inspire interventions, rather than to dictate exactly how they are implemented [31].

Quite often, interventions that start-out with a solid theoretical underpinning, lose their theoretical roots after adapting to real-world necessities, implementation complexities, budget limits, stakeholder feedback, market testing, political tampering, etc.... Then after moving through the process of translating abstract behavioral science principles into concrete intervention materials, such as translating the health belief model into a health app, it can be difficult to make clear links between the foundational theory and applied interventions.

No matter how promising an intervention may have appeared on paper, in practice, they always have the potential to exert unforeseen, and possibly negative outcomes. This is one of the reasons why new behavior change interventions typically undergo stringent monitoring and evaluation, before they are widely disseminated.

Scholars and practitioners, who report that they have disseminated a backfiring technology, can easily feel embarrassed, or worse, find themselves not just stigmatized, but potentially unfunded. Without doubt, there are many practical incentives and disincentives that may motivate people to not publish any information that details how their digital interventions backfired, causing even a small degree of unintended harm, even in marginal population.

We believe that this stigma has created a climate where the existing body of scientific literature may possess a significant degree of publication bias, resulting from too many published studies that only report positive outcomes, and too few studies reporting negative outcomes. This stigma has the potential to create a climate where scientists and practitioners are at greater risk of disseminating harmful interventions.

3   Framework

To aid discussions on intervention backfiring, this section presents two matrices that define categories of backfires while clarifying their potential to undermine the efficacy of behavior change interventions. Figure 1 presents the intention-outcome matrix, which describes different types of outcomes.

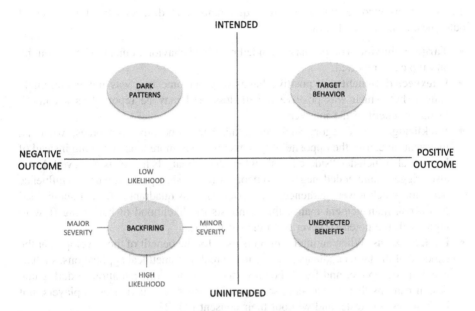

Fig. 1. Intention-Outcome matrix

3.1   Axes of the Intention-Outcome Matrix

The intention-outcome matrix has two axes with four quadrants, which are described below, and illustrated through a fictional binge-drinking reduction intervention.

- **Intended Outcome.** An outcome that was intended by the intervention designer. For example, getting university students to reduce their binge-drinking.
- **Unintended Outcome.** Any outcome that the intervention designer did not intend, whether it is a positive or negative outcome. For example, when a binge-drinking screener accidently motivates some students to adopt other health outcomes, or triggers some students to drink more alcohol after they use it in a competition to see who can achieve the highest binge-drinking score.
- **Positive Outcome.** An outcome that serves the interest of both the intervention designer and the target audience. This is a win-win situation, where both parties benefit. For example, a binge-drinking screener where the target audience achieves reduced alcohol consumption.

- **Negative Outcome.** An outcome that does not serve the interest of the target audience. For example, a binge-drinking screener that causes small segments to drink more alcohol, or exposes them to greater risk.

3.2   Quadrants of the Intention-Outcome Matrix

The intention-outcome matrix has four quadrants, that describes the four types of outcomes, as described below.

- **Target Behavior.** The primary intended positive behavioral outcome being sought, and typically reported.
- **Unexpected Benefits.** A positive behavioral outcome that was not intentionally sought, but which was positive nonetheless, and may be reported as a complimentary benefit of the intervention.
- **Backfiring.** This category includes a number of negative outcomes, when an intervention causes the opposite of the outcome (e.g. more binge drinking instead of less). It also includes "side effects", when the primary behavior is achieved, but it also triggers unintended negative outcomes (e.g. using peer pressure to influence behavior which lowers audiences' self-esteem). This quadrant is further subdivided into a risk management matrix that contrasts the likelihood of backfiring (low to high) with the potential severity (minor to major).
- **Dark Patterns.** When an intervention is used for the benefit of the developer, at the expense of the target audience. This is in the realm of unethical applications, such as coercion, deception, and fraud. For instance, scholars draw attention to dark game design patterns that developers use to provide negative experiences to players, not in their best interests, and without their consent [24, 27].

4   Method

The taxonomy of persuasive backfires presented in this paper was derived through a grounded theory methodology [6, 17], based on a corpus of academic, applied, and personal experiences with backfiring behavior change interventions [3].

We began the process by defining and limiting our selection criteria to interventions that backfire, that cause the opposite behavior, or unanticipated negative consequences that were contrary to the intentions of the program. We excluded flawed interventions that did not contribute towards any outcomes, positive or negative, as these programs constituted poor implementations, not backfires. The first type of flawed intervention includes programs that audiences did not find motivating, as these programs lacked the capacity to achieve significant outcomes. Similarly, we excluded interventions that faced implementation barriers, or created barriers among its target audiences, as it was not possible to assess the outcomes of these interventions.

To gather qualifying sources, we ran a call for references and examples across several academic, professional, and personal networks. The types of references we collected included journal papers, articles, program evaluations, and personal experiences. In total, we collected 47 responses.

We systematically reviewed all sources, and only included submissions that qualified as having demonstrated an unintended negative outcome, or which were presented as having contributed an unintended negative outcome. We also included behavior change interventions that were not implemented within technology per se, but were reasonably implemented in a context that could be applied to online behavior change campaigns or digital products. We also received submissions of backfiring legislation, which is often used in conjunction with communication campaigns, to elicit social change. In total 30 responses were included in our qualitative analysis.

We carried out a qualitative assessment of the corpus, with a view to developing taxonomy of triggers for backfiring interventions.

5   Findings

The findings of our study are presented in Fig. 2, a risk management framework called the likelihood-severity matrix. The four quadrants of backfires include (A) low likelihood and minor severity, (B) high likelihood and minor severity, (C) low likelihood and major severity, and (D) high likelihood and major severity. Through our qualitative assessment of backfires and their potential risks, we have synthesized twelve types of backfires, within six categories: inexperience, fineprint fallacy, personality responses, credibility damage, poor judgment, and social psychology.

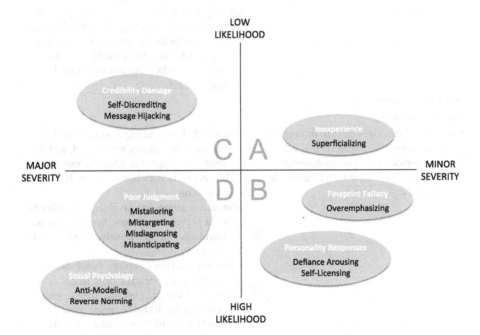

Fig. 2. Likelihood-Severity matrix

The taxonomy of persuasive backfires, presented in Table 1, provides twelve types of backfires within six broad categories.

Table 1. Taxonomy of persuasive backfires

Description	Examples
A: LOW likelihood and MINOR severity	
Inexperience	
Superficializing	
The superficial application of theory, such as copying surface tactics without understanding the underlying strategies, principles, or reasoning.	Research on social media, particularly on Foursquare, looks at driving user motivation through gamification mechanics that compete with intended target behaviors of information sharing [23]. More generally, research that focuses on how gamification elements can drive extrinsic motivation, may cease to be persuasive over the long term, and may potentially deplete intrinsic motivation.
B: HIGH likelihood and MINOR severity	
Fineprint Fallacy	
Overemphasizing	
Motivate people to take action for one strongly emphasized benefit, while omitting (or hiding) harmful factors that are in the fine print.	Stressing "low fat", while still including several unhealthy factors, such as high-sugar, or trans fats. Asking people to take one pill a day to lower their risk of contracting HIV, which causes some groups to engage in riskier sex (and stop using condoms), contributing to an increase in other sexually transmitted diseases [22].
Personality Responses	
Defiance Arousing	
Resistance to messages that are incompatible with a person's self-identity, that can induce unpleasant cognitive dissonance, leading the audience to reject the message, or oppose it.	Guilt and shame messages in anti-drinking ads for drunk drivers are ignored, and in some cases, backfire, when the message is incompatible with how individuals view themselves. Persuasive messaging involving an authority might provoke opposition from groups and individuals who are sensitive or resistant to authorities. One anti-smoking campaign failed due to advocating the message that "teens shouldn't smoke... because they're teens." Youths in the 10th-12th-grade were 12 percent more likely to smoke for each parent-targeted ad they had seen in the last

(*Continued*)

Table 1. (*Continued*)

Description	Examples
	30 days. According to developmental psychologists, teens 15 to 17 years old tend to reject authoritative messages because they believe they are independent, which renders Philip Morris' ad campaign largely useless [16].
	The presence of peer information decreases the savings of nonparticipants who are ineligible for automatic enrollment in a saving plan, while higher observed peer savings rates also decreased savings. Discouragement from upward social comparison seems to drive this reaction [4].
Self-Licensing	
When someone does something good in one area, they sometimes feel like they have a license to misbehave in other.	After donating to charity, people may feel licensed to behave less morally in subsequent decisions [30]. For instance, donating to charity may have a dark side to it, as it negatively affects subsequent, seemingly unrelated moral behavior, such as the intention to be environmentally friendly.
C: LOW likelihood and MAJOR severity	
Credibility Damage	
Self-Discrediting	
When the source disseminates discrediting information, causing a misalignment of source and message credibility.	People report less favorable thoughts and attitudes towards a source, after reading weak arguments presented by a high vs. low expertise source.
	Too much fear mongering may discredit a campaign to the point of disbelief or humor [21].
Message Hijacking	
Third party actors re-contextualize the source's message, bringing a new meaning, which in many cases undermines the intervention by turning it into a public joke.	Creative works designed to cause fear, become a trendy meme with a different meaning, such as humorous cigarette ads of smoking children, reefer madness, fashionable heroin chic [19], or the ad campaign for TV PSA "This is your brain and this is our brain on drugs" which triggered numerous parodies [7].
	England's Beat Bullying Campaign triggered bullying and violence. The campaign was so popular at its launch that supplies of the "Beat Bullying" wristbands quickly sold

(*Continued*)

Table 1. (*Continued*)

Description	Examples
	out. Because of the scarcity of the bracelets, and theme of the campaign, some kids were bullied for wearing the bracelet [11].

D: HIGH likelihood and MAJOR severity

Poor Judgment

Mistailoring

When a tailored messaging system provides information that produces negative outcomes in some users, that could have been avoided with an appropriate message.	A drinking screener showed both low and high drinking students how much they consume in comparison to an average consumption. Those that were above the norm felt encouraged to drink less, while those below received an implied message to drink more. And a boomerang effect [35], when a descriptive social norm was not accompanied by an injunctive social norm in a similar way as described above.

Mistargeting

When a message that was intended for one audience segment is misinterpreted by another group of people.	A one-size-approach to persuasive messaging can deter healthy eating behavior change, leading to a negative change in attitudes towards healthy eating over time. The Playpump program was meant for children to pump water while playing, but resulted in adults using the playground pump, leading to back injuries and other health problems [5].

Misdiagnosing

When a behavior change intervention does not properly diagnose user behavior or psychological processes.	Gaze tracking software, designed to provide proactive help as patients read medical documents, used fixation time as a cue to identify when users were struggling with the material, and might need help. During the trial, the participants with low health literacy had a slower reading rate, causing the system to inappropriately offer help continually, which just annoyed the users, leading to lower comprehension compared to the control condition.

Misanticipating

Changes in policies or directives that lead to unanticipated shifts in beliefs, attitudes or behaviors.	In the Netherlands, the drinking age was changed from 16 to 18, which news stations linked to an increase in drug use among citizens in this age group.

(*Continued*)

Table 1. (*Continued*)

Description	Examples
	Nebraska's "Give Us Your Troubled Child" law backfired, as the Nebraska Safe Haven law enabled parents to drop off kids of any age and the state for the state to take in, resulting in some parents who dropped off grownups [Gra2008].
Social Psychology	
Anti-Modeling	
Demonstrating negative behavior, which exposes people to memory triggers of bad behaviors or temptations, potentially in moments of the greatest susceptibility.	Being exposed to others experiencing the stress of quitting smoking, for example, triggers people to want to smoke. Anti-bad-behavior interventions can remind people of the bad behavior, thus potentially spark their motivation. A cookie company that introduced a 100-calorie packs of snacks, triggered people to eat far more of the small snack packs [28].
Reverse Norming	
Interventions that use examples of popular bad behaviors can establish the bad behavior as a social norm.	An anti-littering program used campaign posters to stress how widespread littering was, accidently contributed to a social norm for littering, by demonstrating how many people were littering. Two separate studies indicated that D.A.R.E. program was ineffective and in some cases, pushed kids toward drug use and lowered self-esteem. Researchers suspected that the intervention's message made some kids want to try drugs as a way of fitting in, stating and the program's message could be misinterpreted by youth as conveying that "peer pressure is around every corner, because everyone is doing drugs but you!" [34].

6 Scientific Considerations

We have authored this paper to initiate a scientific discussion on intervention backfiring, and to encourage scholars to examine this phenomenon in greater depth. We hope this will contribute to more transparency within the academic community, leading to more well-rounded research on persuasive design and its application.

The scientific contribution of this paper includes the persuasive backfiring framework, its two matrices (intention-outcome and likelihood-severity), and taxonomy. These frameworks can be used to define, discuss, and further research behavior change interventions that trigger unintended negative outcomes. Although we have not discussed ethics in this paper, it provides a system to further define ethical and unethical uses of persuasive technology.

Perhaps the most important contribution of this paper, is raising awareness of the elephant in the room, the well-known but rarely discussed fact that applied interventions targeting good outcomes, occasionally produce negative outcomes. It also raises questions on the social stigma attached to the people and organizations that deploy backfiring interventions, and how this may contribute to under reporting negative outcomes, or omitting them altogether.

More concerning, this investigation has identified a potentially large source of publication bias, as we believe that there are many incentives and disincentives, including stigma and embarrassment, that motivate researchers to avoid publishing research on negative outcomes.

We believe that scholars will need to develop innovative new research methods to overcome the research barriers that surround this subject, due to the stigma associated with reporting on interventions that backfire, and the limited ability of scientific studies to identify backfires that are more likely to become apparent in evaluations of real-world interventions, and often informally known by intervention staff but not publicly reported.

For instance, given the ability of technology to employ tailoring techniques, where content can be personalized, persuasive technology scholars are better equipped to undertake research on backfiring psychology, and use this knowledge to advise intervention designers when they need to omit influence principles that may be counterproductive to particular segments.

7   Practitioner Considerations

To assist practitioners, the taxonomy and tools presented in this paper provides a list of risks that can be addressed, if identified before they occur. Moreover, these risks can be used to build more effective interventions, by teaching practitioners how to avoid, mitigate, or manage backfires. The examples in this study suggest that backfires may originate from political tampering during the intervention design phase, evaluations that do not distinguish between groups, overusing a principle to the point of triggering mistrust in a message ("your brain on drugs"), misdiagnosis that leads to subscribing the wrong intervention leading to garbage-in-garbage-out interventions.

However, one ethically questionable practice we discovered was the potential intentional use of backfiring as a dark pattern, designed to deploy an intervention that superficially appears to promote a healthy behavior, but which actually promote unhealthy behavior. When corporations are obliged, or volunteer to carry out public health interventions to warn the public against their product, these corporations can easily benefit from the intentional use of backfiring interventions.

For instance, the "Talk: They'll Listen" campaign is frequently cited as an example of a cleaver antismoking ad campaign that on the outside appeared to be a legitimate antismoking campaign, but which in practice caused an increase in youth smoking [19]. Consequently, policy makers and regulators who empower tobacco, alcohol, and pharmaceutical companies to run their own interventions, need to be fully informed about the potential intentional use, and abuse of backfire-based campaigns, that superficially look effective, but at a deeper level, have been engineered to encourage the opposite effect.

Finally, we believe that backfires are normally present to some degree in all interventions, and that they can never be fully eliminated. It may be more practical to focus on strategies to reduce the riskiest backfires, to manage those that cannot be fully eliminated, and to continually monitor and improve interventions over time.

8 Conclusions

The stigma associated with reporting behavior change interventions that trigger negative outcomes, has relegated the topic of intervention backfiring to an informal observation that is widely known, but rarely discussed or reported. This has created a climate where scholars routinely overemphasize positive outcomes, while failing to report the fact that the same principle, can also lead to unforeseen negative outcomes.

In this paper, we discussed multiple ways how behavior change interventions can backfire. We provided a framework to help facilitate the discussion of this topic, presented tools to aid academics in the study of this realm, and offered advice to practitioners about potential risks. We encourage researchers to build on this work, and take a more systematic look on approaches involving the design of behavior change interventions.

In the future, researchers will need to innovate new ways to study this subject, and extend our scientific and practical knowledge of what pitfalls need to be avoided when designing technology-supported behavior change interventions. We advocate that researchers and practitioners adopt an honest and open attitude towards identifying and removing backfires as soon as possible, and to disseminating strategies to reduce their occurrence, before they cause more harm than good.

References

1. Andreasen, A.: Social marketing in the 21st century. Sage Publications Inc, Thousand Oaks (2006)
2. Bartholomew, L.K., Parcel, G.S., Kok, G., Gottlieb, N.H.: Planning health promotion programs: an intervention mapping approach. Wiley, San Francisco (2011)
3. Beer, M., Eisenstat, R.A., Spector, B.: Why change programs don't produce change (1990)
4. Beshears, J., Choi, J.J., Laibson, D., Madrian, B.C., Milkman, K.L.: The effect of providing peer information on retirement savings decisions. J. Finan. 70(3), 1161–1201 (2015)
5. Chambers, A.: Africa's not-so-magic roundabout (2009). http://www.theguardian.com/commentisfree/2009/nov/24/africa-charity-water-pumps-roundabouts
6. Charmaz, K.: Constructing grounded theory. Sage, Thousand Oaks (2014)
7. Chatterjee, S., Price, A.: Healthy living with persuasive technologies: Framework, is- sues, and challenges. J. Am. Med. Inf. Assoc. 16(2), 171–178 (2009)

8. Crano, W.D., Burgoon, M., Oskamp, S. (eds.): Mass media and drug prevention: Classic and contemporary theories and research. Psychology Press, Mahwah (2001)

9. Cugelman, B., Thelwall, M., Dawes, P.: Online interventions for social marketing health behavior change campaigns: A meta-analysis of psychological architectures and adherence factors. J. Med. Internet Res. **13**(1), e17 (2011). http://doi.org/10.2196/jmir.1367

10. Cunningham, J.A., Wild, T.C., Cordingley, J., Van Mierlo, T., Humphreys, K.: A randomized controlled trial of an internet-based intervention for alcohol abusers. Addiction **104**(12), 2023–2032 (2009)

11. Curtis, P.: Anti-bullying wristband scheme backfires (2004). http://www.theguardian.com/education/2004/dec/08/schools.uk2

12. Davidson, K., Goldstein, M., Kaplan, R., Kaufmann, P., Knatterud, G., Orleans, C., Whitlock, E.: Evidence-based behavioral medicine: What is it and how do we achieve it? Ann. Behav. Med. **26**(3), 161–171 (2003)

13. Embry, D., Biglan, A.: Evidence-based kernels: Fundamental units of behavioral influence. Clin. Child Family Psychol. Rev. **11**(3), 75 (2008)

14. Farvolden, P., Denisoff, E., Selby, P., Bagby, R.M., Rudy, L.: Usage and longitudinal effectiveness of a Web-based self-help cognitive behavioral therapy program for panic disorder. J. Med. Int. Res. **7**(1), e7 (2005). http://www.ncbi.nlm.nih.gov/pmc/articles/PMC1550639/

15. Fogg, B.J.: Persuasive Technology: Using Computers to Change What We Think and Do. Morgan Kaufmann, San Francisco (2003)

16. Fraser, J.: Anti-smoking ads cleverly boost smoking among teens (2006). http://www.naturalnews.com/020996.html

17. Glaser, B.G., Strauss, A.L.: The discovery of grounded theory: Strategies for qualitative research. Transaction Publishers, New Jersey (2009)

18. Graham, J.: Father leaves nine children at Nebraska hospital (2008). http://newsblogs.chicagotribune.com/triage/2008/09/father-leaves-n.html

19. Hastings, G.: Social marketing: why should the devil have all the best tunes?. Butterworth-Heinemann, Oxford (2007)

20. Healey, B., Zimmerman, R.S.: The new world of health promotion: New program development, implementation, and evaluation. Jones & Bartlett Learning, Sudbury (2009)

21. Hinkley, K.: 5 Ridiculous Anti-Drugs Posters (2014). http://www.talkingdrugs.org/5-anti-drugs-campaigns

22. Holpuch, A.: Truvada has been called the 'miracle' HIV pill–so why is uptake so slow (2014). http://www.theguardian.com/world/2014/sep/18/truvada-mircle-pill-prevent-hiv-controversy

23. Kietzmann, J.H., Hermkens, K., McCarthy, I.P., Silvestre, B.S.: Social media? Get serious! Understanding the functional building blocks of social media. Bus. Horiz. **54**(3), 241–251 (2011)

24. Kirkland, A., Metzl, J.M. (eds.): Against health: How health became the new morality. NYU Press, New York (2010)

25. Kotler, P., Roberto, N., Lee, N.: Social marketing: improving the quality of life, 2nd edn. Sage Publications Inc, California (2002)

26. Lenert, L., Munoz, R., Perez, J., Bansod, A.: Automated e-mail messaging as a tool for improving quit rates in an internet smoking cessation intervention. J. Am. Med. Inf. Assoc. **11**(4), 235–240 (2004)

27. Linehan, C., Harrer, S., Kirman, B., Lawson, S., Carter, M.: Games against health: a player-centered design philosophy. In: Proceedings of the 33rd Annual ACM Conference Extended Abstracts on Human Factors in Computing Systems, pp. 589–600. ACM (2015, April)

28. London, L.: Guiltless Girls: Unpacking 100-calorie Snacks (2009)
29. Marshall, A., Leslie, E., Bauman, A., Marcus, B., Owen, N.: Print versus website physical activity programs A randomized trial. Am. J. Prev. Med. **25**(2), 88–94 (2003)
30. Meijers, M.H., Verlegh, P.W., Noordewier, M.K., Smit, E.G.: The dark side of donating: how donating may license environmentally unfriendly behavior. Social Influence, 1–14 (2015). doi:10.1080/15534510.2015.1092468
31. Michie, S., Abraham, C.: Interventions to change health behaviours: evidence-based or evidence-inspired? Psychol. Health **19**(1), 29–49 (2004)
32. O'Keefe, D.: Persuasion: Theory and Research. Sage Publications Inc, London (2002)
33. Prochaska, J.O., Velicer, W.F.: The transtheoretical model of health behavior change. Am. J. Health Promot. **12**(1), 38–48 (1997)
34. Reaves, J.: Just Say No to DARE (2001). http://content.time.com/time/education/article/0,8599,99564,00.html
35. Schultz, P.W., Nolan, J.M., Cialdini, R.B., Goldstein, N.J., Griskevicius, V.: The constructive, destructive, and reconstructive power of social norms. Psychol. Sci. **18**(5), 429–434 (2007)
36. Stibe, A.: Towards a framework for socially influencing systems: Meta-analysis of four PLS-SEM based studies. In: MacTavish, T., Basapur, S. (eds.) PERSUASIVE 2015. LNCS, vol. 9072, pp. 172–183. Springer, Heidelberg (2015)
37. Stibe, A.: Advancing typology of computer-supported influence: moderation effects in socially influencing systems. In: MacTavish, T., Basapur, S. (eds.) PERSUASIVE 2015. LNCS, vol. 9072, pp. 253–264. Springer, Heidelberg (2015)
38. Webb, T., Joseph, J., Yardley, L., Michie, S.: Using the internet to promote health behavior change: a systematic review and meta-analysis of the impact of theoretical basis, use of behavior change techniques, and mode of delivery on efficacy. J. Med. Internet Res. **12**(1), e4 (2010). http://doi.org/10.2196/jmir.1376

Captology and Technology Appropriation: Unintended Use as a Source for Designing Persuasive Technologies

Alina Krischkowsky[✉], Bernhard Maurer, and Manfred Tscheligi

Center for Human-Computer Interaction, Department of Computer Sciences,
University of Salzburg, Salzburg, Austria
{alina.krischkowsky,bernhard.maurer,manfred.tscheligi}@sbg.ac.at

Abstract. In this paper we theoretically reflect upon persuasive technology usage under the light of technology appropriation. The intended usage of technology often fails, meaning that the designers' intended use is not always translated into user behavior. This is also true for persuasive technology, since technology will always be used within a context involving users' own intentions that may not always be anticipated by designers. This clashes with Fogg's framing of captology, which explicitly focuses on endogenous intent, i.e., a persuasive intent that is designed into a technology. With this paper we open up an initial theoretical discourse around these two concepts, highlighting how the design of persuasive technologies can be informed by existing knowledge around technology appropriation. This is done by reflecting upon three identified 'action points': (1) learning from appropriation, (2) designing for appropriation, and (3) designing for personal differences and ambiguity of interaction.

Keywords: Technology appropriation · Captology · Intentionality · Unintended use

1 Introduction

In this paper we open up a discourse around the design and use of interactive persuasive technology (PT) by reflecting upon conceptualizations around technology appropriation and unintended use. Since *persuasion requires intentionality* (e.g., [1, 2]), we argue that these technological 'built-in' intentions will always be used within a context involving users' own intentions that may not always be accordingly anticipated by designers. Therefore, we discuss in how far *designing for the unexpected* [8], in terms of unintended use, can be a valuable source for designing PTs. In particular we will reflect upon Fogg's captological design [2] and on technology appropriation in terms of related design perspectives and principles. In doing this theoretical reflection, we highlight that also unintended use of PT does not necessarily have to be a sign of 'failure' but rather a sign that the technology has become "the user's own" (e.g., [8, 17]). Such phenomena need to be named and taken seriously and not neglected by considering them 'side effects' [2]. Especially, for the design of PTs the study of unintended use is critical to understand the manifold ways of how technology can be appropriated, to also counteract more systematically undesired negative consequences.

© Springer International Publishing Switzerland 2016
A. Meschtscherjakov et al. (Eds.): PERSUASIVE 2016, LNCS 9638, pp. 78–83, 2016.
DOI: 10.1007/978-3-319-31510-2_7

2   Intended and Unintended Use

The following section details related work on PT and intentionality complemented with remarks on technology appropriation and unintended use to outline the very characteristic foundations of these two concepts.

2.1   Intended Use and Persuasive Technology

As already defined in Foggs' early work [1], PT is an "interactive technology that changes a person's attitudes or behaviors" (p. 225). A central aspect of this definition is that persuasion always *implies an intent* to change attitudes and/or behaviors. So to say, persuasion requires intentionality (e.g., [1, 2]). The concept of *captology* (i.e., the study of computers as PT [2]) specifically focuses on planned persuasive effects of technology and not on potential side effects, i.e., that persuasive *intent is designed into a computing product*, also referred to as– "built-in"– persuasive intent [2].

   However, Fogg's work has also been criticized (e.g., [3, 4]). For example, Johnson [4] emphasizes that captological design neglects user-centered design philosophies, since it excludes *unintended consequences* and instead focuses on attitude and behavior changes that are intended by the designer. Here, Atkinson argues that an "ethical design impasse is created" ([3], p. 171), since responsible user-centered design necessities and a sound examination of intended *and* unintended consequences of technology usage are missing. Verbeek [6] agrees with that and highlights that unintended consequences need to be fundamentally incorporated into design decisionmaking processes by better understanding and predicting them. These complementary viewpoints illustrate to explicitly include unintended use of PTs in research, design and theoretical reflections thereof to emphasize their innovation potential, but also systematically counteract undesired negative consequences.

2.2   Unintended Use and Technology Appropriation

Verbeek talks about the *uncertainty* that surrounds eventual effects of PT, as persuasion cannot be seen as an intrinsic property of technologies [6]. Therefore, technologies may be approached as entities that have no fixed identities, rather embody *interpretative flexibility* [16] and/or *multistability* [7]. These approaches towards understanding technologies in their actual contexts of usage, derive from various research disciplines and theorists, such as e.g., phenomenology [7], or mediation theory [6]. The theoretical core idea is that technologies need to be *interpreted* and *appropriated* by the user in order to be used [6]. There exist many examples of unintended use, coming from people's everyday life experiences and practices, but also from observations in various research disciplines, such as HCI (e.g., [17]). Technology that is used differently than initially intended by the designers and not simply what they gave to them [9], may not be a sign of 'failure' rather than a sign that the technology has become "the user's own" (e.g., [8, 17]). In regard to 'failing' technologies, Dix [8] and Carroll [9] counter that "design can never be complete" as it is impossible to design for the unexpected, but that "you can design to allow the unexpected". Thus, users complete the design as they adapt and appropriate it [9], fitting them into their working practices [10].

3   Deriving an Informed Basis: Appropriation and Persuasion

An important question deriving from this discourse around persuasion and appropriation is, in how far these concepts clash or complement with each other? In this section, we discuss this question on basis of their theoretical *foundations*.

Captological design focuses on planned persuasive effects and not on potential side effects [2]. Simply said, if a technological artifact is designed with an intent in mind to change a specific attitude or behavior (e.g., persuade drivers to change their driving style towards a more economic one), and you observe in your studies that your intended attitude and behavior change is met (e.g., people adopted your designed fuel-saving technology to drive more economical), your design has worked out. But what happens if the planned outcome is different than intended (e.g., no or different attitude/behavior change adopted)? We agree that unintended consequences categorically do not belong with having been persuaded [3]. However, is it also a sign of failure from a design perspective? In many disciplines, appropriation is considered as a positive phenomenon in system design and a source for technological innovations [8, 9]. Atkinson [3] and Berdichewsky et al. [5] state that it is central for the persuasive discipline itself to show (moral) responsibility and name such phenomena, i.e., side effects that are neglected in captological design.

Thereby, appropriation holds several advantages, such as, situatedness, dynamics and ownership [8]. *Situatedness* means that the end point of design is the *intervention* [11], and not just an artefact or an artefact and its immediate ways of interacting with it. It is rather the way it changes the environment in which it is set [8]. Therefore, in designing PTs, we cannot expect to understand each usage context fully and meet every possible need to change a certain behavior or attitude. It can rather be about the general changes/interventions (also unintended) a new technology brings into a given usage context that may be seen as initial leverage points to innovate and (re-)design. Concerning *dynamics*, it is critical for the design process, to envision that usage environments and needs change. Over time, the use context of technology may change (e.g., a persuasive app that was designed for individual use, is used by multiple users). The technology therefore needs to be responsive to this change (e.g., explicitly allowing for collaborative use). With appropriation a certain sense of *ownership* evolves. When designing technologies with a specific intent, people using these systems may feel a loss of control, i.e., not doing things their own way. This aspect has already been discussed in persuasive literature (e.g., [3, 5]), in terms of moral and ethic questions (e.g., human autonomy) surrounding PT design and use. In contrast, appropriation argues for ownership, to allow people to do things their own way to raise positive feelings that can be as important as the things that can be achieved with the very technology [8]. Therefore, designing *situated* and *dynamic* PTs that also allow for *ownership*, hold the potential to create technologies that persuade by being situated in peoples practices.

4   Action Points

Based on this general discussion around appropriable PTs that allow for situatedness, dynamic use and ownership, the following section details action points of how we can leverage the users' different ways of appropriating PTs and thereby, complete the design through their actions. This is done by outlining how designers and users of PTs can learn from appropriation and unintended use practices as well as how designers can apply appropriation principles to fit the users' respective appropriation 'needs'.

Learning from Appropriation and Unintended Use. The knowledge on how a user appropriates a specifc design or artifact is a valuable source for reflection for both, the user (i.e., learning from own behaviour) as well as the designer (i.e., learning based on the user's unintended use in context). By deliberately designing for open-ended use, the act of appropriation itself can become a reflective practice for the user, leading to new layers a persuasive design can address. For instance, technology can allow for confronting the user with his/her appropriations (i.e., how s/he uses the technology differently on a daily basis). This confrontation can be used by designers of PT as a way to induce behaviour change by allowing the user to reflect upon his/her own actions and usage appropriations.

We further argue for open ended persuasive designs in order to address long term persuasive goals, rather than short term. PT that is *appropriable* can potentially be more deeply rooted in a user's everyday practices. In that sense, persuasive techologies that are integrated into users' everyday routines, by the users themselves, can also become natural for the user, making such technologies inherently part of their lives to address long term persuasive goals. In that sense, technologies can become mediatory artifacts constantly adapting and communicating with the user.

Designing for Appropriation: Intended vs. Unintended Use. There exist several design approaches with a strong focus on appropriation, such as "continuous design and redesign" [14], "continuing design in use" [13], and metadesign "designing for design after design" [15]. What unites all of these approaches is that the main challenge for designers is to design *malleable technologies* that can be adapted to users' organizational, social and personal practices to harvest users' needs in order to improve its design [9]. The main question that arises is– How can we balance intentionality (for persuasion purposes) with open, flexible and dynamic design to allow for unintended use (for appropriation purposes)? We believe that designing appropriable PTs is a challenge, but the fact that design for appropriation is possible is made most clear by realizing that some sorts of design make appropriation difficult or impossible [8]. This might be true for PT as well. In the following we outline some major design principles from appropriation literature that can provide an initial step towards designing appropriable PTs.

Interpretation allowed! (e.g., [6–8, 16]) It is important that not everything in a system or product does have a fixed meaning. It is rather critical to include elements where users can add their own meanings, contextualize their own interactions, to make them adaptable to their own needs and surroundings of interaction.

Provide visibility! (e.g., [8]) It is central that the systems' functioning is clear to the users so that they can anticipate likely effects of their actions. This is how users are empowered to make the system do what they would like. This is particularly relevant for technologies when the effects of actions become visible at different time.

Reveal Intentions! (e.g., [8]) Appropriation can be used to subvert systems (i.e., deliberately using something different than intended). This is of particular relevance for persuasion, as designers may not try to prevent such subversion but aim to expose the intention behind the system. This supports users in choosing appropriations that may subvert the system rules but still preserve the intent. This means that persuasion may work in its inherent usage and not exclusively with the given functions.

Learn! (e.g., [4, 8]) A user's appropriation practices can lead to new technologies that incorporate these adaptations created by the user, supporting the development of new innovative technologies. In observing and documenting in our research the many different ways in which technology has been appropriated, technology may be re-designed or new technologies emerge to support newly discovered uses and resulting behaviors. This form of co-design, has often been criticized as being lacking in persuasive and specifically captological designs.

By considering interpretative flexibility, visibility and the exposure of intentions in the design of PTs, we argue that users may be given the opportunity to complete the design and persuasive intent with their own actions and appropriations.

Designing for Personal Differences and Ambiguity of Interaction. Besides allowing for appropriated use based on e.g., everyday practices of a user, we further argue for allowing appropriation and unintentionality on an interactional level. As physical action is an important component of human cognition and self-awareness, it is strongly related to how a human creates reason and perceives himself within the environment. This notion of *thinking through doing* [12] is for instance very prominent in body-based interactions. However, every body is different and individual movement differences are a matter of personal traits. Embracing this ambiguity of interactions can be a promising source for interaction designs of PT. If a PT allows for body-based interactions (e.g., interacting via a physical artifact), a user's personal way of doing and interacting with it can potentially foster the act of appropriation, leading to higher user engagement. Ideally, the act of using PT can then become a matter of self expression, which makes such technology much more likely to be adopted and used on a daily basis. This presents new design opportunities for PT that are deeply embedded into the user's everyday practices and routines.

5 Conclusion and Future Work

With this paper we took an initial step towards *designing for appropriable PTs*. In our discussion around persuasion and appropriation and our three derived 'action points' we have highlighted how conceptualizations around appropriation can potentially be a source for the design of PTs. Nevertheless, with this theoretical discourse new important questions emerge, such as, how to balance precise persuasive intent and open-ended design at the same time? Such questions will be part of our future work, aiming to derive concrete principles for the design of appropriabale PTs on basis of empirical 'over time' research and theoretical reflections thereof.

Acknowledgements. The financial support by the Austrian Federal Ministry of Science, Research and Economy and the National Foundation for Research, Technology and Development is gratefully acknowledged (Christian Doppler Laboratory for Contextual Interfaces).

References

1. Fogg, B.J.: Persuasive computers: perspectives and research directions. In: Proceedings of the CHI, pp. 225–232. ACM (1998)
2. Fogg, B.J.: Persuasive Technology: Using Computers to Change What We Think and Do. Morgan Kaufmann, Amsterdam (2003)
3. Atkinson, B.M.: Captology: A critical review. In: IJsselsteijn, W.A., de Kort, Y.A., Midden, C., Eggen, B., van den Hoven, E. (eds.) PERSUASIVE 2006. LNCS, vol. 3962, pp. 171–182. Springer, Heidelberg (2006)
4. Johnson, R.R.: Book reviews: Persuasive technology. JBTC, J. Bus. Tech. Commun. **7**, 251–254 (2004)
5. Berdichewsky, D., Neuenschwander, E.: Toward an ethics of persuasive technology'. Commun. ACM **42**(5), 51–58 (1999)
6. Verbeek, P-P.: Persuasive Technology and Moral Responsibility: Toward an ethical framework for persuasive technologies. In: Proceedings of PERSUASIVE 2006, Springer (2006)
7. Ihde, D.: Technology and the Lifeworld. Bloomington/Minneapolis, Cambridge (1990)
8. Dix, A.: Designing for appropriation. In: Proceedings of the BCS-HCI 2007. UK, pp. 27–30 (2007)
9. Carroll, J.: Completing design in use: Closing the appropriation cycle. In: Proceedings of the ECIS 2004, Turku, Finland, 11 p. Paper 44 (2004)
10. Dourish, P.: The appropriation of interactive technologies: Some lessons from placeless documents. JCSCW **12**(4), 465–490 (2003)
11. Dix, A., Finlay, J., Abowd, G., Beale, R.: Interaction design basics, 3rd edn. Human Computer Interaction. Prentice Hall, Upper Saddle River (2004)
12. Klemmer, S.R., Hartmann, B., Takayama, L.: How bodies matter: Five themes for interaction design. In: Proceedings of the DIS 2006, pp. 140–149. ACM (2006)
13. Henderson, A., Kyng, M.: There's no place like home: Continuing design in use, pp. 219–240. Lawrence Erlbaum, USA (1991)
14. Jones, J.C.: Continuous design and redesign. Des. Stud. **4**(1), 53–60 (1983)
15. Ehn, P.: Participation in design things. In: Proceedings of the Participatory Design 2008, pp. 92–101 (2008)
16. Bijker, W.E., Pinch, T.J.: The Social Construction of Facts and Artifacts: Or How the Sociology of Science and the Sociology of Technology Might Benefit of Each Other. MIT Press, Cambridge MA (1987)
17. Bødker, S., Christiansen, E.: Poetry in motion: Appropriation of the world of apps. In: Proceedings of the ECCE 2012, pp. 78–84. ACM (2012)

Prevention and Motivation

Self-Reflecting and Mindfulness: Cultivating Curiosity and Decentering Situated in Everyday Life

Ralph Vacca[✉] and Christopher Hoadley

Educational Communication and Technology, New York University, New York, USA
{ralph.vacca,tophe}@nyu.edu

Abstract. Research on the use of mobile to promote mindfulness states is still relatively nascent, especially when exploring how such states can be cultivated in
everyday life, outside of meditation-based approaches. In this study we investigate the
design of a mobile app that seeks to cultivate mindfulness states situated in everyday
life. Using reminders to prompt self-reflection and breathing exercises to prompt body
awareness, we sought to address the overarching question – how can we design
towards mindfulness situated in everyday living and how might it change what we
mean by mindfulness? Our findings suggest that mobile-based approaches can
promote curiosity and decentering through self-reflection, and that the valence and
likelihood of experiencing certain mental events may influence how self-reflection
is experienced, which in turn influences curiosity and decentering factors of mindfulness states.

Keywords: Mindfulness · Situated context · Self-reflection · Curiosity ·
Decentering · Emotional health · Persuasive design · Mobile learning

1   Introduction

Traditionally, mindfulness focuses on complete freedom from suffering and cultivating
positive qualities of the mind characterized by a state of altruistic omniscience. Wester-
nized adoption of mindfulness is largely removed from the spiritual origins and focused
on the therapeutic benefits – happiness and wellness. Despite these differences, both
share a characterization of mindfulness as a transient state of non-appraisal in which
mental experiences and sensory information are meta-cognitively monitored without
evaluation or interpretation [1, 2]. Furthermore, both share a view of mindfulness
training as a cultivation of dispositional traits that eventually will impact all aspects of
one's everyday life [3].

Building on the momentum of the quantified-self and persuasive technology movement is the opportunity to use mobile devices to support mindfulness as a practice that
is situated in everyday life. Mobility is increasingly being understood as the mediation
of one's relationship with situated contexts such as location and those around us [4].

In this study we investigate the design of a mobile app that seeks to activate and
support mindfulness states situated throughout a person's everyday life. Using reminders
to prompt self-reflection and breathing exercises to prompt body awareness, we sought
to address the overarching question – how can we design towards mindfulness situated

© Springer International Publishing Switzerland 2016
A. Meschtscherjakov et al. (Eds.): PERSUASIVE 2016, LNCS 9638, pp. 87–98, 2016.
DOI: 10.1007/978-3-319-31510-2_8

in everyday living and how might it change what we mean by mindfulness? Specifically we sought to explore how self-reflection throughout one's day serves as a mediating process that influences the way one experiences curiosity and decentering – two factors commonly used to operationalize a mindfulness state [5].

2 Related Work

2.1 Mindfulness States

Mindfulness can be understood both as a dispositional trait and as a temporary state that can be induced. The two perspectives are interlinked in that consistent induction of mindfulness states may lead to long-term changes in mindfulness as a dispositional trait [6]. When understanding mindfulness as a state, two factors of curiosity and decentering are often used to operationalize the construct [5]. Lau et al. [5] characterize curiosity as present-moment awareness with an investigative interest, while decentering is defined as reflecting a shift from identifying personally with thoughts and feelings to relating to one's experience of a wider field of awareness. In other words, decentering is about seeing one's thoughts and feelings as passing mental events in the mind rather than reflections of reality [7].

There is debate as to how such states can be cultivated that stem largely from one's interpretation of what a mindfulness state actually is. For instance, as we mentioned, the curiosity factor of a mindfulness state is characterized as being present-moment aware- ness with an investigative interest. There however are differences in the extent to which such awareness is unencumbered by language or conception. For instance, Buddha's earliest teachings describe mindfulness as a form of moment-to-moment application of bare attention that does not linguistically or conceptually elaborate one's observed experience [8]. This may stand in contrast to approaches to mindfulness that see aware- ness as a form of dealing with the narratives themselves such as therapeutic interventions that advocate for forms of managing the interpretations (e.g., acceptance) we assign through mindfulness-like approaches [3, 9]. Furthermore, ongoing work on under- standing the neurological underpinnings of mindfulness indicate that early stage mind- fulness practitioners may experience top-down attentional control processes (i.e., conceptual), while more experienced practitioners are able to attenuate in a more non- conceptual experiential manner [10].

2.2 Self-Reflection as a Mediating Process

In the quantified-self movement, self-monitoring is instrumental to changes in behavior. By shifting awareness to patterns of behavior one can better self-regulate either through increased motivation, deeper insights, or other persuasive aspects. While there are a variety of semantic variations in terminology, self-reflection can be considered a speci- alized subset of self-monitoring focused on internal mental events rather than behaviors or sensory data.

Adopting the Self-Reflection and Insight Scale (SRIS) operationalization of self- reflection we are defining self-reflection as having certain characteristics. First, while self-reflection can be seen an involuntary process as is the case with rumination that is correlated with a variety of mood disorders [11] we are viewing self-reflection as a voluntary effortful process. Second, the focus of self-reflection is understood as one that is conceptual – there is a top-down attentional focus that involves language and appraisal, rather than a focus on experiential attention. We are assuming self-reflection involves dealing with the contents of mental events (conceptualization). Third, self-reflection is being seen as free from any regulatory or problem-solving orientation. In the SRIS instrument, the second factor of insight captures one's ability to understand and make sense of their thoughts and emotions, while self-reflection seeks only to capture one's awareness of such mental events.

2.3   Designing for Self-Reflection

There are a variety of design approaches to promoting self-reflection while situated in everyday life. Reminders to self-reflect on current mental events or particular ones are a popular persuasive approach. Examples include, Mood Panda's [12] reminders to track current moods and Conscious app's [13] initial daily directive to self-reflect on and ongoing reminders to reengage effort to self-reflect on that particular directive. Another approach goes beyond tracking and attempts to provide guidance on the self-reflective process, e.g., the Mindfulness App [14] prompts users to engage in short 1-minute guided meditations. Lastly, there is an approach that does not attempt interject into the everyday experience of the user, but provides an on-demand library to help mediate one's interaction with their situated context. In the Buddhify mobile app [15], users can select from meditations categorized by goals and context (e.g., traveling or feeling sick).

3   Study Design

3.1   Theoretical Framework

Our study's goal was to obtain a rich understanding of how specific design embodiments in our tool influence curiosity and decentering through self-reflection.

In designing our tool, we laid out a conjecture map that outlined key design embodiments, their relation to mediating processes, and their relation to our target outcomes (Fig. 1). The relationship we anticipated between embodiments and mediating processes are our design conjectures, and the relation between mediating processes and outcomes are our theoretical conjectures. The objective of specifying design conjectures is to trace the observed effects back to the embodiments. This can be challenging in that each conjecture is implemented in tools and activities in ways that their operation is not isolated – in turn making the study of each of the pieces separately not possible [16]. In short, our design seeks to provide specific mental events for users to self-reflect on and explore how situating this self-reflective process in everyday life in a particular way may influence how mindfulness states are experienced.

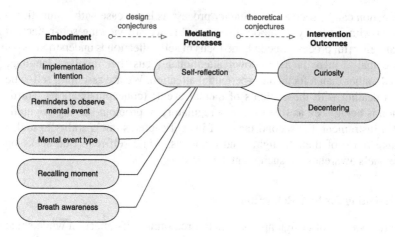

Fig. 1. Conjecture map of mobile tool design

3.2 Mobile Mindfulness App Design

The mobile app engages users in five different challenges each targeting different mental event. All of the challenges shared the same design embodiments but they differed in the specific mental event targeted (see Table 1).

Table 1. A list of challenges, properties, and sequence of interactions

Mental Event	Valence	Scope	Sequence of Interactions
Gratitude	Positive	Broad	Recall moment of gratitude in your mind
			Focus on breathing for 15 s
Conflict	Negative	Relational	Recall moment of conflict
			Focus on your breath for 15 s
Self-Compassion	Positive	Broad	Recall moment of self-compassion in your mind
			Focus on breathing for 15 s
Self-Criticism	Negative	Broad	Recall moment of self-criticism
			Focus on breathing for 15 s
Envy	Negative	Narrow	Recall moment of envy in your mind
			Focus on breathing for 15 s

Given we are viewing the self-reflective process as conceptual, the type of mental event is especially relevant. A review of mindfulness-based interventions [3, 17] and prior pilot testing led us to outline five different mental events categorized by valence and scope. Valence describes whether the mental event is likely to be linked to a positive or negative affective state. Scope describes how broad or narrow the mental event is likely to be characterized by the user. For instance, self-criticism is a broad mental event

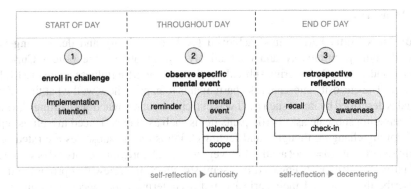

Fig. 2. The daylong life cycle of a challenge start and completion

that can encompass other events such as envy. In addition we have a relational scope that is both narrow and entails focusing on "conflict" with another person.

As illustrated in Fig. 2, a challenge is started by the user at the beginning of the day and entails setting the intention to observe a specific mental event (e.g., self-criticism) by accepting the challenge.

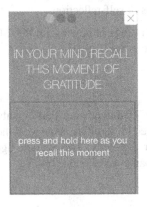

Fig. 3. Check-in. Step 1 – Recalling moment.

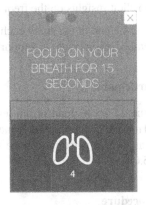

Fig. 4. Check-in. Step 2 – Focus on breath.

After accepting the challenge, users are prompted throughout the day via reminders to make an effort to observe that mental event. No action needs to be taken on part of the user when the mental event is observed. At the end of the day, the user is prompted to check-in, which consists of two-steps. First they are prompted to recall one moment where they observed the mental event (Fig. 3), and second to focus on their breath for 15 s and let that mental event recalled go as they shifted their focus (Fig. 4). The attentional shift to breath is a common attentional control exercise used in mindfulness activities to promote decentering [18]. While throughout the day the reminders seek to prompt self-reflection and curiosity on specific mental events, the end of the day interaction seeks to use the observed mental events to engage users in a decentered form of self-reflection.

3.3   Measures

Mindfulness State. Participants' achieved levels of curiosity and decentering was assessed both quantitatively and qualitatively. Quantitatively the 6-item Curiosity subscale and 7-item Decentering subscale of the Toronto Mindfulness Scale (TMS) [5] was used. The curiosity subscale asks participants to express how well what they experienced is described by items such as "I was curious about my reactions to things", while the decentering subscale asks participants items such as "I experienced myself as separate from my changing thoughts and feelings". Items on the subscales are rated on a 5-point Likert scale (0 = "not at all", 4 = "very much"). Scores on the subscales summed. Qualitatively, participants engaged in a semi-structured interview that prompted them to describe the details of their curiosity and decentering experiences with interview questions adapted from the TMS subscale questions.

Self-Reflection. Self-reflection for each challenge was measured primarily through a semi-structured interview that focused on the how self-reflection was experienced. In addition, the 12-item self-reflection subscale (SRIS-SR) of the Self-Reflection Insight Scale (SRIS) [19] was used. Self-reflection items include; "It was important to me to try to understand what my feelings mean". The items are on 7-point scales (1 = Strongly Disagree, 7 = Strongly Agree). Lastly, we added some customized survey questions that sought to elicit insights on the frequency of moments of self-reflection.

Utility. At the end of the study each user completed ratings of how useful the different design embodiments were to supporting self-reflection (See Table 3).

3.4   Participants

We recruited 11 participants from several New York City universities. Participants were required to have never previously meditated or engaged in cognitive behavioral therapy, as well as have a personal iPhone they can use for the study. The average age was (M = 25.09, SD = 3.86), and 7 out of the 11 participants were female (64 %).

3.5   Procedure

Participants were asked to complete an initial survey when signing up to ensure they had not engaged in any form of meditation or cognitive-behavior therapy prior to this experience. Each user was prompted to complete all of the five challenges over one week, and complete a survey each time a challenge was completed. The survey included questions that span the TMS and SRIS-SR measures, as well as customized questions that focused on the frequency of self-reflection. The order of the challenges completed by users was counterbalanced to minimize any learning effects. After completing all of the challenges, users completed a utility survey and engaged in an hour-long semi-structured interview. The interview protocol was structured to address each of the design and theoretical conjectures.

4   Results

This mixed method study was structured as sequential explanatory [20] in which the first phase was to analyze our quantitative data so as to inform subsequent semi-structured interviews conducted with all of the eleven participants (Table 2).

4.1   Phase I: Quantitative Analysis

Curiosity, decentering and SRIS-SR scores for each mental event type were all normally distributed, as assessed by Shapiro-Wilk's test ($p > .05$). In addition, when running a repeated measures ANOVA on curiosity, decentering, and SRIS-SR, we used Greenhouse-Geisser correction. For curiosity, post hoc tests using the Bonferroni correction revealed that conflict significantly differed from every other mental event type in curiosity ($p < .0005$). In addition envy differed from gratitude ($p < .05$) and self-compassion ($p < .05$). For decentering, post hoc tests using the Bonferroni correction revealed that all of the challenges differed from each other by mental event type ($p < .0005$), except between self-compassion and self-criticism. Lastly, for SRIS-SR post hoc tests using the Bonferroni correction revealed that all of the challenges differed from each other by mental event type on SRIS-R scores, except for Gratitude and Self-Compassion ($p < .0005$).

Table 2. Summary of Quantitative Analysis

Mental Event	Curiosity	Decentering	SRIS-SR
All	$(F(2.677, 26.768) = 186.315, p < 0.0005)$, partial $\eta2 = .96$	$(F(2.113, 21.130) = 382.560, p < 0.001)$, partial $\eta2 = .975$	$(F(2.890, 28.898) = 1481.631, p < 0.001)$, partial $\eta2 = .993$
Self-Criticism	$M = 27.00, SD = 2.19$	$M = 19.64, SD = 1.80$	$M = 64.55, SD = 2.16$
Envy	$M = 26.09, SD = 2.46$	$M = 16.82, SD = 1.94$	$M = 62.09, SD = 1.51$
Self-Compassion	$M = 27.18, SD = 2.23$	$M = 19.45, SD = 2.29$	$M = 66.91, SD = 1.70$
Gratitude	$M = 27.18, SD = 2.23$	$M = 27.36, SD = 2.15$	$M = 66.64, SD = 2.24$
Conflict	$M = 19.45, SD = 2.29$	$M = 13.91, SD = 1.81$	$M = 49.55, SD = 2.11$

The two self-reflection in-action (SR-InAct) questions served the purpose to inform subsequent interview questioning only, rather than be used as part of an inferential analysis. As such only the means were calculated. Negative thinking ($M = 3.91, SD = 1.221$) and gratitude ($M = 3.91, SD = .701$) were slightly above neutral. Self-compassion had the highest mean ($M = 4.45, SD = .688$), and envy ($M = 1.36, SD = .505$) and conflict ($M = 1.27, SD = .467$) were on the lower end.

The mean ratings on the utility of the various design embodiments were 4 or above, indicating that no embodiment did not contribute to self-reflective practices. In looking at the response rate of end-of-day check-ins that required recalling the moment and engaging in breath awareness, about 96 % of end-of-day checkin reminders led to a completed challenge, while the remaining were incomplete and required an repeated enrollment in the challenge – two challenges in the entire study.

Table 3. Utility for Design Conjectures

Question	Rating
By accepting the challenge I felt I was setting an intention to self-reflect	M = 4.18, SD = .60
Setting an intention to self-reflect made it more likely I would self-reflect	M = 4.09, SD = .70
Without the reminders I would have not self-reflected throughout the day	M = 4.18, SD = .75
My self-reflection experience was different based on the mental event	M = 4.27, SD = .46
Recalling a moment was easier when I self-reflected throughout the day.	M = 4.45, SD = 52
Focusing on breathing was helpful in changing the focus of my attention	M = 4, SD = .77

4.2 Phase II: Qualitative Analysis

The eleven semi-structured interviews were transcribed and analyzed using analytic codes that were directly mapped to the five design conjectures and two theoretical conjectures illustrated in Fig. 1. Each coded interview was treated as a case with the unit analysis as each user's single experience with the mobile app. Cases were individually analyzed for themes and concurrently arranged in a word table for cross-comparisons and shared themes [21] across the seven different conjectures. From the word table a review of themes was conducted and a list of the major themes contributing to the initial research questions were outlined and are discussed below.

5 Discussion

The goal of this study is to better understand how specific design embodiments enacted self-reflection and in turn influenced curiosity and decentering experiences. While overall users scores on the TMS and SRIS-SR indicated high levels of curiosity and self-reflection, and varied levels of decentering, we focused on how such processes were experienced, and how specific embodiments shaped these experiences.

5.1 Perceived Control

The theme of perceived control is about the extent to which users felt they could handle the degree of self-reflection asked by the challenges. All of the users felt strongly that initially accepting the challenge felt like they were formally setting the intention to self-reflect. In addition, users felt "strongly" or "very strongly" that setting an intention for the day was essential to feeling they would self-reflect.

In our interviews, the length of the intention (i.e., day), and clarity on what was expected was highlighted as important to their perceived control over self-reflection. For instance one user shared that he, "would have lost steam if I was committing to something for more than a day, but I took it one day at a time." Another user shared she, "liked how simple it seemed at first" and another user said, "I could understand what I was supposed to do, like, if I see it, just acknowledge I observed it."

The use of reminders played into this perceived control in that forgetting was consistently mentioned, as a reason why they thought self-reflecting throughout the day would be challenging. Over 90 % of users felt strongly that without the reminders they would not have self-reflected throughout the day on specific mental events. This is line with research that suggests that when situated in everyday contexts there may be a lack of cognitive resources that can serve as an obstacle to challenging automatized cognitive habits, such as not being aware of specific mental events [22].

The implications for design suggest there is value in the use of reminders to prompt situated self-reflection in general. In addition, our findings suggest that short temporal commitments (e.g. daylong) and clear implementation intentions may help create a strong sense of control over being able to self-reflect throughout one's often busy and attention-demanding day. In addition, the use of reminders when motivation obstacles are not apparent may be effective in supporting one's perceived sense of control and in turn strengthen one's intention to observe internal mental events.

5.2   Likelihood of Opportunities to Observe

Across all of the challenges curiosity scores were high yet we did notice differences in self-reflection scores (SRIS-SR). The pattern was that challenges that targeted narrow mental events had lower self-reported engagement in self-reflection. In other words, there seemed to be difficulty with self-reflecting on mental events we categorized as "narrow." Mean scores of our self-reflection in-action question asking users to rate the degree to which they self-reflected throughout the day supports this findings. At the lower end of all the challenges was envy ($M = 1.36$, $SD = .505$) and conflict ($M = 1.27$, $SD = .467$).

In our interviews users consistently shared that self-reflecting was hard for envy because it did not seem to come up too often in their day-to-day interactions. One user did state that outside of the study he began to notice mental events he would characterize as "envious." One user shared that, "I feel like I used to feel envy a lot, but now I have this job and I'm not about that." Another user described the challenge as, "looking for something and [I] didn't know if I was making it happen because I was looking for it." In other words, for most users envy just did not occur too often and as a result they experienced difficulty in self-reflecting and rated the activity of recalling observed moments challenging.

However, in exploring why curiosity levels remained high despite low self-reflection scores we understood that for this narrow mental event, the reminders served less as reminders to observe, but more as an invitation to think deeper on what they might be missing or how they may be interpreting events. In other words, as one user put it, "I just didn't notice moments of envy. But then I was like, maybe I'm just not realizing their envy, you know? So I just started thinking back, like maybe I'm missing something. Maybe I'm just totally not labeling it right." Other users shared similar sentiments of addressing the difficulty with self-reflecting on envy by retrospectively looking back and trying to see if they were incorrectly characterizing certain thoughts and feelings they had. The low scores on the SRIS-SR subscale which removes motivation from picture [23] was, most likely, sensitive to challenges in observing, while the curiosity subscale picked up on the investigative aspect of one's reaction to the challenge. We noticed the same thematic pattern with the mental event type, conflict, which we labeled as "relational", although to a lesser degree.

The implications for design here are that personalization or on-demand interactions may better address differences in the likelihood of engaging in particular kinds of mental events. In addition, future research on how low likelihood mental events may positively impact motivation to self-reflect may be worth exploring.

5.3   Self-Regulation Impulse

In our phase I quantitative analysis we saw variations in decentering scores between challenges by mental event type. The post-hoc analyses did not yield any additional insight in that all of the types significantly differed from each other. In looking at means scores we noticed that gratitude (a positive valence event type) hovered above all the rest ($M = 27.36$, $SD = 2.157$). Our initial thought was that all positive valence types might have higher decentering scores, yet in the middle were self-criticism and envy and self-compassion with means all hovering around 18, and the lowest decentering score was the conflict challenge ($M = 13.91$, $SD = 1.814$).

From our interviews what emerged was a theme of self-regulation impulse that was connected to how negative the user felt the particular mental event was. For instance, one user shared, "I felt like the point of the gratitude one was to feel good, but I didn't see what the point of the other one – the criticism one. I was just wanting to, you know, change it." This is in contrast with another user who described their experience on self-reflecting as, "I was okay just sitting with that thought and moving on."

All of the users shared the sentiment that focusing on self-criticism made them want to be proactive in some way. This is inline with research that suggest there may be two different kinds of self-reflection – one that is problem focused (PF) and the other that is self-focused (SF) [23]. In describing how this impulse to self-regulate influenced their sense of thoughts as passing or as separate from themselves, users repeatedly described feeling attached to negative thoughts, while being able to let go of positive ones. For instance one user shared, "In the gratitude one I felt it in my breath and I moved on. But in the other one. The critical one. I was like, I should stop doing that." We sought to understand why self-compassion, which we labeled as positive, did not fall into our hypothesized pattern that positive valence mental events did not elicit strong impulses to self-regulate. Users shared that they felt self-compassion overlapped with self-criticism in that many were self-compassionate about mistakes or things they were saying to themselves. This indicates that the valence of mental events may be more complicated to clearly delineate as positive or negative.

In discussing the conflict challenge with users, which had the lowest decentering score was the conflict challenge ($M = 13.91$, $SD = 1.814$), there was by far dominant focus on problem-solving rather than acknowledging the presence of specific mental events. This suggests that prompting users to self-reflect on relational instances, such as conflict between people, may bring the focus to problem solving and exacerbate impulses to self-regulate.

The implications for design are that focusing on mental events that are likely to induce negative affect, may benefit from embedded emotion regulation activities that can leverage impulse to self-regulate. In addition the findings also suggest the need to explore differentiated interactions to support decentering. Given all five mental event types used the same recall and breathing exercises, perhaps extended or guided decentering activities are needed to counteract ones desire to self-regulate.

5.4 Shifting Attention Through Body Awareness

Overall breath awareness was described easy to engage in. In our utility ratings, most users reported that, "Focusing on breathing was helpful in changing the focus of [their] attention." Interviews indicated that body awareness provided a general sense of calm and detachment before dealing with negative mental events. One user stated, "I felt like I had to remember something annoying or shameful, and then just let it go by focusing somewhere else." Another described it as, "the breathing was like at school when you have to take a minute before you do something you'll regret. Except here I think you do it so you could just be okay with what went down." The design implication here is that body awareness may be a powerful design embodiment in shifting attention during an end-of-day reflection and leading to a sense of "letting go" and "being with it", which are in line with decentered experiences.

6 Conclusions and Future Work

A limitation of this study is the limited data points on users' engagement with the challenges and mental event types. An increased number would have provided a larger lens and reduction in confounding situational factors (e.g., a rough day at work) in the data. Furthermore, there was no experimental design that may have allowed for different causal claims to be made about specific design embodiments. In addition, the use of SRIS-SR and TMS have their limitations. SRIS-SR is not written as a state-based retrospective instrument, and TMS is intended for primarily meditation-based experiences. Lastly, there was limited control over situational factors during sample selection (e.g. heavy commuters, demanding work schedules).

Future studies may want to explore the potential for such situated approaches to harness self-regulatory impulses to connect to more traditional forms of cognitive behavioral strategies such as cognitive reappraisal. Recent research has made the case that mindfulness states may support cognitive reappraisal [24]. Furthermore, an experimental design comparing different forms of decentering, and reflection prompts may provide deeper insights into how variations in language, frequency, and body awareness interactions can influence curiosity and decentering through self-reflection.

References

1. Van Dam, N.T., Earleywine, M., Borders, A.: Measuring mindfulness? An item response theory analysis of the mindful attention awareness scale. Pers. Individ. Dif. **49**, 805–810 (2010)

2. Bodhi, B.: What does mindfulness really mean? A canonical perspective. Contemp. Buddhism. **12**, 19–39 (2011)
3. Kabat-zinn, J.: Mindfulness-Based Interventions in Context: Past. Present, and Future **10**, 144–156 (2003)
4. Sharples, M., Taylor, J., Vavoula, G.: A theory of learning for the mobile age. In: Sage Handbook of Elearning Research, pp. 221–247 (2010)
5. Lau, M., Bishop, S.R., Segal, Z.V., Buis, T., Anderson, N.D., Carlson, L., Shapiro, S., Carmody, J., Abbey, S., Devins, G.: The toronto mindfulness scale: development and validation. J. Clin. Psychol. **62**, 1445–1467 (2006)
6. Garland, E.L., Hanley, A., Farb, N.A., Froeliger, B.: State Mindfulness During Meditation Predicts Enhanced Cognitive Reappraisal. Mindfulness (N. Y) (2013)
7. Teasdale, J.D., Moore, R.G., Hayhurst, H., Pope, M., Williams, S., Segal, Z.V.: Metacognitive awareness and prevention of relapse in depression: empirical evidence. J. Consult. Clin. Psychol. **70**, 275–287 (2002)
8. Kuan, T.: Mindfulness in Early Buddhism: New Approaches Through Psychology and Textual Analysis of Pali. Routledge, Chinese and Sanskrit Sources (2007)
9. Hofmann, S.G., Asmundson, G.J.G.: Acceptance and mindfulness-based therapy: new wave or old hat? Clin. Psychol. Rev. **28**, 1–16 (2008)
10. Chiesa, A., Serretti, A., Jakobsen, J.C.: Mindfulness: top-down or bottom-up emotion regulation strategy? Clin. Psychol. Rev. **33**, 82–96 (2013)
11. Watkins, E., Brown, R.G.: Rumination and executive function in depression: an experimental study. J. Neurol. Neurosurg. Psychiatry **72**, 400–402 (2002)
12. MoodPanda: MoodPanda (2015). http://www.moodpanda.com/
13. Makan Studios: Consciouss (2014). http://www.consciousday.com/
14. Mindapps Inc.: The Mindfulness App (2014)
15. Everywhere, M.: Buddhify (2015)
16. Sandoval, W.: Conjecture mapping: an approach to systematic educational design research. J. Learn. Sci. **23**, 18–36 (2014)
17. Cullen, M.: Mindfulness-based interventions: an emerging phenomenon. Mindfulness **2**, 186–193 (2011)
18. Tang, Y.-Y., Posner, M.I.: Attention training and attention state training. Trends Cogn. Sci. **13**, 222–227 (2009)
19. Grant, A.M., Franklin, J., Langford, P.: The self-reflection and insight scale: a new measure of private self-consciousness. Soc. Behav. Personal. an Int. J. **30**, 821–835 (2002)
20. Creswell, J., Clark, V.P.: Choosing a mixed methods design. In: Designing and Conducting Mixed Methods Research, pp. 53–106. Sage Publications (CA) (2007)
21. Yin, R.: Case Study Research: Design and Methods. Sage Publications, Thousand Oaks (2009)
22. Holland, R.W., Aarts, H., Langendam, D.: Breaking and creating habits on the working floor: a field-experiment on the power of implementation intentions. J. Exp. Soc. Psychol. **42**, 776–783 (2006)
23. Grant, A.M., Unit, C.P., Wales, S., Franklin, J., Langford, P., Psychology, C.: The self-reflection and insight scale: a new measure of private self-consciousness. Soc. Behav. Pers. **30**, 821–836 (2002)
24. Garland, E.L., Hanley, A., Farb, N.A., Froeliger, B.: State mindfulness during meditation predicts enhanced cognitive reappraisal. Mindfulness **6**, 234–242 (2013)

Alcohol Behaviour Change: Lessons Learned from User Reviews of iTunes Apps

Omar Mubin[1]([✉]), Abdullah Al Mahmud[2], and Muhammad Ashad Kabir[3]

[1] Western Sydney University, Parramatta, Australia
o.mubin@westernsydney.edu.au
[2] Swinburne University of Technology, Melbourne, Australia
aalmahmud@swin.edu.au
[3] Charles Sturt University, Bathurst, Australia
akabir@csu.edu.au

Abstract. Mobile based persuasive technology can help us to shape positive behaviour and induce habit cessation. This paper reports on the preliminary content analysis of the comments made by users on a set of 18 iTunes apps that were designed to attempt to reduce the over consumption of alcohol and ultimately cut down drinking. In total 204 comments were retrieved from the set of 18 applications using data generated from a custom batch script. Our main results from the content analysis show that an efficient user interface is imperative to facilitate the user acceptance of persuasive mobile systems that attempt to inhibit consumption of alcohol. Furthermore, we noted more positive comments towards apps that adopted a self control behavioural change strategy, particularly as they followed a subtle and not abrupt interaction style. We conclude our analysis by providing a list of design recommendations for mobile apps that can assist in inhibiting alcohol consumption. Our analysis indicated that customisation and the possibility of maintaining incremental milestones were amongst the more sought after app features.

Keywords: Alcohol · Behaviour change · Mobile computing · Mobile apps · iTunes

1 Introduction

Binge drinking, drink driving, alcohol related violence, alcohol related illness are some of the many ill effects of the over consumption of alcohol [17]. Various intervention strategies operate on a governmental level or through non-governmental organisations with the ultimate aim of promoting awareness and reminding people of the side effects of consuming alcohol in large amounts. In addition, technology (such as computing, mobile, smart systems, etc.) has the potential to transform how we deliver alcohol interventions and promote behaviour change from harmful alcohol for example [21]. In today's digitally connected world with a high penetration of smart phones, mobile technology can be utilised as an efficacious tool as it provides users with the right information at the right

© Springer International Publishing Switzerland 2016
A. Meschtscherjakov et al. (Eds.): PERSUASIVE 2016, LNCS 9638, pp. 99–109, 2016.
DOI: 10.1007/978-3-319-31510-2_9

time allowing them to make informed decisions; in particular within the health domain [19]. This ultimately promotes sustained behaviour change. Newer and newer mobile apps are emerging day by day and they can provide obvious merits to change behaviour by providing appealing interfaces and appropriate features. Persuasive technology or captology is broadly defined as a stream of technology that is designed to change attitudes or behaviors of the users through persuasion and social influence, but not through coercion [7]. According to BJ Fogg [6] technology can persuade users by adopting certain guidelines; for example: increasing self efficacy, providing tailored information, triggering decision making, guiding users through a process, etc. In sum the goal of persuasive technology is to initially provide motivation and consequently the ability to change behaviour [8]. Technologies have had a significant impact in alleviating various social issues (obesity, well being, sustainability, environmental awareness, etc.).

Accessing information and support for alcohol related issues through technology deviates away from traditional rehabilitation procedures and therapy as it can be done autonomously, anonymously and conveniently. The option of remaining anonymous is important in sensitive areas such as substance abuse because it is often easier to get information anonymously via an interactive computing program, than face another human being [7]. Furthermore, the accessibility of information is not confined to a physical location nor is it tied to a specific time-frame. A self-administered and stand-alone intervention helps to eliminate various barriers such as the stigma of attending a treatment facility, the high cost of treatment, and scheduling and transportation issues. Currently there are mostly web/desktop-based interventions in place to assist in persuading individuals to reduce their consumption of alcohol and inform them on the effects of alcoholism [3]. The downfall with web/desktop-interventions is firstly their feasibility and inability to be conveniently accessed at the end-users own discretion. Secondly, customisation is usually low for such web based interventions - personalisation is now being considered as an integral component of mobile based behavioural change applications [11]. Consequently, it is imperative to build efficacious intervention programs (possibly mobile based and on the go) to stimulate or help sustain positive behaviour change for drinkers who do not connect with support service as there is evidence that mobile intervention is suitable to recover from alcoholism [12].

We have noticed that governmental organisations such as the National Health Service England (NHS) [15] are slowly beginning to recognise and advocate the importance of providing mobile apps for promoting reduced consumption of alcohol. However, little is known about the effectiveness of such apps especially for behaviour change and user insights are relatively unexplored [5]. As the target of those apps are a specific user group, it is very crucial to acknowledge their feedback in order to judge the quality of those apps. It has been observed that some mobile apps are not designed according to the established rules so that they can effectively change a particular behaviour. For example, a study of iPhone apps for smoking cessation found that certain apps are not designed based on the recommended guidelines for smoking cessation [1]. Similar violations of design principles can be seen in apps from other domains [22]. Within Human Computer

Interaction (HCI) and Mobile Computing the role of mobile apps in promoting health and well-being is an acknowledged and promising research area. However more recently [18] efforts are being dedicated in achieving a deeper understanding of the implications of health monitoring through mobile applications, more specifically recognising that the solution is not in simply providing digital information but rather carefully designing the visualisation, presentation and modality of the information. In sum, although researchers have begun to understand behavioural change techniques that result in a reduction of alcohol consumption through mobile apps [13]; it is still necessary to look for user preferences and opinions concerning those and other similar mobile apps.

End user review is very important in order to understand users' perception of a particular product. It has been found that end user reviews play a vital role in order to buy items from web stores such as Amazon [14]. End user reviews appear on app store as ratings, comments and sometimes with visual marks of goodness or badness, which may influence the number of downloads of those apps. We are not aware of any study which particularly focused on understanding mobile app reviews on different apps designed to change alcohol consumption. Such an investigation can provide us with some answers as to what design features are the most efficient in incurring behavioural changes towards alcohol intake. There are some studies which have investigated mobile apps in order to understand the process of user ratings and user opinions [9]. Using analysis of user reviews on social media (specifically iTunes, youtube, etc.) to determine and elicit user insights, comments, feedback and complaints is slowly gathering interest in the field of Human Computer Interaction and Mobile Computing [10]. With the proliferation of Apple devices such as the iPhone and the popularity of the App Store (as evidenced by 100 billion app downloads [2]) we proceeded with iTunes as the platform of choice for our analysis.

As the first step in our design process towards creating a persuasive mobile application (app) to control the consumption of alcohol we aim to understand the impact of existing mobile applications to support the abstinence of over consumption of alcohol. We also aim to realise what particular design features and persuasive strategies are most preferred by the users. In order to determine such insights from users we extracted comments from iTunes on a set of short listed existing mobile applications of varying persuasive strategies that were aimed to control drinking behaviour of its users. The comments were then analysed using content analysis. In conclusion we discuss design guidelines and recommendations for developing such mobile apps and attempt to ground our findings through an overview of commercial apps recommended by the NHS in the UK which are meant to control alcohol consumption.

2   Method

Our research methodology was primarily based on the prior work of [4] where the authors conducted a needs assessment to examine mobile smart-phone apps that promoted alcohol behavior change. Furthermore, in their research a meta level categorical analysis of iTunes apps designed to mitigate and inhibit alcohol addiction was conducted to understand the various behavioural strategies they employ to control drinking behaviour. However, an analysis on user opinions, feedback and insights was missing and they did not present any user interface guidelines to inform the design of such mobile apps which is vital given the explosion in the number of smart phones. Therefore, we build on top of the work of [4] by conducting content analysis on a set of user reviews on relevant iTunes apps with a goal of identifying recommendations to inform the design of mobile apps that inhibit the over consumption of alcohol.

2.1   App Selection

The apps were retrieved through iTunes by utilising a set of predefined keywords. We utilised the following set of keywords to search for applications: alcohol self help (4), alcohol abstinence (3), alcohol recovery (53), substance abuse (24), quit drinking (31), alcohol harm reduction (73), quit alcohol (22), alcohol moderation (0), alcohol anonymous (65). All keywords were adapted from those discussed in [4]. The number of unique applications retrieved for each keyword are provided in brackets. There maybe additional keywords that could have been employed in the search however it is our opinion that through the existing list of keywords a fairly exhaustive set of apps was retrieved. In fact the appearance of an app via specific keywords was not mutually exclusive and apps would be listed for a number of different keywords.

In the work of [4], two primary categories of apps were considered for analysis; firstly apps which facilitated alcohol consumption and secondly apps which provided an intervention. Overall, in iTunes there are a number of applications relevant to alcohol consumption however our focus was on applications of mainly a persuasive type that can change the behaviour of people in a positive way both in the long term and short term. Therefore we ignored any app that would facilitate alcohol consumption (such as recipe apps, etc.) or that would provide general information about alcohol without providing the feature of assisting in overcoming a drinking habit. Categorisation of an app into one of these categories was enabled by reading the basic description of the app in iTunes and through the definitions of each description in [4] it was ensured that this was a mutually exclusive process. This filtration resulted in a set of 26 applications. In order to automate the extraction of comments, we wrote a simple batch script that would query the iTunes API for the comments on each app on the basis of an app ID. 8 apps were depicted by the iTunes API as not having any registered comments.

Each application from the set of 18 remaining applications was then categorised into one of the following evidence-based subcategories as suggested in [4,5]: (1) motivational or counselling and (2) self coping or self control. Motivational or counselling applications would provide insightful feedback to drive behavioural changes whereas applications employing self control or self coping strategies utilised mainly metrics such as the Blood Alcohol Concentration (BAC) to provide information to the user with little or no initiative towards decision making. The number of apps that adopted a self control behavioural change strategy were 6 in number. The intervention strategy employed by the app (or simply the category of the app) was the independent variable of our analysis as we wished to ascertain which of the two strategies were the most effective and preferred by the users.

2.2 Coding Process

In total 204 comments (excluding comments that were junk, spam or not in English) were retrieved from the set of 18 applications using data generated from the script on March 27, 2015. 29 comments were from self control apps - see details in Table 1. The average length of a review was 35.4 words. The maximum length was 225 words and the minimum length was 2 words. The entire process

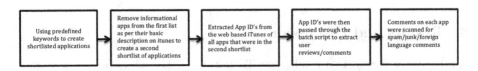

Fig. 1. Sequence of steps/process of shortlisting apps and comments

Table 1. Details of the chosen apps which were used to analyse user reviews

Name of App	Keyword used on iTunes	Category of App	# of Comm-ents	Name of App	Keyword used on iTunes	Category of App	# of Comm-ents
Self Help	Alcohol Self Help	Self control Self coping	1	Step Away	Alcohol Reduction	Motivational Counselling	16
Substance Abuse	Alcohol Self Help	Self control Self coping	4	How to Stop Drinking Alcohol	Alcohol Reduction	Motivational Counselling	1
Stop Drinking With Andrew Johnson	Alcohol Reduction	Motivational Counselling	36	Quit n Save	Alcohol Reduction	Motivational Counselling	1
iRecovery	Alcohol Reduction	Motivational Counselling	13	I am Sober	Alcohol Recovery	Motivational Counselling	50
Quit That	Alcohol Reduction	Motivational Counselling	25	Addicaid	Alcohol Recovery	Self Control Self Coping	21
Addiction Counter	Alcohol Reduction	Self Control Self Coping	1	New to Recovery	Substance Abuse	Self Control Self Coping	1
Saying When	Alcohol Reduction	Motivational Counselling	3	Addiction Avert	Substance Abuse	Motivational Counselling	12
Sober Tool	Alcohol Reduction	Motivational Counselling	11	No Go	Quit Drinking	Self Control Self Coping	1
Quit Drinking Hypnosis	Alcohol Reduction	Motivational Counselling	7				

of shortlisting apps and comments is summarised in a block diagram (see Fig. 1). Each comment was treated as one unit of data. Each comment was then coded to determine:

1. valence (positive, negative or irrelevant) towards the effectiveness of the behavioural change strategy and feedback by the user in actually being able to carry out a behavioural change in their life.
2. valence (positive, negative or irrelevant) towards the application features, design, user interface, usability, etc.

   In order to verify our coding scheme two authors separately coded $\approx 20\%$ of the comments. Cohen's Kappa for valence for behavioural change strategy ($\kappa = 0.69$) and for valence for application features ($\kappa = 0.65$) was computed which indicated moderate agreement. Discrepancies in coding were resolved after discussion.

3   Results and Discussion

A table of the categorised results (see Table 2) from the coding is provided summarising the total number of coded comments across the two valence types and the category of the application. A Chi-Square Test revealed that there was a significant but weak association between valence attribution towards the application features and the category of apps ($\chi^2(N = 204,2) = 9.64$, p $= 0.008$, Cramer $V = 0.22$). Apps that adopted a self control paradigm elicited significantly fewer negative comments on the application features as compared to apps that followed motivational strategies (Z $= -2.5$). A second Chi-Square Test revealed that the category of apps did not have a significant association with the valence attribution towards the effectiveness of the behavioural change strategy employed by the app ($\chi^2(N = 204,2) = 1.62$, p $= 0.45$).

Table 2. Table summarising total number of coded comments

		Valence RE effectiveness of the behavioural strategy			Valence RE application features		
		Positive	Negative	Irrelevant	Positive	Negative	Irrelevant
Category of	Motivational	82	8	85	82	41	52
application	Self control	10	2	17	22	1	6

One of the main trends observed in our analysis was that in general users preferred the user interface and design features of self control apps as compared to apps that followed a motivational strategy. Prior work [5] has depicted similar trends (albeit in health-based behavioural change applications), primarily due to the user feeling agitated by over prompting or by an over zealous system. It can be suggested that in such situations the user would desire control and edit rights over the addiction control plan and strategy. Some of the negative comments on the features of a motivational style of behavioral change referred to the demanding nature of such applications, for example: *"I have tried this app several times it did nothing for me except give me some anxiety from the fast pace and demanding tone used it gave me no positive results at all"* or to the inability of the strategy convincing them to incur a behavioural change, for example: *"It hasn't really helped me to stop drinking"*. Further research is required to determine if the preference of the design features of self control and self coping style of applications was due to a cause and effect relationship with user interface inadequacies. It would not be naive to assume that implementing motivational apps would be more challenging than apps of simple self reporting or self recording nature. In our overview of the iTunes comments we noticed that many users thought that motivational apps were *"slow"*, *"useless"*, *"inaccurate"*, etc. The difficulty in implementing persuasive applications that facilitate behavioural change explicitly and directly are known to be a technical challenge [20]; primarily due to real time monitoring requirements.

Many users preferred the simplicity in design of the self control and self coping style of apps as indicated in the following comment: *"The app is intuitive and the design is bright and refreshing - nothing clinical or scary about it"*. It goes without saying that simple, engaging and motivational interaction (i.e., the user interface) is imperative for the success of a persuasive mobile application - as also emphasised in [16]. There were only 3 comments which were coded to be positive in terms of the evaluation of their behavioural change strategy and negative in terms of their application features. Overall, when an app had a usable interface most users were positive about the prospects of being able to change their behavior (only 1 comment which indicated otherwise).

3.1 Design Recommendations

We analysed user comments across both categories of apps to elicit specific yet emerging patterns and we also extracted design features that were preferred and recommended. A number of acquired design features that we present as design recommendations are now listed with some sample comments:

- Customisation with respect to layout, options, features, alerts, plans, etc. was one of the key guidelines. Ultimately users wished to have the ability to modify both user interface and behavioral strategy aspects at their own will (*"personalisation feature is great and very effective"*).
- Real time feedback was also deemed to be important, as users wished to visualise the result of their behavioural changes instantly (*"The app provides immediate accountability"*).
- The most preferred mode of interaction was relaxing, gradual, not abrupt and soothing intervention. This was a key feature found in most self control apps as the following comments illustrate: (*"It not only helps me to relax and fall asleep, but it has helped to reduce my desire for alcohol"*) and (*"This app has such a soothing and intuitive design"*).

- Incremental goals and targets also allowed users to set short term objectives and perceive success on their completion: (*"I love getting the alert every night telling me I am one more day sober"*) and (*"I love the milestones. I set each new one as my wallpaper"*). This feature (i.e. milestones, daily goals, etc.) was one of the most popular and sought after and was one of the key elements appreciated in self control apps.
- Many users thought social interaction and the ability to communicate progress through social media was important, as evidenced by the following: (*"The only thing I wish it did was allow me to post to a social network my progress, but I worked around that by taking screenshots and posting those"*) and (*"Unless I'm missing it, I'm really surprised that I can't tweet or post anywhere for that matter directly from app"*).
- The ability to control other cravings besides alcohol through the same app was also a desired aspect: (*"Would be really nice if I could change it from alcohol to something else"*). Though we have seen several apps for alcohol behaviour change a few apps were more generic. For example, they could be used for multiple purposes such as smoke cessation, cutting down alcohol consumption or quitting other bad habits.

As a final step in our analysis we sourced apps from the National Health Service (NHS) England Health Apps Library [15] to benchmark, compare, ground and contrast our findings. The Health Apps Library is aimed at people living in England who want to use apps to manage their health; and health professionals who may want to recommend an app to someone if needed. When we searched the library we found in total eight apps which were associated with the keyword alcohol and which have been reviewed by clinicians in the UK to ensure that they are safe and trustworthy. Out of those eight apps there were three apps, which were not related to alcohol behavior change rather they were either for general health tracking or for creating awareness for other people. The apps, which are related, to track or cut down alcohol consumption were 1. Leaf-your discrete drink tracker, 2. DrinkCoach, 3. Change4Life drinks tracker, 4. Type 1 diabetes friend, and 5. Drink meter. No user reviews were found for those apps except for Change4Life drinks tracker. That particular app had a 4.5 start average rating and had the following features: a. track drinks each day, b. view drinking levels over a week or a fortnight to spot when someone is at an heightened risk, c. learn more about the specific risks, d. get daily tips and feedback, e. add daily notes, f. share with friends via Facebook or Twitter. In general users found the app motivational and one person had been using it for two years. We noticed that the overall goal of these five apps was to help people drink within the safe limits rather than motivate them to completely quit. Clearly these five apps were of a self control type relying on the user to him/herself manage their alcohol intake. This is consistent with our earlier findings that motivational apps are not widely implemented or deployed yet, probably due to user interface or user perception issues.

3.2 Limitations and Future Work

There are a number of limitations of our study some of which are inherent to the structure and setup of iTunes. The retrieval of comments for a particular app through the iTunes API did not synchronise with what was seen as the comments for that API through the iTunes website/software. In this paper, we have only considered one source (i.e., the API) and aim to merge the two sources in our future research. However, we did notice that the sample size of comments retrieved from the API were much larger in number than what was being seen through the iTunes software/website. The actual number of downloads and popularity of an app is also a measure that cannot be retrieved through iTunes. The popularity can also not be determined by the level of usage of an app; we cannot tell from a particular comment if that particular user is an expert or a novice user of that app.

Furthermore, it is evident that self control apps were fewer in number and hence the corresponding set of comments was smaller than motivational apps. We aim to address this constraint by considering Android apps found on Google Play. The limited number of user reviews across apps in general was one of the reasons why we did not restrict the extracted reviews to a specific time period. Another interesting observation while searching the apps was that we found a number of varying behavioural change strategies (beyond the two we discussed: motivational and self control) in the apps which were aimed to change behaviour. In the future, it will be equally interesting to extend our analysis to a wider variety of persuasive strategies. We would also like to acknowledge the possibility that some apps could comprise of both motivational and self control features. That may actually be quite beneficial allowing further opportunity for users to customise their interaction. In our sample of 18 apps we did not observe any to merge both types of behavioural strategies.

Although some comments were quite large we did not observe any comment which had a merge of positive and negative emotions; most users were very assured as to how they evaluated either the interface or the behavioural strategy of the app. However the subjectivity of the coding process must be acknowledged. One of the key limitations of our process of content analysis was that we did not benchmark or crosscheck the accuracy of the comments made on an app by actually analysing its interface. Despite a number of limitations we are of the opinion that our design recommendations, trends and lessons can be of help for future implementations of apps that attempt to counter the over consumption of alcohol.

4 Conclusion

In this paper we have presented the preliminary content analysis of the comments made by users on both self control and motivational type iTunes apps that were designed to attempt to reduce the over consumption of alcohol and ultimately cut down drinking. Our main results show that an self control apps are more popular and were rated more positively primarily due to being less invasive and more supportive of customisation. Users also found issues in the user interface of motivational apps which may be due to the difficulty in implementing such apps and sourcing real time information. The most sought after and preferred feature was the ability of apps to support incremental progress using elements such as daily milestones and goals. We have also summarised some key design guidelines as a prospective checklist which would be useful for other researchers and mobile app designers to incorporate in systems that aim to inhibit the consumption of alcohol.

References

1. Abroms, L.C., Padmanabhan, N., Thaweethai, L., Phillips, T.: iphone apps for smoking cessation: a content analysis. Am. J. Prev. Med. **40**(3), 279–285 (2011)
2. App. Store (2015). http://www.theverge.com/2015/6/8/8739611/apple-wwdc-2015-stats-update
3. Bewick, B.M., Trusler, K., Barkham, M., Hill, A.J., Cahill, J., Mulhern, B.: The effectiveness of web-based interventions designed to decrease alcohol consumptiona systematic review. Prev. Med. **47**(1), 17–26 (2008)
4. Cohn, A.M., Hunter-Reel, D., Hagman, B.T., Mitchell, J.: Promoting behavior change from alcohol use through mobile technology: the future of ecological momentary assessment. Alcohol.: Clin. Exp. Res. **35**(12), 2209–2215 (2011)
5. Dennison, L., Morrison, L., Conway, G., Yardley, L.: Opportunities and challenges for smartphone applications in supporting health behavior change: qualitative study. J. Med. Internet Res. **15**(4), e86 (2013)
6. Fogg, B., Cuellar, G., Danielson, D.: Motivating, influencing, and persuading users: An introduction to captology. Hum. Comput. Interact. Fundam. **9**, 109–122 (2009)
7. Fogg, B.J.: Persuasive technology: using computers to change what we think and do. Ubiquit. **2002**(December), 5 (2002)
8. Fogg, B.J.: A behavior model for persuasive design. In: Proceedings of the 4th international Conference on Persuasive Technology, pp. 40. ACM (2009)
9. Hoon, L., Vasa, R., Schneider, J.G., Mouzakis, K.: A preliminary analysis of vocabulary in mobile app. user reviews. In: Proceedings of the 24th Australian Computer-Human Interaction Conference, OzCHI 2012, pp. 245–248. ACM, NY, USA, New York (2012)
10. Khalid, H., Shihab, E., Nagappan, M., Hassan, A.: What do mobile app. users complain about? a study on free ios apps (2014)
11. Masthoff, J., Vassileva, J.: Tutorial on personalization for behaviour change. In: Proceedings of the 20th International Conference on Intelligent User Interfaces, pp. 439–442. ACM (2015)
12. McTavish, F.M., Chih, M.Y., Shah, D., Gustafson, D.H.: How patients recovering from alcoholism use a smartphone intervention. J. Dual Diagn. **8**(4), 294–304 (2012)
13. Michie, S., Whittington, C., Hamoudi, Z., Zarnani, F., Tober, G., West, R.: Identification of behaviour change techniques to reduce excessive alcohol consumption. Addict. **107**(8), 1431–1440 (2012)
14. Mudambi, S.M., Schuff, D.: What makes a helpful review? a study of customer reviews on amazon. com. MIS Q. **34**(1), 185–200 (2010)
15. NHS Health Apps Library (2015). http://apps.nhs.uk/apps/alcohol/

16. Oinas-Kukkonen, H., Harjumaa, M.: Persuasive systems design: Key issues, process model, and system features. Commun. Assoc. Inf. Syst. **24**(1), 28 (2009)
17. Organization, W.H., et al.: Global status report on alcohol and health-2014. World Health Organization (2014)
18. Panel Mobile HCI 2015 (2015). http://mobilehci.acm.org/2015/panel.html
19. Toscos, T., Faber, A., An, S., Gandhi, M.P.: Chick clique: persuasive technology to motivate teenage girls to exercise. In: CHI 2006 extended abstracts on Human factors in computing systems, pp. 1873–1878. ACM (2006)
20. del Valle, A.C.A., Opalach, A.: The persuasive mirror: computerized persuasion for healthy living
21. Wang, K.C., Hsieh, Y.H., Yen, C.H., You, C.W., Chen, Y.C., Huang, M.C., Lau, S.Y., Kao, H.L.C., Chu, H.H.: Soberdiary: A phone-based support system for assisting recovery from alcohol dependence. In: Proceedings of the 2014 ACM International Joint Conference on Pervasive and Ubiquitous Computing, pp. 311–314. ACM (2014)
22. Wolf, J.A., Moreau, J.F., Akilov, O., Patton, T., English, J.C., Ho, J., Ferris, L.K.: Diagnostic inaccuracy of smartphone applications for melanoma detection. JAMA Dermatol. **149**(4), 422–426 (2013)

Persuasive Strategies to Improve Driving Behaviour of Elderly Drivers by a Feedback Approach

Perrine Ruer[✉], Charles Gouin-Vallerand, and Evelyne F. Vallières

LICEF Research Center, Télé-Université du Québec, Montréal, Canada
{pruer,cgouinva,evallier}@teluq.ca

Abstract. We are witnessing a growing aging population who wishes to live independently. In a driving context, the elderly want to maintain an active lifestyle, but they may suffer from impairments due to aging. New intelligent transportation systems can be beneficial for drivers to assist them with driving. Hence, new intelligent technologies have to be accepted and have to persuade the driver of adopting safer driving behaviours. In this paper, we present a persuasive driving feedback for elderly drivers. The feedback objectives are to evaluate the drivers' perception of the driving fatigue and to compare it with their driving behaviour. Our first results from an exploratory field experiment with twenty elderly drivers support the use of the feedback with that category of drivers relative to fatigue perception. The originality of this paper is to enable progress in the area of persuasive technologies applied to road safety and for elder people.

Keywords: Elderly drivers · Persuasive technology · Feedback · Contextual information · Road safety

1 Introduction

Aging is a growing phenomenon in almost all countries of the world. The percentage of people of 65 and older will more than double between 2010 and 2050 [1]. Elder people want to continue to drive to maintain their independence, even more so for elderly drivers living in rural or remote areas. Mobility is fundamental to them because it allows them to maintain an active aging. Thus, it is in the best interest of societies to maintain elderly adults driving as long as they can safely do so. In the last decade, there has been much attention given to technologies focusing on elderly drivers' mobility [2]. Indeed, the development of transport technologies can address their mobility need by allowing them to use safely their personal car as long as possible. For the past few years, there has been a growing interest in intelligent vehicles. A notable initiative on intelligent vehicles was created by the U.S. Department of Transportation with the mission of preventing highway crashes [3].

Technologies can be useful as countermeasures to driving fatigue among elderly drivers, as long as they induce behaviour changes. Persuasive technologies have this feature. The association of persuasion strategies to technology is essential because persuasive technologies can help changing user's behaviour. To do so, it is essential to take into account the characteristics of elderly people and to educate them on how to

© Springer International Publishing Switzerland 2016
A. Meschtscherjakov et al. (Eds.): PERSUASIVE 2016, LNCS 9638, pp. 110–121, 2016.
DOI: 10.1007/978-3-319-31510-2_10

use technology and when [2]. However, in the road safety scientific literature, there is a lack of knowledge about persuasive technology applied to elderly drivers.

Therefore, this paper presents a persuasive system that was designed for helping elderly drivers to manage their fatigue at the wheel. The paper is structured as follow. Section 2 presents an overview of persuasive technologies, in light of elderly drivers and driving self-regulation. In Sect. 3, we present our methodology to design the persuasive system. Section 4 reports our first results. Finally, Sect. 5 concludes with the limits of this exploratory study and suggestions for future research in that field.

2 Related Works

2.1 Persuasive Technologies

In [4], Fogg defines persuasion as "an attempt to change attitudes or behaviours or both (without using coercion or deception)" (p. 16). The aims of persuasive technologies are to induce attitude change and behavioural outcomes. Changing these outcomes is central (e.g. reinforce attitudes, act of complying, etc.). And the concept of motivational affordance (motivation to use the system) is affiliated with psychological outcomes and target behaviours. All persuasive technologies focus on these final effects. The results can be positive (partially or fully), negative or with no effect [5].

Oinas-Kukkonen and Harjumaa [6] define the context analysis as the grouping of the persuasion's intent, the understanding of the persuasion event and the definition or recognition in the use of ongoing strategies. First, persuasive technology involves a voluntary change by the user of his/her behaviours [4]. Indeed, persuasive systems have to influence, motivate or convince the user to take action. Besides the intent, the event of persuasion and the strategy have to be considered for the design and the use of a persuasive technology. The event concerns the usage and the user of the persuasive system. First, the usage (or the context of use) refers to the problem domains' attributes (for instance, promotion of health or ecological consumption). Then, an analysis of the user is also important. Indeed, there are individual differences between people on how to interpret information. For instance, there are differences in cognitive processes between younger and elder people. These differences have an impact on the persuasion strategy which is defined as the message and how it is delivered [5, 6]. Once the context analysis has been determined, the next phase is to design the persuasive system. To do so, the information content and the software functionalities need to be understood to design and evaluate the software system persuasiveness.

2.2 Existing Persuasive Technologies in the Automotive Context

During the last 30 years, there has been growing progresses in the domain of in-vehicle technologies. These technologies are likely to have used persuasive strategies. The best-known persuasive technologies in automotive context are eco-driving technologies [7, 8]. In 2015, persuasive technologies have been designed in order to improve users' safe driving behaviours and their motivation. There are two basic workings. The first one is to give real-time feedback to a current individual driving behaviour, for instance such as recommendations. The second basic working is to accumulate information about a driver behaviours and to give an accumulated feedback to the driver [7].

The most prevalent persuasive systems in automotive context are in-car interfaces and mobile systems, like smartphone applications [7, 9]. Persuasive systems integrated in a vehicle give real-time feedback with optical advices (for instance, a bar chart or pictograms can appear on the dashboard to give a driving behaviour feedback). The inconvenience of in-car technologies is that it is not installed in many cars, even though in the next few years, we expect they will be increasing. As for persuasive mobile systems, several applications have been developed to give driving feedback to the user after the driving. The example presented by Schätzl [7] was an application which gives information about speed curve over time and abrupt accelerations and decelerations. The disadvantages of using mobile app is that it has to be downloaded, or to be manually started before each driving session and it can be used only with a compatible smart-phone [9].

Nevertheless, persuasive technologies affect the driving behaviour and have a positive influence, for instance on the fuel consumption [7]. Persuasive technologies can promote driver behaviour and improve road safety, provided that the persuasive technologies address appropriately the drivers' characteristics and are well-accepted by them [9]. Indeed, acceptance of technology is necessary, in order to avoid rejection by the user [8]. But technologies could also improve the quality of life by overcoming age-related deficits [10].

In sum, persuasive technologies can not only improve driving safety, save resources, protect the environment but they can also improve the quality of life of elderly drivers by overcoming age-related deficits.

2.3 Elderly Drivers

Elders have specific driving characteristics. They are prudent, drive at low speed and respect the traffic laws and their driving style is low risk taking [11]. Their main causes of accidents are errors which are defined as judgment and observation failures dangerous to other drivers [12]. When driving, a lot of information is asked from the driver in a time constraint (for instance: changing direction, insertion in traffic, intersection, etc.). Elderly drivers have difficulties to manage the unexpected and accidents happen when they are making decisions under this time constraint [12].

Drivers have to respond rapidly to risks, which requires good abilities like attention, perception, motor abilities, information treatment, etc. With aging, some physiological impairments appear and have negative impacts on driving skills [13]. The cognitive skills are affected and lead to a longer reaction time, a diminution of attention, and a shorter memory [14]. Physical abilities are worsening with a deterioration of psycho-motor skills, development of arthritis, which causes neck problems, or also the vulner-ability of the body [10]. And sensory functions decline with a diminution of visual acuity, diminution of hearing or even, perceptual ability [14, 15]. These impairments are common among the elderly with normal aging. In addition, there is an increase of diseases, associated with medication in-take and a higher risk of accidents. Medication alters the driving skills and reduces sensorimotor performance (for example: decreased alertness, impaired vision, etc.) [10]. Therefore, some authors propose license restrictions to manage elderly drivers' safety [16], even though empirical research has clearly showed that driving cessation had adverse negative consequences [10, 15, 17] as it is a stressful experience having a negative impact on their quality of life.

2.4 Driving Fatigue Self-Regulation

Fatigue is one cause of elders' accidents. Fatigue refers to a transitional state between wakefulness and sleep leading to sleep if it isn't interrupted [18]. Different models and theories have been proposed in order to explain the safe and risky behaviour of elderly drivers. Among them, a multifactorial model by Anstey and her colleagues [14] suggests that both self-monitoring beliefs about one's driving capacity and one's real capacity to drive safely are predictors of driving behaviour. Self-monitoring is determined by cognition, whereas the capacity to drive safely is determined by the sensorial, physical and cognitive variables. For instance, the driver whose capacity to drive safely is reduced due to a visual deficit, while at the same time his or her beliefs about the capacity to drive match his or her real capacities, then the driver is susceptible to self-regulate and drive safely. However, if that same driver is unaware of the deficit, decides to ignore it or overestimates his or her visual capacities, that driver is susceptible to have unsafe driving behaviours.

Research has shown that elderly drivers, like other groups of drivers, continue to drive even though they are drowsy or nodding off [19]. Furthermore, drowsy or fatigued drivers use different strategies in order to keep awake, such as opening the window, putting on the radio, talking to passengers, stopping to eat, to exercise or to relax, without napping or sleeping. Yet, these strategies are the least efficient ones in order to counter fatigue at the wheel, while the most efficient strategies, such as stopping to nap or sleep or asking a passenger to drive, are generally avoided even though drivers know they are the efficient ones [20, 21].

Persuasive technologies can be applied to feedback concerning specific driving behaviours, for instance, those relative to fatigue, and for a category of persons, such as elder people.

2.5 The Applicability of a Design Persuasive Method Through a Real Driving Feedback

The design method we chose to apply to the development of a real driving feedback is the Persuasive Systems Design (PSD) Process Model, proposed by Oinas-Kukkonen and Harjumaa [6]. The advantages of this methodology are its usefulness to study feedback with users in real-life contexts and its applicability to on-road situations.

Oinas-Kukkonen and Harjumaa have established a set of design principles that have been classified in four categories adapted partially from Fogg's work [4, 6]. They are primary task, dialogue, system credibility, and social support. For each of them, Oinas-Kukkonen and Harjumaa give the design principles, the requirements and offer implementation examples. Primary task is defined by the authors as "the carrying out of the user's primary task". For instance, the design-principle self-monitoring in the automotive context would be that the system should provide a feedback of the driving performance (speed, braking, vigilance, etc.). The users can track their performance or status, through a tool (in-car interface or mobile phone application), to improve decision making.

Dialogue is the user's feedback, via verbal-information or other kinds of summaries to support and help the users to move closer to their target behaviour. An example of the application of the praise principle to an elderly driver would be an image or some words to motivate the person to adopt a better driving style. The other goal could be to increase safe driving for the driver and the community (i.e. other drivers).

As for the system credibility, it allows designing a system that could be more convincing for the users. For example, the fact that feedback can be transmitted to the point of view of some authorities, such as a government transport ministry, could have more persuasive power.

The fourth category, social support is about designing a system that will motivate the users by leveraging social influence. An example of the social learning principle applied to feedback for elderly drivers is a shared event log for encouraging good behaviours.

3   Methodology

In our study, the intent is to persuade the elderly driver to manage appropriately his/her fatigue on his/her subsequent conduct of the vehicle. We did a pilot study to evaluate the perception of the driving fatigue with elderly drivers and compared it with their driving behaviour. To do this, we did experimental work and we measured perceived fatigue, speed, sleep habits, etc. During the experimentation, each participant drove around 50 km on a closed driving circuit with the LiSA car (in French: *Laboratoire intelligent de Sécurité Automobile*. In English: Intelligent Laboratory on Automobile Safety) (Fig. 1). Participants were asked to respect a 60 km/h limit.

For the event, we took into account the driving context and the driver. In the context of our research, we used an instrumented vehicle, the LiSA, a Nissan Versa 2008. The car is equipped with a data logger AIM Evo4 which can collect data on speed, steering wheel movements, acceleration, braking, 3-axis acceleration and GPS location from the car embedded computer. LiSA also includes an eye tracking faceLAB 5.0 system, a Microsoft Kinect (with a head tracking software [22]) camera and several other cameras to monitor the driver. Finally, all the data are recorded by a computer installed on-board. Thus, LiSA is able to collect a wide range of contextual information.

To complete the contextual information on the user profile, questionnaires were filled before, during and after the experimentation to collect sociodemographic variables, such as age, gender, driving experience, opinions toward safe driving, etc. Moreover, in the context of our experiment, we collected the driver's level of perceived fatigue by using a scale ranging from '0' not at all fatigued to '10' very much fatigued at four times during the experimental session. Each participant was asked his or her level of fatigue just before starting driving (Time 1), after 15 min

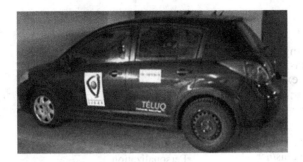

Fig. 1. The LiSA instrumented vehicle

of driving once the experiment had started (Time 2), after 30 min (Time 3), and when the driving experiment ended (around 45 min) (Time 4). The focus of the experiment was to measure the level of perceived fatigue, not the physiological level of fatigue. A 45-minutes driving task on a monotony road low (e.g., 60 km/h) has been found to induce fatigue in prior laboratory experiments [18] and a field experiment pretest. The pretest shows a significant increase in the assessed fatigue level for the majority of the participants, without reaching a hazardous level.

Finally, in the present study, the data analysis strategies adopted was the use of a tool with data mining and statistical evaluation algorithms. For example, one algorithm transforms the data on the most common measure by aggregating the data from sensors with an higher sensing frequency by computing the average values [23]. We also use a quasi-monotonic segmentation algorithm [24] to reduce the noise and compute the relevant acceleration and deceleration behaviours of the participants. We used it to allow an easy visualization of the data collected. This tool was used first to test algorithms offline and to stock the contextual information collected for each participant. We applied this tool to all data collected from the field experiment. The tool enabled us to visualize the collected data with graphs and maps. It then proposed a feedback solution to promote awareness of the fatigue impact on driving (particularly speed) and bring the drivers to better manage their fatigue and, ultimately, change their driving behaviours accordingly.

For designing the feedback, we selected the most suitable persuasive design principles from Persuasive Systems Design (PSD) Process Model [6]. Following an analysis of the persuasion context, in terms of intent, event and strategy, systems qualities were applied to the design of the feedback (Fig. 2). We explain each of them in the next page.

The goal of this intervention was to provide participants with information on their driving style relative to fatigue. The feedback consisted of three pages. The first one showed illustrations, in the form of readily understandable pictograms and graphs. The second page gave a written description of the driving experiment and definitions (in order to facilitate understanding of terms that could be perceived too technical) and a short summary for those who were less interested in too detailed explanations. Finally, in the third page, different sections explained in more detail the first page's illustrations, including one section comparing the driver data to scientific research in the field. These sections may be viewed as a kind of dialogue with the driver. We included praise, for those who had identified well their fatigue, and suggestions, for those who perceived it

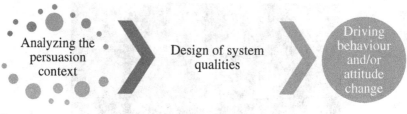

- Intent:
  - Persuade the elderly driver about his/her driving and his/her fatigue perceived
- Event:
  - Driving context and driver information
- Strategy:
  - A Data Analysis Tool

- Primariy task support:
  - Tailoring
  - Personalization
  - Self-monitoring
- Dialogue support:
  - Suggestion
- System credibility:
  - Trustworthiness
  - Real-world feel
- Social support:
  - Social comparison

Fig. 2. Phases adapted from PSD process model

less well. For praise, words were used to provide personal feedback information based on the user good driving behaviours. And for the suggestions, the feedback proposed different comparison between the speed limit and driver's speed, between perceived fatigue and driver's speed, etc.

A fictitious example of the first page with illustrations is presented in Fig. 3.

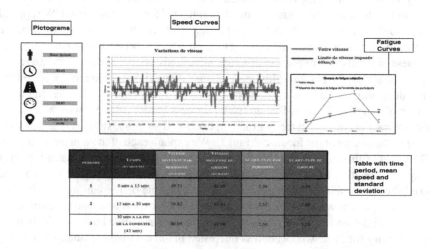

Fig. 3. Fictitious example of the feedback first page for one participant

In this example, at the top left, there are pictograms depicting participant gender, driving time, kilometers travelled, mean speed and type of activity. Because of the exploratory nature of the study we selected different pictograms in order to verify which ones were evaluated as most useful and easily understandable. The content of the information was tailored according to the context in which the experimental driving was done and in line with the interests of elder people. And each feedback is personalized depending on the driving behaviour.

At the center of the example, the graph depicts the participant speed during the 45 min experiment and the graph on the far right, the perceived level of fatigue of the participant and his or her the reference age group at four moments during the driving period. These curves allowed a better fit to the reality of the driver experience, for system credibility. Because objectives information from real-world context is obtained through data coming from sensors into the instrumented vehicle and questionnaires, the tool can be viewed as trustworthy and without bias.

The table at the bottom of the page indicates mean speed and standard deviation every 15 min, for the participant and for the reference age group allowing social comparison and some form of social support. Each elder person can compare his/her driving performance with his/her age group's reference, mainly for speed and fatigue. After the design of our feedback, we tested it with elderly drivers.

4   First Results

Twenty older drivers participated in the experiment and received the feedback. Because two of them were unreachable for the phone interview, the results presented here are for the eighteen participants who completed the whole experiment. The mean age was 66,7 years old (SD = 6,43). All participants had a valid driver's license and they declared a satisfactory medical condition during the phone recruitment. To complete the self-declared medical condition and before the driving, each participant did a screening test, the Useful Field of View (UFOV) test. This test is designed for people aged 55 and older and is recommended as a control measure for the ability to drive [25]. During the experiment, the measures taken were perceived fatigue, speed, etc. Each participant drove around 50 km on a close driving circuit with the LiSA car. At the end, we offered each participant his/her driving feedback. As the tool was offline, feedback was given either in electronic format or in paper format if the person had no access to internet. The eighteen participants received a financial compensation of 30 $ and 10 $ CAN respectively for their participation in the driving experiment and phone interview.

After a few weeks, participants were contacted by phone to answer a phone interview. Nine questions dealt with the design of the feedback and ten with the participants driving performance and the impact of the feedback received about the driving. Initially, we wanted to know if the participants were satisfied with the information received through the feedback, if the information met their expectations and if they had taken the time to read all the information received. Secondly, it seemed important to check whether the feedback received corresponded to what they remembered and had retained from the experience (e.g. speed, perceived fatigue, etc.). Thirdly, we wanted to know if they found the feedback useful and if it had had an impact on their subsequent driving and management of driving fatigue. The results are presented under the following categories: (1) satisfaction, expectations, information and memory and (2) usefulness of the information received and changes in behaviour.

About satisfaction, expectations, information and memory, the vast majority of participants said they were satisfied or very satisfied with the information received (88.2 %) and over half of the participants (58.8 %) indicated that the information met their expectations. Three in four participants (75 %) found that the speed curve, shown in the graph, corresponded to their memory, and almost all (88 %) found that the figure showing fatigue perceived during the experiment represented what they had felt. Table 1 presents the mean score and standard deviation for each categories.

Table 1. Mean score and Standard Deviation (SD) for satisfaction, expectations, information and memory

	Satisfaction	Expectations	Information	Memories	
				Speed curves	Fatigue curves
Mean	4,35/5	3,64/5	9,11/10	4,35/5	4,29/5
SD	0,86	0,93	0,92	0,86	0,84

Relative to the usefulness of the information received and behaviour changes, the comparison with the reference age group was considered useful by all participants and the general impression of feedback, content and graphic presentation was very positive (Table 2). Despite the positive impression left by the feedback, only about one in two (52.9 %) said that it had an impact on their driving afterwards and 70 % of participants said that it would have an impact in the future. Three out of five (64,7 %) believed that this feedback would foster better management of their fatigue in the future.

Table 2. Mean score and Standard Deviation (SD) for usefulness of the information received and behaviour changes

	Usefulness of the information	Behaviour change		
		Impact on the driving afterwards	Impact on the driving in the future	Impact on their fatigue management
Mean	4,58/5	2,47/5	2,64/5	2,94/5
SD	0,50	1,41	1,32	1,29

About the feedback design, fourteen participants said they read the feedback (the three pages) and found it very useful, relevant and understandable. Finally, as for the other feedback elements, which one they most and least liked. The fatigue curve was the most liked and the least liked was the pictograms.

5   Discussion and Conclusion

Overall, persuasive technology in automotive context promotes safety for drivers. With the aging, elder people are more concerned about driving fatigue on the wheel. Persuasive technologies appear as a solution to help them to improve their behaviour and drive safely. We proposed in this paper the results of an exploratory study of a persuasive technology designed for elderly drivers, in the form of feedback. The goal of the feedback was to promote awareness of the fatigue impact on driving (particularly speed) and bring the drivers to better manage their fatigue and, ultimately, driving behaviours. We tested it with twenty elderly drivers after an experimentation of 45 min driving time. Eighteen elder persons answered a phone interview about the satisfaction, expectations, information and memories and about the usefulness of the information received and changes in behaviour. The preliminary results are encouraging. The feedback as conceived for elderly drivers was well received and was considered useful. 70 % of participant said that the feedback would have an impact on their driving behaviour in the future. The design of persuasive feedbacks for elderly drivers seems promising as our results suggest that some elderly drivers appreciate receiving constructive information on their driving.

However, further works are needed. Firstly, we proposed the feedback between one and two months after the driving session, and the interview took place several weeks after the feedback was given. It would be important, in a future study to verify if feedback given to elderly drivers on their driving has inducing real changes in their driving behaviours and/or in their attitude toward driving fatigue. In addition, in our current experiment, the number of participants was relatively small. It would be important in future research to increase the number of elder participant substantially.

Secondly, the feedback design for elderly should be further improved. For example, some of our participants suggested an improvement could be done by increasing the size of curves in the illustrations. They didn't see well due to vision problems. Others proposed different colors than those we had used like a darker green color to accentuate contrasts. So, the design has to be considered because it might play a role in persuading.

Furthermore, it would be interesting to expand and test feedback which would include other real-world information, such as physiological data (blinking movement, heartbeat, etc.) or the environmental context (weather, traffic, etc.). Some driving behaviours due to fatigue are associated with environmental context, for instance, monotony road or night condition. The objective would be to increase context awareness and induce more behavioural changes among elderly drivers when fatigued at the wheel, using efficient persuasive tools designed specifically for that category of drivers.

Acknowledgments. We want to particularly thank the Canadian Automobile Association (CAA) Foundation, Section of the Quebec Province, for funding the research works behind this paper.

References

1. Sivak, M., Schoettle, B.: Recent changes in the age composition of drivers in 15 countries. Traffic Inj. Prev. **13**(2), 126–132 (2012)
2. Reimer, B.: Driver assistance systems and the transition to automated vehicles: A path to increase older adult safety and mobility? Publ. Policy Aging Rep. **24**(1), 27–31 (2014)
3. Emery, L., Srinivasan, G., Bezzina, D., Leblanc, D., Sayer, J., Bogard, S., Pomerleau, D.: Status report on USDOT project – an intelligent vehicle initiative road departure crash warning field operational test. In: 19th International Technical Conference Enhanced Safety of Vehicles, Washington DC (2005)
4. Fogg, B.J.: Persuasive Technology: Using Computers to Change What We Think and Do. Morgan Kaufmann Publishers Inc., San Francisco (2003)
5. Hamari, J., Koivisto, J., Pakkanen, T.: Do persuasive technologies persuade? - a review of empirical studies. In: Spagnolli, A., Chittaro, L., Gamberini, L. (eds.) PERSUASIVE 2014. LNCS, vol. 8462, pp. 118–136. Springer, Heidelberg (2014)
6. Oinas-Kukkonen, H., Harjumaa, M.: Persuasive systems design: key issues, process model, and system features. Commun. Assoc. Inf. Syst. **24**(1), 28 (2009)
7. Schätzl, J.: How Effective are Persuasive Technologies in Automotive Context? Persuasive Technologies and Applications (2015)
8. Meschtscherjakov, A., Wilfinger, D., Scherndl, T., Tscheligi, M.: Acceptance of future persuasive in-car interfaces towards a more economic driving behaviour. In: Proceedings of the 1st International Conference on Automotive User Interfaces and Interactive Vehicular Applications, pp. 81–88. ACM (2009)
9. Vaezipour, A., Rakotonirainy, A., Haworth, N.: Reviewing in-vehicle systems to improve fuel efficiency and road safety. Procedia Manuf. **3**, 3192–3199 (2015)
10. Eby, D.W., Molnar, L.J.: Has the time come for an older driver vehicle? (2012)
11. Gruau, S., Pottier, A., Davenne, D., Denise, P.: Les facteurs d'accidents de la route par somnolence chez les conducteurs âgés: Prévention par l'activité physique. Recherche-Transports-Securite 79, 134–144 (2003)
12. Assailly, J.P., Bonin-Guillaume, S., Mohr, A., Parola, A., Grandjean, R., Frances, Y.M.: Les conducteurs âgés en bonne santé font plus d'erreurs et d'oublis que d'infractions: Enquête auprès de 904 volontaires. La Presse Médicale **35**(6), 941–947 (2006)
13. Oxley, J., Langford, J., Koppel, S., Charlton, J.: Senior Driving Longer, Smarter, Safer: Enhancement of an Innovative Educational and Training Package for the Safe Mobility of Seniors. Technical Report, Monash University Accident Research Centre, Monash Injury Research Institute (2013)
14. Anstey, K., Wood, J., Lord, S., Walker, J.G.: Cognitive, sensory and physical factors enabling driving safety in older adults. Clin. Psychol. Rev. **25**(1), 45–65 (2005)
15. Owsley, C., Mcgwin, G.: Vision and driving. Vision. Res. **50**(23), 2348–2361 (2010)
16. Langford, J., Koppel, S.: Licence restrictions as an under-used strategy in managing older driver safety. Accid. Anal. Prev. **43**(1), 487–493 (2011)
17. Rakotonirainy, A., Steinhardt, D.: In-vehicle technology functional requirements for older drivers. In: The 1st International Conference on Automotive User Interfaces and Interactive Vehicular Applications, pp. 27–33. ACM, New York (2009)
18. Thiffault, P., Bergeron, J.: Monotony of road environment and driver fatigue: a simulator study. Accid. Anal. Prev. **35**(3), 381–391 (2003)
19. Beirness, D.J., Simpson, H.M., Desmond, K.: The Road Safety Monitor 2004: Drowsy Driving. Traffic Injury Research Foundation, Ottawa, Ontario (2005)

20. Gershon, P., Shinar, D., Oron-Gilad, T., Parmet, Y., Ronen, A.: Usage and perceived effectiveness of fatigue countermeasures for professional and nonprofessional drivers. Accid. Anal. Prev. **43**, 797–803 (2011)
21. Vanlaar, W., Simpson, H., Mayhew, D., Robertson, R.: Fatigued and drowsy driving: a survey of attitudes, opinions and behaviours. J. Saf. Res. **39**, 303–309 (2008)
22. Kedowide, C., Gouin-Vallerand, C., Vallieres, E.F.: Recognizing blind spot check activity with car drivers based on decision tree classifiers. In: 28th AAAI Conference on Artificial Intelligence (AAAI 2014), Québec (2014)
23. Ruer, P., Gouin-Vallerand, C., Zhang, L., Lemire, D., Vallières, E.F.: An analysis tool for the contextual information from field experiments on driving fatigue. In: Christiansen, H., Stojanovic, I., Papadopoulos, G.A. (eds.) Modeling and Using Context. LNCS, vol. 9405, pp. 172–185. Springer, Heidelberg (2015)
24. Lemire, D., Brooks, M., Yan, Y.: An optimal linear time algorithm for quasi-monotonic segmentation. Int. J. Comput. Math. **86**(7), 1093–1104 (2009)
25. Clay, O.J., Wadley, V.G., Edwards, J.D., Roth, D.L., Roenker, D.L., Ball, K.K.: Cumulative meta-analysis of the relationship between useful field of view and driving performance in older adults: Current and future implications. Optom. Vis. Sci. **82**(8), 724–731 (2005)

Creating Awareness of Sleep-Wake Hours by Gamification

Ezgi Ilhan[1(✉)], Bahar Sener[2,3], and Hüseyin Hacihabiboğlu[4]

[1] Department of Industrial Design, Atilim University, Ankara, Turkey
ezgi.ilhan@atilim.edu.tr
[2] Department of Industrial Design, Middle East Technical University, Ankara, Turkey
[3] School of Engineering, University of Liverpool, Liverpool, UK
bsener@metu.edu.tr
[4] Department of Modeling and Simulation, Middle East Technical University, Ankara, Turkey
hhuseyin@metu.edu.tr

Abstract. Gamification can be used to motivate people to carry out hard-to-perform tasks. It can help in changing undesirable habits and in improving a person's subjective well-being. Sleep-wake behaviors are important determinants of day-to-day well-being. This study aims to find out whether it is possible to modify sleep-wake habits using gamification. To this end, a gamified alarm clock app, *Sleepy Bird*, was designed and tested in a user study with thirteen participants using gamified and thirteen participants using non-gamified versions for two weeks. The results indicate that the participants of the gamified version were more motivated to start the day at required times than the participants of the non-gamified version. The participants of the gamified version were also observed to have made desirable modifications to their sleep-wake habits.

Keywords: Gamification · Sleep-wake habits · Habit modification · Subjective well-being

1   Introduction

As one of the critical dimensions of subjective well-being, management of sleep-wake habits of people is an area that can benefit from gamification. Waking-up and sleeping at required hours can be considered as difficult-to-perform tasks (at least for some). This study aims to find out whether it is possible to modify sleep-wake habits and improve people's subjective well-being using gamification. A gamified alarm clock app, *Sleepy Bird*, was designed and tested in a user study to investigate whether the app can create positive feelings and better awareness of sleep-wake habits.

1.1   Gamification

The popularity of gamification derives from the popularity of playing games. The Global Games Market Report [17] indicates that globally, 1.2 billion people had played games by 2014. Playing has the power to trigger new behaviors against previous habits [3]. Gamification is a useful strategy that can influence people positively in the activities that they ignore, find boring, tiresome or even difficult to achieve. Gamification is based

A. Meschtscherjakov et al. (Eds.): PERSUASIVE 2016, LNCS 9638, pp. 122–133, 2016.
DOI: 10.1007/978-3-319-31510-2_11

on the usage of game design elements in non-game contexts [6]. It has the potential to persuade people to take actions about undesirable but necessary activities [2] making them more appealing to people by creating *extrinsic* and *intrinsic* motivations [21]. An extrinsic motivation [16] satisfies needs with tangible outcomes such as reputation, titles, money and real rewards, whereas an intrinsic motivation symbolizes the satisfaction from an interesting and enjoyable activity. The success of a gamified tool comes from the satisfaction of intrinsic motivation and self-defined goals of players [21]. In this study, gamification is used as a motivation tool to regulate sleep-wake habits of people in order to improve their well-being.

1.2 Sleep-Wake Habits

Sleep-wake habits play an important role in happiness and long-term well-being. The more efficiently the subject sleeps, the higher the emotional, psychological and social well-being becomes. Thus, if sleep problems are reduced, both emotional and psychological well-being will improve [8, 9].

Sleep duration is also related to psychological health. Although it may differ for different age groups, nominal adequate sleep duration is 6 to 8.5 h. Optimal sleepers are known to have lower rates of incidence for depression due to possessing higher amounts of mastery, self-confidence and social relations, whereas insufficient sleep causes depression, stress and both physical and cognitive fatigue during the following day [15] and is known to deteriorate the learning performance of adolescents [19].

There are examples of mobile apps or alarm clocks that use gamification to track people's sleep-wake habits, and to ease waking-up times and prevent snoozing. For instance, '*Gun O'Clock*' aims to wake people up with a game which the user has to shoot the clock with a toy gun; or the users of '*Helicopter Alarm Clock*' need to catch a flying helicopter and put it on its nest to stop the alarm [4]. '*Zeo Sleep Manager*' is another example that tracks sleep cycles using wearable devices [14]. It has sensors on its headband to measure the electrical current during sleep phases. Then, it wirelessly sends the information to the mobile platform to make users aware of their sleep-wake habits and health conditions.

Some of the apps come with gamified features as well. People need to follow instructions offered by the mobile apps in order to go-to-bed, wake-up on time or to have enough sleep. '*Early Bird*', developed for Starbucks, tries to persuade people to start their day on time with feedback messages and a reward system on a social platform [20]. When people use this alarm app without snoozing, it gives achievements to users. The achievement system is implemented with points, stars, social sharing and a cup of coffee, which is available for an hour after getting out of the bed.

Existing hardware/software solutions either compel people to wake-up at adjusted hours or use wearable electronics rather than using the power of persuasive design. Without using persuasive design and a '*fun factor*' effectively, gamified apps remain inadequate in influencing sleep-wake habits in a profoundly positive way. Tracking sleep through an app can help people to become aware of their sleep-wake habits. This can help to improve their sleep-wake behaviors positively in the long run [11].

2   Methodology

With the evidence from literature that sleeping and waking-up are important everyday behaviors and that gamification could potentially increase subjective well-being, the present study explored the effects of gamification on the attainment of the following goals: (1) increasing the motivation of participants for waking-up, (2) creating better awareness of sleep-wake habits, and (3) creating positive attitudes towards sleeping and waking up at optimal times.

The study required an understanding of people's existing sleep durations and waking-up times. A mobile alarm clock app, which allows remote data collection, was considered to be an appropriate tool to track sleep-wake habits of the participants. A specially designed gamified alarm clock app–*Sleepy Bird*– was used to track and collect sleep-related data in order to determine the effects of gamification.

2.1   Development of the Mobile App

Sleepy Bird was designed specifically for the present study, by modifying an existing popular game with alarm features. It was considered that in platform games, the quantitative progression of players can be observed easily. *Flappy Bird* [7] is a popular game which was downloaded up to 3 million times per day. Owing to this popularity, *Flappy Bird* was selected as a starting point for a gamified alarm clock app.

For the technical development of the app, Java language and `libgdx` graphics library were used. The entire *Flappy Bird* game was redesigned and redeveloped for the Android platform with embedded alarm functions, feedback, and calculations.

Both a gamified (G) and a non-gamified (N-G) version of *Sleepy Bird* were used in the study. The differences between the versions can be seen in Table 1. Since gratifying feedback was suggested to motivate participants intrinsically, both versions of the app offered personal feedback messages and insights about wake-up times, snooze actions, and sleep durations.

Table 1.   Differences between G and N-G versions of *Sleepy Bird* app

Gamified Version (Experiment Group)	Non-Gamified Version (Control Group)
Alarm time and sound	Alarm time and sound
Going to bed hour and sleep duration	Going to bed hour and sleep duration
Feedback about wake/sleep actions	Feedback about wake/sleep actions
Revised *Flappy Bird* game	N/A
Game elements (e.g. visual elements, lives, points, feedbacks, leader board)	N/A

As *Sleepy Bird* aimed to create positive feelings while starting the day, color choices and graphics design were carefully made. The *Sleepy Bird* character was designed to have a big red eye to emphasize its level of drowsiness. The game also used light to set an ambience, informing participants that the sun had risen that morning.

The app was designed with a Turkish language interface to fit the target user group of the study. At the top of the game screen, the score and remaining lives were displayed (see Fig. 1). For the gamified version, *Sleepy Bird* was designed to have four buttons on the main screen, which were grouped into two with color coding. OYNA (*play*) and (EN İYİLER) (*leader board*) buttons were related to gaming; ALARM KUR (*set alarm*) and UYKUYA DAL (*sleep*) buttons were related to sleeping-waking up. For the non-gamified version 'play' and 'leader board' were removed.

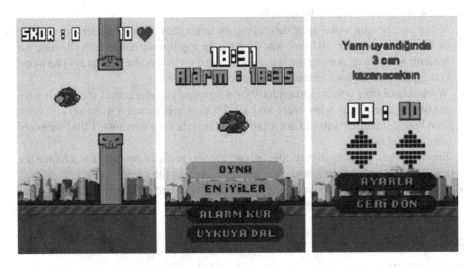

Fig. 1. Example screenshots from '*Sleepy Bird*'

The game provided personal feedback messages when, for example, the participants set the alarm or wanted to sleep. The messages aimed to create awareness about sleep-wake habits and were shown in red color to draw attention. If the feedback message was relatively long, a pop-up screen opened just as *Sleepy Bird* communicated with the users about their action.

The *Sleepy Bird* character appeared on the main screen to remind users to set their alarms for the following day and not to sleep late in order to wake-up easily next morning. Depending on the wake-up time set by the participants, the app showed them the score award for the next day. In order to record the sleep duration, the users needed to tap on the sleep button. After the alarm went off and awakened them in the morning, they played the game whenever they wanted during the day. The interface enabled the participants to check the leader board as a way to self-assess their standing among other players. The non-gamified version only required setting the alarm and sleep hours.

Decisions Behind the Design of 'Sleepy Bird'. In the development process of the app versions, the following considerations were taken into account:

- ideal wake-up time was set to be between 6.00-8.00 am and at least 1.5-2 h before the work time [5].
- adequate sleep duration was set as 7 h for the target group [22].
- game elements such as points, lives and leader boards were used to motivate participants [13].
- continuous feedback messages about personally required sleep-wake hours were provided [16].

The game rules were set as:

- The game gave '10 lives' by default.
- When participants woke-up at their optimum hours they won the maximum number of lives. Reward with '30 lives' was found as an appropriate solution to alleviate the tradeoff between enhancing the fun and keeping the value in the gameplay. The worst condition of wake-hour rewarded the user with '3 lives'.
- Work/school time was important for the background calculations of the app. It gave maximum game lives when there was a 1-2 h time gap between wake-up and work start hours. If participants did not wake-up at the right time they lost '1 life' for every 5 min of delay.
- Snoozing the alarm negatively affected participants in the competition. Each time the participants snoozed the alarm, they fell 25 m back in the game.
- If participants went to bed too early or too late, the speed of *Sleepy Bird* (character) increased to make the game more difficult.

2.2 Data Collection Tools

Data were collected via pre-use questionnaire (delivered prior to the use of the app), post-use questionnaire (delivered on the completion of the predetermined usage period), and usage logs. The pre-use questionnaire aimed to select and group the participants according to their scores. The post-use questionnaire aimed to collect usage-related information. The questionnaires also helped to compare relevant data between G and N-G versions of the app. Sleep-wake habits, moods and awareness levels were collected. Four scales were implemented in the questionnaires to collect personal evaluations. These were Epworth Sleepiness Scale (ESS), Pittsburgh Sleep Quality Index (PSQI), Morningness-Eveningness Questionnaire (MEQ), and Delighted-Terrible Scale.

2.3 Selection and Distribution of the Participants

The call for recruiting participants was made via word of mouth, e-mails and social media channels. Eligible participants were required to fit the following criteria:

- using of an alarm to wake-up.
- being within the age group of 18–35 (with similar sleep-wake habits).
- possessing average awaking difficulty.
- having a mobile phone running on Android platform.
- having no particular aversion to the *Flappy Bird* game.

A pre-use questionnaire was sent to qualifying volunteers. Candidates without sleep-related problems or with serious medical problems were excluded from the study. Selected participants were divided into two groups to use either G or N-G versions of the apps. Since the game in the app was a modified form of *Flappy Bird,* participants' approaches to the game played a significant role in deciding the group divisions. If participants had positive attitudes towards *Flappy Bird*, they were assigned to the G version of the app. If they were not interested in *Flappy Bird*, they were given the N-G version. An equal number of participants were allocated to each group. In total, 26 participants took part in the study (13 G; and 13 N-G users). Prior to finalizing the details of the main study, as a piloting, different user groups utilized the app in different time periods during the development stages. This helped to detect and correct possible functional errors, to improve the app's performance, choose appropriate statistical analysis methods, and decide on the number of participants that would be recruited for the study.

3   Results and Analysis

The results of the pre-use questionnaire, computer logs and post-use questionnaire were analyzed as described in the following sections.

3.1   Pre-use Questionnaire

The pre-use questionnaire is organized in three parts to assess the suitability of the candidates for the study and then to collect relevant information about them.

(i) **Part 1.**   In Part 1, the Epworth Sleepiness Scale (ESS) was used to gather information on the candidates' subjective evaluations of sleep levels [12]. A total score was evaluated as participants having 'average sleep problems' (scores between 4 to 9); 'sleep problems' (10–14); and 'requiring professional medical help' (15 +). If the score was medium level (4–14), the participants were considered to have the right level of sleep problem to take part in the study. In the ESS results, the minimum total score was 4, and the maximum score was 13, with a mean score of 7.76 within the selected group of participants. Of the volunteers, six received ESS scores lower than 4, and were not included in the tests as they presented no sleep problems.

(ii) **Part 2.**   In this part, the participants' sleep, work and snooze behaviors were evaluated. Some questions included in this part were adapted from the Pittsburgh Sleep Quality Index (PSQI) to obtain information about participants' subjective sleep-wake evaluations [18]. This part of the study aimed to assess pre-use sleep patterns of the participants. They were also asked the time of the day that they start working, to correctly calculate their appropriate wake-up hours. It was observed that 92 % of the participants started their school or work between 8.00–10.00 am.

(iii) **Part 3.**   This part of the questionnaire focused on the participants' personal assessments about their wake-up attitudes and motivations. The questions regarding sleep-wake habits were obtained using the Morningness-Eveningness Questionnaire (MEQ) [10]. The

26 participants assigned scores ranging from 1 to 5 (1 being 'strongly disagree' to 5 being 'strongly agree') to each of the following six questions. All scores given in brackets are out of 130 (the sum of G and N-G = 26 × 5).

- Q1 asked whether participants believed it was easy to wake-up in the morning, and the answers showed the lowest total score (54/130).
- Answers to Q2 proposed that G app would help to wake-up more easily (*81/130).
- Q3 (63/130) and Q4 (74/130) focused on the degree of being wakeful or tired after waking-up.
- Q5 received the highest total score (99/130) indicating that the participants had positive feelings when they started the day at a correct time.
- Q6 received a high score (87/130) implying that G app would motivate participants to start the day at a correct time.

The results of Part 3 of the pre-use questionnaire are later compared with counterparts from the post-use questionnaire, to examine whether a positive change in participants' attitudes could be established.

3.2   Computer Logs

Computer logs were used to collect each of the 26 participant's sleep-wake actions quantitatively. After the installation of *Sleepy Bird* on their phones, the usage data were automatically gathered in a database, and all the actions taken in the app were remotely recorded in the system. The logs were related to wake-up time, sleep time, sleep duration and number of snooze actions.

The participants were required to set the alarm clock every day for the next morning before going to bed. When the alarm setting was forgotten, participants' data were not useful for the evaluations of that day. Therefore, at 10.00 pm every evening, reminders about alarm-setting were displayed by both versions of the app.

At the end of the study, a total of 325 samples (i.e. number of total actions related to wake-up hours, sleep duration, and number of snoozes) were gathered from the participants. Data comparisons were made based on the app version (G or N-G), and each participant's habits relative to the first- and second-half usage periods and the usage time (weekend or weekdays). Differences between the following were determined:

- number of snoozes,
- wake-up time (deviation from *personalized* optimum time),
- going to sleep time (deviation from *personalized* optimum time),
- sleep durations (deviation from *personalized* optimum duration).

The usage frequency between G and N-G versions showed a slight difference: G alarm provided a total usage data of 170 (52.3 %) samples, whereas N-G alarm provided a total of 155 (47.7 %) data.

Analysis Strategy for the Logs. In order to analyze the computer logs, data were analyzed in SPSS to find out: the mean, range, minimum and maximum values of wake and sleep time, snooze actions, sleep durations, and difference from optimum cases.

In order to establish the presence of any statistically significant values, a full factorial ANOVA model was obtained. The model included (i) game version, (ii) first and second half of usage; and, (iii) weekend vs. weekday usage as variables. All the tests were designed with 95 % confidence interval to have a margin of error less than 5 %, to reach a high level of reliability.

(i) Game version. An important goal for the study was to investigate the possible effects of gamification. Table 2 summarizes a descriptive statistics of snooze numbers, difference from optimum wake/sleep time and difference from sleep durations for G and N-G versions. The mean of snooze numbers (0.74) and difference from optimum sleep duration (which is 0) of the G version (24.33 min) was lower than mean values for the N-G version (46.33 min). Moreover, going-to-sleep time was closer to optimum (which is 0) for the G version, with a mean deviation of -11.75 min, whereas it was -36.85 min for the N-G version.

Table 2. Group statistics of actions by app version (G/N-G) for 26 participants

	Version*	Total no. of Samples	Mean	Std. Deviation	Std. Error Mean
Snooze	G	170	**0,74**	**1,373**	0,105
	N-G	154	**1,19**	**1,604**	0,129
Difference_optimum_wake	G	170	13,18	56,324	4,320
	N-G	154	9,77	59,607	4,803
Difference_optimum_sleep	G	169	**-11,75**	**84,303**	6,485
	N-G	150	**-36,85**	**76,252**	6,226
Difference_optimum_duration	G	169	**24,33**	**88,391**	6,799
	N-G	149	**46,33**	**84,928**	6,958

*G: gamified; N-G: non-gamified.

In order to see whether there was a statistically significant difference of sleep-wake habits between the G (experiment) and N-G (control) users, one-way ANOVA was used. The difference was statistically significant for three actions according to post-hoc comparisons. As can be observed from Table 2 (text in **bold**), *Sleepy Bird* resulted in significant differences between the G and N-G versions in terms of snooze action; go-to-sleep hours; and sleep durations.

Both subjective questionnaire evaluations and computer log results showed that wake-up hours changed in a positive way for participants of the G version. Participants of N-G also changed their wake-up hours with the help of feedback from the app. Participants of G version (7.24 h) became closer to optimum sleep durations (7 h) than participants of N-G version (7.46 h) at the end of the study. Going-to-sleep time changed in a personally-positive way for participants of both G (from 01.13 am to 00.19 am) and N-G versions (from 00.32 am to 23.53 pm).

(ii) First and Second Half of Usage Period. Since the participants used the apps for different numbers of days, the median value was different for each participant. The app usage ranged from 8 to 22 days between the participants. Average values of the date set (i.e. wake-up time, sleep time, sleep durations, snooze numbers) of the first half of the usage period was compared to that of the second half. In the second half, mean values for the tested dependent variables approached zero. Thus, all of the actions had a positive progression in the duration of the study.

For G users, all the mean values became closer to zero in the second half, which indicated the optimal case. At the beginning of tests, participants snoozed the alarms more (0.99 times in average), woke–up later (17 min later than their personalized optimum time), slept earlier (15.49 min earlier than their personalized optimum time), and slept more (32.86 min more than their personalized optimum durations). According to post-hoc comparisons, gamification resulted in statistically significant differences in terms of snooze action ($p = 0.008$) between first half usage of gamified and second half usage of gamified versions.

(iii) Weekend vs. Weekdays. Participants used *Sleepy Bird* most frequently on Tuesdays and Wednesdays (18 %) and least frequently on Saturdays (9.5 %). The alarm was set 70 times (21.8 %) during the weekends compared to 250 times (78.2 %) in school/work days. For G users, 133 action data events on weekdays and 37 action data events at weekends were collected. According to post-hoc comparison results, differences in the snooze action while using the gamified version of *Sleepy Birds* was statistically significant ($p = 0.036$) between weekdays and weekend usage. For N-G users, 120 data events in weekdays and 34 data events at weekends were gathered. According to post-hoc comparisons, the N-G version of *Sleepy Bird* caused statistically significant results in terms of difference from optimum going-to-sleep time ($p = 0.035$) between weekdays and weekend.

3.3   Post-use Questionnaire

The post-use questionnaire enabled data comparisons between G and N-G versions of app users in response to whether a gamified alarm app created positive feelings and awareness for sleep-wake habits.

(i) Part 1. This part revealed the emotional experience related to the usage of the app. Delighted-Terrible Scale [1] (one question to select one of the facial expressions) was used to measure short term subjective well-being after the usage of *Sleepy Bird*. One participant (4 %) felt very delighted due to *Sleepy Bird*. Six participants (23 %) felt delighted during usage and 15 participants (58 %) pointed out that they felt happy due to this special alarm design. Four participants (15 %) felt neutral. The average feeling for the gamified version was between a delighted and happy, whereas the average feeling for the non-gamified version was between a happy and neutral.

(ii) Part 2. This part was used to measure changes in participants' awareness levels regarding their sleep-wake habits after the usage of the app. It consisted of four questions focusing on: wake-up hours (Q1), sleep durations (Q2), the interval between waking-up and starting to study/work (Q3), and number of snoozes (Q4). G users scored a total of 177 points, whereas N-G users scored 124 points, indicating that awareness levels of sleep-wake habits reached a higher level for the participants of G version. Q2: in relation to participants' awareness on sleep duration, both G and N-G users scored a total of 80 points, which was the maximum score received within this part of the questionnaire. Q3 & Q4: total scores for both questions were identical for G and N-G users (75). This indicated that the *Sleepy Bird* app helped to increase participants' awareness for the time interval between wake and work time, and snooze action. Q1: total score for this question had the minimum value (71), which was about awareness level to start the day at correct hours.

When results were analyzed in SPSS using a t-test, awareness levels on sleep-wake habits between G and N-G showed some statistically significant differences for all of the questions (Q1: $p = 0.010$; Q2: $p = 0.042$; Q3: $P = 0.004$; Q4: $p = 0.011$). Participants of the G version gained a significant awareness as a result of app usage.

(iii) Part 3. This part was used to analyze participants' self-evaluations of their wake-up attitudes and motivations after using *Sleepy Bird*. In contrast with the same part (Part 3) of the *pre-use* questionnaire results, the scores were higher in total as indicated in Table 3 (text in **bold**). G users evaluated themselves as relatively more successful, more motivated and feeling more positive in terms of waking-up at early hours. These participants gave the highest score to Q1 (54 points), indicating how much they thought that they were waking-up at the correct time in the morning. G group also scored higher than N-G for Q5 (52) and Q6 (50) in the post-use questionnaire indicating that the app made them feel psychologically better and more motivated to wake-up at required hours. Q2 (40) showed that G group could not wake-up so easily during app usage. Score of Q3 and Q4 (36) showed that G group did not feel that awake, well-rested and lively after getting out of the bed.

Table 3. Total scores received for six questions in pre- and post- questioannires

No.	Pre-Questionnaire		Post-Questionnaire	
	G	N-G	G	N-G
Q1	27	27	**54**	**49**
Q2	45	36	40	**41**
Q3	31	32	**36**	**34**
Q4	37	37	36	33
Q5	53	46	52	43
Q6	49	38	**50**	**44**
Total Score	242	216	**268**	**244**

Although the total scores for G and N-G groups increased in the post-use questionnaire, only one question was calculated at the statistically significant level. According to separate t-test analysis, Q1 showed a significant change in G ($p = 0.00$) and N-G ($p = 0.001$) groups. Moreover, the total score of questions for both groups ($p = 0.012$) showed statistically significant changes between pre-use and post-use of the app. This result showed that the app provided motivation and positive attitudes on sleep-wake habits, especially for (Q1) waking-up at correct hours.

(iv) Part 4. This part was used to understand participants' tendency to change their sleep-wake habits as well as their suggestions for new app features. Open-ended questions were used to collect participants' comments on positive and negative aspects of *Sleepy Bird*. In total, 17 participants (65 %) stated that a gamified app would change sleep-wake behaviors in the long term. The 'leaderboard' was interpreted as the most attractive part for competition. Example comments from the participants of the gamified version were:

- "I decreased my snooze habit for the game success. I confess that I dismissed the alarm of *Sleepy Bird* once and set the alarm of my phone again in order not to lose game lives in the app." (Participant 8)
- "During the usage period, the app said to me that I will be either fresh or fatigued the following day. When it said that I will be fresh, I was really fresh. Conversely after the notification of tiredness, I felt tired the next day." (Participant 13)

4   Discussion and Conclusions

This paper investigated the practical outcomes of gamification informed by domain knowledge in sleep medicine. It provided a broader attention to the relationship between gamification, and sleep-wake habits. The aim was to examine whether gamification can create motivation and awareness to improve sleep-wake habits, so as to positively influence subjective well-being in the long term.

The study utilized gamification with a shift from *an extrinsic reward system* to *an intrinsic feedback system*. *Sleepy Bird* app was designed to focus on 'intrinsic motivations' with its gratifying feedback system. With its feedback and notifications, the app gave information on optimum wake and sleep hours to improve users' awareness of sleep-wake habits. The results revealed that gamification can be useful for the creation of positive feelings and better awareness about sleep-wake habits. Gamification also helped the study participants to start their day at required hours, since the app notified them about their required sleep-wake hours and sleep durations. A gamified alarm app also encouraged participants to not snooze their alarms.

The results provide insights for game developers. Computer logs allowed collection of game-related data concerning the numbers of game lives, game points and top scores. Time, sequence and frequency of actions taken by 'players' can be tracked through such an app design. The feedback messages about competition and leaderboard results were useful ways to concentrate users' attention to their sleep-wake habits indirectly so that they may become better in the game.

References

1. Andrews, F.M., Withey, S.B.: Social Indicators of Well-being: Americans' Perceptions of Life Quality. Plenum Press, New York (1976)
2. Baranowski, T., Buday, R., Thompson, D.I., Baranowski, J.: Playing for real: Video games and stories for health-related behavior change. Am. J. Prev. Med. **34**(1), 74–82 (2008)

3. Chan, K.: Playing in traffic: Pervasive gaming for commuters. In: Paper presented at the Interactive Entertainment, New Zealand, 22 November 2011

4. Chou, Y.: How gamification can help you get out of bed by "killing" time. Retrieved from http://www.yukaichou.com/product-gamification/gamification-bed-killing-time/ #.VCgqz_l_sUg (2012). Accessed 10 October 2014

5. Ciftci, B.: Personal communication (Associate Professor at Department of Thoracic Medicine in Sanatoryum Hospital, Ankara, Turkey), 24 February 2014

6. Deterding, S., Sicart, M., Nacke, L., O'Hara, K., Dixon, D.: Gamification: Using game design elements in non-gaming contexts. In: Proceedings of the CHI 2011, Vancouver, Canada, pp. 2425–2428. ACM (2011)

7. Gayomali, C.: A quick guide to flappy bird, the super-addicting, incredibly popular game. Retrieved from http://www.fastcompany.com/3025959/fast-feed/a-quick-guide-to-flappy-bird-the-super-addicting-incredibly-popular-game (2014). Accessed 14 September 2014

8. Gray, E.K., Watson, D.: General and specific traits of personality and their relation to sleep and academic performance. J. Pers. 70(2), 177–206 (2002)

9. Hamilton, N.A., Gallagher, M.W., Preacher, K.J., Stevens, N., Nelson, C.A., Karlson, C., McCurdy, D.: Insomnia and well-being. J. Consult. Clin. Psychol. 75(6), 939–946 (2007)

10. Horne, J.A., Ostberg, O.: A self-assessment questionnaire to determine morningness-eveningness in human circadian rhythms. Int. J. Chronobiol. 4(2), 97–110 (1976)

11. Hurd, R.: 8 Best sleep tracking apps and devices now that Zeo is gone. Retrieved from http://dreamstudies.org/2013/07/16/best-sleep-tracking-apps-devices/ (2013). Accessed 7 July 2014

12. Johns, M.W.: A new method for measuring daytime sleepiness: The Epworth Sleepiness Scale. Sleep 14(6), 540–545 (1991)

13. Montola, M., Nummenmaa, T., Lucero, A., Boberg, M., Korhonen, H.: Applying game achievement systems to enhance user experience in a photo sharing service. In: MindTrek 2009 Proceedings of the 13th International MindTrek Conference: Everyday Life in the Ubiquitous Era, pp. 94–97. ACM, New York (2009)

14. Orlin, J.: Sleep tracking startup Zeo says goodnight. Retrieved from http://techcrunch.com/2013/05/22/sleep-tracking-startup-zeo-says-goodnight/ (2013). Accessed 7 June 2014

15. Roberts, R.E., Roberts, C.R., Chen, I.G.: Functioning of adolescents with symptoms of disturbed sleep. J. Youth Adolesc. 30(1), 1–18 (2001)

16. Ryan, R.M., Deci, E.L.: Intrinsic and extrinsic motivations: classic definitions and new directions. Contemp. Educ. Psychol. 25(1), 54–67 (2000)

17. Schutte, W.: Global games market report infographics. Retrieved from http://www.newzoo.com/infographics/global-games-market-report-infographics/ (2013). Accessed 15 March 2015

18. Smyth MSN, C.: The pittsburgh sleep quality index (PSQI). N.Y. Univ. Coll. Nurs. 29(6), 1–2 (2012)

19. Wolfson, A.R., Carskadon, M.A.: Sleep schedules and daytime functioning in adolescents. Child Dev. 69(4), 875–887 (1998)

20. Young, K.: Starbucks early bird offers discounted coffee for the dedicated. Retrieved from http://www.trendhunter.com/trends/starbucks-early-bird (2012). Accessed 12 September 2014

21. Zichermann, G.: Intrinsic and extrinsic motivation in gamification. In: Paper presented at the Gamification Summit, San Francisco, 27 October 2011

22. Zohar, D., Tzischinsky, O., Epstein, R., Lavie, P.: The effects of sleep loss on medical residents' emotional reactions to work events: A cognitive-energy model. Sleep 28(1), 47–54 (2005)

Methods and Models

Cicero: Middleware for Developing Persuasive Mobile Applications

Antonello D'Aloia[1], Matteo Lelli[1(✉)], Duckki Lee[2], Sumi Helal[3],
and Paolo Bellavista[1]

[1] Department of Computer Science and Engineering,
University of Bologna, Bologna, Italy
{antonello.daloia,matteo.lelli4}@studio.unibo.it,
paolo.bellavista@unibo.it
[2] Creative Innovation Center, Advanced Convergence R&D Lab,
LG Electronics, Seoul, South Korea
csleedk@gmail.com
[3] Mobile and Pervasive Computing Lab, University of Florida, Gainesville, USA
helal@cise.ufl.edu

Abstract. We present Cicero – a middleware solution to support developers design and implement persuasive mobile apps. Based on the Action-Behavior Model (ABM), Cicero provides developers with powerful class libraries and collaboration methodology to streamline the development of mobile persuasive apps without requiring a steep knowledge of behavior science theory or venturing into domain-specific knowledge and artifacts. Cicero guides the developers in following the ABM steps, provides APIs for cyber sense and cyber influence, and embodies the necessary model computations including measuring end-user compliance and response to influence and persuasion. Cicero also facilitates the engagement of domain experts in a clearly defined collaborative role. Here we also originally detail the design and implementation of an Android version of the Cicero middleware and we present a use case to practically exemplify how Cicero can facilitate the application developers' work.

Keywords: Persuasive computing · Middleware · Mobile app development · Android · Sensing · Actuation · Situation · Activity recognition

1 Introduction

Mobile smart technologies and products have become extremely pervasive and are an essential part of our daily lives. Their almost ubiquitous presence is influencing us and has begun to change our way of life and behaviors, either intentionally or unintentionally. Among the many digital gadgets and products, smartphones and smart watches are the most popular personal devices that we use today. They are getting much attention lately as potentially powerful persuasive tools that could change human behavior due to their accessibility, sensibility, connectivity, and triggerability.

However, recent research work in the field has shown that it is not easy to create persuasive mobile apps without adequate knowledge of behavior and persuasion theory.

© Springer International Publishing Switzerland 2016
A. Meschtscherjakov et al. (Eds.): PERSUASIVE 2016, LNCS 9638, pp. 137–149, 2016.
DOI: 10.1007/978-3-319-31510-2_12

In addition, assessing user behavior response to persuasive influencing factors is another non-trivial challenge. App developers usually lack such knowledge and, therefore, to bridge this gap, we propose Cicero – a middleware and associated toolkit to support developers in designing and programming persuasive mobile apps. Based on the Action-based Behavior Model (ABM) [4, 5] and situation-based user compliance assessment algorithms [1–3], Cicero is designed to provide developers with powerful class libraries and a programming/collaboration methodology to streamline the development process of persuasive apps without requiring a steep knowledge of behavior and persuasion theory or venturing into domain-specific knowledge and artifacts. Cicero guides the developers in following the ABM model, provides API for cyber sense and cyber influence, and embodies the necessary model computations including the effective measurement of end-user response to influence and persuasion.

The remainder of the paper is structured as follows. In Sect. 2, we briefly de-scribe the ABM model and discuss related work. Section 3 describes how Cicero is designed as a mobile efficient specialization of the general ABM. Cicero Android implementation follows in Sect. 4, together with a use case in Sect. 5. After reporting experimental performance results of our Cicero middle-ware, conclusive remarks and directions of future work end the paper.

2 Background

Existing behavior theories and models are not adequate to mobile intervention [6]. In order to fully utilize mobile technologies, behavior models are required to have dynamic, regulatory system components to guide rapid intervention adaptation based on the individual's current and past behavior and situational context [6]. ABM is designed to meet these requirements by providing adaptive iterative process based on domain-specific behavior assessment. ABM provides specific step for a cyber system to follow to persuade a user to change behavior. ABM also gives technological guidelines on how a cyber system should act to provide persuasive influence by providing specific cyber actions, which could be easily converted to APIs that developers understand and utilize to create apps. We briefly describe ABM here. Further explanation on the specific choices and inner workings of the ABM can be found in [4, 5].

ABM [4, 5] is a persuasion template designed by incorporating relevant persuasion theories into a "cyber model" that app developers can understand and utilize in a broad range of applications that require persuasion. As shown in Fig. 1, the model consists of a cyber system (cyber sense and cyber influence) and a set of user actions.

Each step contributes and relates to one or more of the three elements of persuasion: motivation, ability

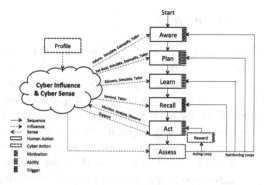

Fig. 1. Action behavior model

and trigger [7]. The cyber influence affects and helps the user to take each action within ethical guidelines [8]. As the user works toward her goals, the cyber sense monitors, analyzes and observes her actions. After the initial rounds of steps, the Assess action evaluates the achievements of the goals and either rewards or rolls the user back through reinforcement loops to the appropriate model step based on the measured deficits of each action. For positive achievements, the Reward action may give intrinsic, extrinsic, or virtual rewards to reinforce the motivation.

A specific definition of situation that involves contexts, activities, and device interactions, which was introduced in [3], is utilized by cyber sense. Based on this definition, Situation-based Assess Tree (SAT) [1, 2] is defined as a formalism, structure, and algorithm for domain-specific behavior assessment under the ABM model.

The Cicero middleware implements a strictly mobile specialization of ABM where cyber sense and influencing are limited to Android smart phones/watches. Cicero also implements the Assess step through an optimized, cloud-based implementation of the SAT algorithm as detailed in the following.

2.1 Related Work

Despite the increasing number of applications with persuasion features, only few middleware and frameworks nowadays exist to support and streamline persuasive app development. Moreover, some middleware solutions are specific for mobile crowd-sensing lacking underlying persuasion theory. In this section, we analyze related work on persuasion middleware, paying specific attention to their cyber sense influence capabilities, and to their differences and similarities with our work.

Code In The Air (CITA) [10, 11] is a system developed in the Networks and Mobile Systems group at MIT that simplifies the development of complex tasking applications via a Web interface. CITA enables non-expert end users to easily express simple tasks on their smartphones, and more sophisticated developers to code complex tasks by writing purely server-side scripts in JavaScript. It is worth mentioning that CITA can sense and recognize a number of low-level activities such as isWalking, isDriving, enterPlace, and leavePlace. In addition, CITA allows developers and users to compose lower-level activities using logical predicates to create high-level activities. Regarding the ability to persuade the user, CITA provides limited support in the form of triggers and reminders. It uses an asynchronous message delivery service to trigger users' task fulfillment.

Funf [12] initially developed at the MIT Media Lab is another extensible sensing and data processing framework for Android devices. It aims to help developers create applications that need mobile sensing easily without having to access low-level APIs, but with no support of cyber influence and rich persuasion features. There are also some commercial applications similar to CITA and Funf, most notably Tasker[1], which allows users to perform tasks based on contexts such as time, date, location, event, input gestures, or using information provided by other applications. If compared with CITA and Funf, Tasker provides richer sentience as it is capable of providing sensor

---

[1] http://tasker.dinglisch.net/.

values and more articulated/complex contexts, which are richer, modular, and easily extensible in an app-specific way by developers.

The Pervasive Middleware for Activity Recognition (PEMAR) framework [13] aims to increase the level of physical activity by creating a middleware for active games on mobile devices. PEMAR can to recognize human motions based on human activities and their contexts, but it lacks as well as an underlying theory of persuasion, though games are used as a method of persuasion.

Google recently released Google Fit [14] - an open platform that allows users to control their fitness data, and supports developers build health and fitness apps. It also targets manufacturers and aims to influence their future device designs to take advantage of. With Fit and the Google Play services location APIs[2], developers should be able to easily create health and wellness applications. Nevertheless, without proper support for persuasion, developers have to create a lot of persuasion-related code behavior from scratch, which is time consuming and involves a steep learning curve.

MoST [15] is a smartphone sensing library developed at the University of Bologna. From the functional point of view, it is very similar to Google Play services location APIs, but it is open source, lightweight, modular, and more efficient in terms of resource usage, in particular battery.

Finally, DailyAlert [16] is a generic mobile persuasion toolkit for smartphones that generalizes and automates persuasion as a service for mobile applications. It follows the thin-client design to reduce power consumption on users' devices and to simplify integration with mobile applications. Although DailyAlert is a complete persuasive toolkit, similar to Cicero, it is not based on explicit theoretical foundation and models.

3 Cicero Design

To design a mobile technology specialization (or translation) of ABM, its cyber sense, cyber influence, and its Assess Tree algorithm, we limit the cyberspace and its devices to Android smartphones/tablets and Android Wear. The set of available sensors on these devices are identified and explicitly made accessible to our middleware. Similarly, following a pyramid design methodology [9] as shown in Fig. 2, a rich set of potential activities and contexts are defined and explicitly supported in the middleware. Together, they constitute the second layer of the pyramid. It is impor-

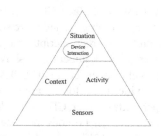

Fig. 2. Cicero design pyramid

tant to note that information about activities could be used to recognize applicable contexts (hence the larger representation of Activity compared to Context in this layer). Finally, in the top of the pyramid, programmable situation structures that may utilize any of the predefined contexts, activities or device interactions are supported. Situations are key to implementing the Assess step in the ABM.

---

[2] https://developers.google.com/android/reference/com/google/android/gms/location/package-summary.

It is worth noting that device interaction is co-located with the situation layer because interactions with end users (e.g., through screen views, flash LED, vibration, or integrated speakers) are often coordinated based on materialized situations.

3.1 Sensors

Most Android smartphones/watches have built-in sensors capable of providing high precision/accuracy raw data to measure motion, orientation, low-level activities, and various environmental conditions. We divide such sensors into three broad categories: motion sensors (used to measure acceleration and rotational forces along three axes, such as accelerometers, gyroscopes, and vector sensors), environmental sensors (for various environmental parameters, such as humidity and pressure), and position sensors (used to measure the physical position of a device, such as GPS or Wi-Fi)[3].

3.2 Activity

Cicero maximizes the leverage of existing Android features especially Google Play Services, by offering rich APIs such as ActivityRecognitionAPI and the FusedLocationProviderAPI for managing motion and position sensors[4]. Combined, they help recognize several user activities including still, tilting (device angle related to gravity change significantly), on foot, walking, running, on bicycle, in vehicle, and unknown.

To support a broader set of activities, we used additional libraries and APIs offered by the Android platform including SensorManager[5], which is used to manage environment sensors, TelephonyManager[6], which is used to sense the device status, and MediaRecorder[7] used to detect sounds around the user. We have supported the following activities based on these APIs in Cicero: *"walking"*, *"running"*, *"still"*, *"calling"*, *"going to < Loc>"*, *"being at < Loc>"*, and *"near < Loc>"*. Developers are provided with a very simple interface to register and detect occurrences of activities.

3.3 Context

In addition to the above activity recognition features, situations as defined in ABM need more details – contexts and device actions. Context is determined by wiring (combining) data that derive from different sensors. We denote gathered sensor data with the symbol $SE_k(x)$ which represents the sensed data by the kth sensor. Using AND, OR, and NOT operators, we define the following three context models:

---

[3] http://developer.android.com/guide/topics/sensors/sensors_overview.html.

[4] https://developers.google.com/android/guides/overview.

[5] http://developer.android.com/reference/android/hardware/SensorManager.html.

[6] http://developer.android.com/reference/android/telephony/TelephonyManager.html.

[7] http://developer.android.com/reference/android/media/MediaRecorder.html.

(1) Locational Model: context combines sensor data collected in different locations, (2) Snapshot Model: context combines sensor data collected in different points in time, and (3) Value Model: context as in (1) and (2) but defined over ranges of values rather than specific single sensor values. This model is more practical to use in real-world applications. Context under Value Model can be expressed as follows:

$$C = SE_1(v_a, v_b) \; op \; SE_2(v_a, v_b) \; op. . .op \; SE_k(v_a, v_b)$$

Where v_a and v_b represent the two extremities of the range of a given sensor SE_i.

3.4 Situation

By recognizing different activities, contexts, and device actions, it is possible to recognize the occurrence of predefined situations that will enable the SAT assessment algorithm and the ABM Access step. We utilize a simple quorum-based decision method to recognize situations: if two or more elements of a situation are true (out of three, i.e., device action, context, and activity), the situation is considered to have occurred [3].

4 Cicero Implementation

In this section, we further explain the main characteristics of Cicero and its components. Cicero works on mobile devices and in a layer underlying persuasive apps. For the developer, Cicero is a middleware and a tool that simplifies the development process of persuasive applications. For the end-user, Cicero is a run-time under which Cicero-based apps execute. Developers can create persuasive applications by setting cyber sense and cyber influence and, in general, by setting and programming each step in ABM. This includes setting goals and contents relative to the Aware and Learn steps, setting suggestions and reminders relative to the Recall step, and setting Rewards based on available incentives. End users are transparently guided by ABM and its steps: they can use the app by setting goals, checking their own progress, interacting with reminders, and obtaining rewards.

The Cicero architecture, shown in Fig. 3, consists of two main managers: sentience manager and cyber manager. The former is concerned with sensing in general and allows the developer to select contexts and activities to monitor. The cyber manager works to facilitate the developer's work to set and program the various steps in ABM. In addition, it is concerned with recognizing situations and monitoring the progression of the various steps. Periodically, the cyber manager would evaluate how the user conforms to the settings of the model (progress towards goals) through the SAT algorithm. SAT evaluations are done in the cloud whereas all other processing of the cyber manager is done on the hosting mobile device. We give the design/implementation details of each manager below.

4.1 Sentience Manager (SM)

SM accesses and gathers sensor data using listeners and filters data in order to evaluate the achievement of goals. SM implements the Act step of ABM, thus it is initialized and processed by the cyber manager. In order to manage the different sensors, SM is further divided into several components:

- Location: used to manage position sensors. This component is based on FusedLocationProviderAPI (an efficient module integrated in Google Play Services).
- Motion: related to the motion sensors. This module can detect in background the user's activities using ActivityRecognitionAPI offers by Google Play.
- Environment: for handling environmental sensors, such as amplitude or lightness.
- Social: related to social activities such as making or receiving phone calls, and the frequency of such activities.
- TimeService: service to manage and filter sensed data about time context.

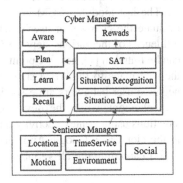

Fig. 3. Cicero architecture

These components, in order to manage gathered data, interact with an Android service running in the background that allows filtering data and the assessment of the goals achievement. In order to do that, this service owns a pool of objects, each of which is waiting to be concurrently updated from related components in SM regarding a particular situation.

Another important responsibility of SM is sending events to the cyber manager in order to detect the different situations that drive the SAT algorithm evaluation.

4.2 Cyber Manager (CM)

CM implements the ABM steps except for the Act (which is managed by SM). For Aware, Plan, Learn, and Recall steps the developer can set own activities into adapters offered by Cicero. Aware and Learn steps should inform and educate the end user, thus they have to show influential contents. Cicero facilitates for such content to be placed by a domain expert into a shared Google Drive folder accessible to the user through the app. This enables the collaboration and participation of the domain experts, for example physical therapists or doctors, who know best what content are appropriate, and who are capable of using something as simple as Google Drive (but not any more complex than that). The Plan step, depending on the goal-setting theory, should guide the user during the configuration of variables that characterize the goals. After the Plan step is set, CM initializes the SM using the scanning classes and SM's own initialization services.

Reminding the user is a very important aspect of persuasive apps so the user can behave and converge towards the set goals. Thus, Recall step is realized by Cicero using Android Notification triggered according to set schedules at configuration time, and by SAT through reinforcement loops. Cicero sends notifications only when the device is active to ensure user's attention is secured. When the device is locked the notification is queued and sent as soon as the user unlocks the device.

The last module of CM is the Assess step that implements the SAT algorithm to evaluate the changes in user's behavior and compliance (response to the persuasive influences of the various steps). SAT tree is shown in Fig. 4. While the details of SAT can be found in [1], here we point only to the facts that internal nodes in the level below the root maps to the ABM steps, while the lowest level nodes which are positive or negative user behaviors are essentially situations. Domain experts prescribe (describe) the behaviors, while the developers use Cicero to implement behavior nodes into situations using context, activity and device interactions. Evaluation is currently hosted in the cloud as a Google App server, offering an Assess service. In fact, the domain expert can configure all variables of SAT by an online service.

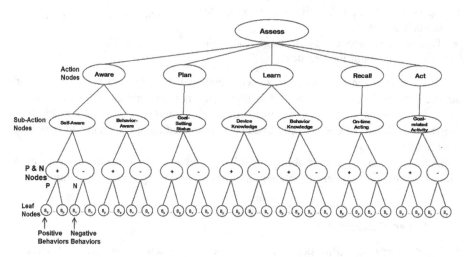

Fig. 4. Situation based Access Tree (SAT)

5 Cicero Use Case

In order to better describe Cicero and to demonstrate its benefits to developers, we present a contrived use case in which we use Cicero to develop a mobile application to help obese individuals lose weight. We present the use case and analyze how using Cicero greatly eases the development tasks and reduces the total work effort required by the developer. We describe the use case scenario and then describe the steps taken in developing the application.

Scenario. San Raffaele is a local clinic which cares for numerous patients with obesity related diseases. Clinic executive board decided to tap into mobile technology to help reduce the impact of obesity among its patients and to better manage their chronic conditions. San Raffaele contracts with a local software firm to develop a mobile app for this purpose. The firm assigns Michael a chief mobile app developer. Recognizing that his firm never possessed experience in user empowerment and persuasion theories, he researched how a mobile application may be able to motivate users. Then, after a brief search he finds Cicero, a middleware to support his team in developing the persuasive mobile app to the local clinic.

Application. Following Cicero's footsteps, Michael realizes that the app needs to include an Aware step to make users aware of why it is so important to walk in order to improve health. He follows Cicero guidelines and understands that content in this step needs to be provided by the domain experts. Michael communicates with the San Raffaele clinic and obtains a list of hyperlinks that provide awareness about this topic as well as other information needed by other steps such as Plan step. Next, Michael realizes that a user Profile needs to be captured (see Fig. 1). He implements the Profile one-time step that prompts the users to insert personal information including the location of their gym in order to be able to tailor the application to their needs. Next, Michael completes the Plan step which sets a target schedule and instructs the users about the proper way to walk (e.g., it is not healthy walking under a bright sunlight midday), showing a list of links to useful web pages or videos (Learn step).

The final tasks in the development process involves collaboration and communication with San Raffaele's experts to obtain descriptions of the negative and positive behaviors which the developer will map into P- and N-nodes as per the SAT tree structure in Fig. 4. Once these nodes are created, the application is essentially complete and is able to sense users' motions and locations which automate the recognition of contexts, activities and eventually situations. This allows the SAT tree to assess changes in users' behaviors. Lack of response to persuasion automatically invokes reinforcement loops. By rolling back the non-compliant user to the appropriate previous step. Also, based on the Plan step, the application automatically sends to users reminders in order to assist them in reaching their set goals. Michael gets a firsthand experience with Cicero and sees how it makes it extremely easy and fast for him to develop the first prototype of the app to demo it to San Raffaele. As will be shown below, Michael did not have to write the application from scratch, to the opposite, by relying on Cicero, he ended up coding only small sections of code.

Implementation. The first task for Michael is to code four Android Activity classes, one for each related ABM step. Then Michael sets these Activities in the Cicero middleware, using the related `setActivityAdapter` method of CM. After that, Cicero will start them when it is appropriate. For instance, Michael creates an Activity called `AwareActivity` that shows the users a list of hyperlinks about the importance of walking. Michael is free to develop that Activity as he wishes, such as using a list of links to web pages or integrating it with documents stored in a shared Google Drive folder. After that, he informs Cicero that his `AwareActivity` is the Activity that implements the ABM Aware step, using the `setAssessActivityAdapter` method. It is important to notice here how Cicero streamlines development and provides valuable reusable code yet at the same time allows the developer some freedom and flexibility. Indeed, developers can use reusable Android Activity, only setting them in the CM, allowing simplicity of use and reusability.

Next, we show how situations are defined and created. In dealing with delicate pathologies (e.g., Diabetes or Bipolar diseases), collaboration between the developer and domain experts (who are an authority in deciding on positive and negative behaviors) is required. In particular, developers have to engage domain experts, asking for behaviors that should be usefully tracked in that pathology. Situations must also be categorized or mapped into sub-action nodes. The domain expert does not need to understand the working of the SAT tree but should be fully aware of the concept of positive and negative behaviors and also of the meanings of the ABM steps. Situations related to this use case are shown in Table 1. They are described in simple phrases that involve a metric or two (e.g., 20 min, daily, or a specific location). These phrases should be the output from the domain expert. Cicero natively supports all the situations identified, therefore, Michael can develop his application completely using the middleware.

Table 1. Situations setup in the San Raffaele use case

Action Node	Sub-action node	P-or-N Node	Situation
Aware	Behavior-Aware	P Node	P1: Walk more than before
		N Node	N1: Walk less than before
Plan	Goal-Setting Status	P Node	P2: Complete set goals
		N Node	N2: Do not set goals
Learn	Behavior Knowledge	P Node	P3: Do not walk in bright sunlight
		N Node	N3: Walk in bright sunlight
Act	Goal-related Activity	P Node	P4: Walk 20 min daily
			P5: Go to gym twice a week
		N Node	N4: Walk < 20 min daily
			N5: Do not be at the gym twice in a week

Now that situations are clearly defined, it is time for Michael to implement the situation and to build up the SAT using his implementation. In order to do that, Michael calls suitable methods of CM. For example, in order to add the P4 situation in Table 1, Michael invokes the method addGoalRelatedActivityPNode of CM passing in, among other parameters, ActivityName.Walking, ContextName.Duration, and 20 min as reference value. Then, Cicero creates the related Leaf Node, adds it to the SAT tree, and starts the sensing thread of user motions. This will begin the SAT algorithm evaluation of user responses.

After all situations are added to SAT tree, Michael programs some notifications to be displayed occasionally when the user switches on the device. In this way, the user is more involved than popping out a notification when he or she is not actively using the smartphone. Michael only creates the notification messages (subclass of Android Notification) but Cicero schedules them according to the developer's preferences (Profile), such as frequency or preferred times. Moreover, other recalls based on situations are possible. Which notifications Michael implements is a matter of design choices and developer creativity.

By completing the steps described above, developers have a ready-to-test and use application. Clearly, it implies a great saving in time and amount of written code if compared to creating the same application from scratch. Indeed, to develop from scratch a quite complex application as in our use case, a developer would have to code dozens of classes, not to mention the amount of time to research and understand theories about persuasive technologies/applications. Nevertheless, relying on Cicero, the same developer has to write just few classes, where only about few tens of code lines relate to the interaction with Cicero to fully develop the persuasive application.

6 Some Experimental Performance Results of the Cicero Middleware

To assess the performance of Cicero in different conditions, we utilized the use case as a driver for several evaluations. An application developed relying on the use case was used daily for a week by a 25-years-old user. The device used was a smartphone Nexus 5 featured by Android 6.0. By using Android Debug Bridge[8] and Dev Tool[9] by Android Studio, we have thoroughly analyzed CPU and RAM usages. In particular, considering the Act step, which is the only one that runs in the background, the CPU usage reached a peak of 2 %, but demonstrated to be lower on average; the used RAM was 19 MB with an assigned heap of 24 MB.

Battery is recognized as the most challenging resource for many types of mobile devices. The Cicero battery consumption was measured by using Trepn Profiler to assess the level of consumed energy[10] of the mobile device: by using daily profiling that mimics the usual daily behavior of the considered target users, we have found a battery consumption of 7 % on average per day. Cicero is also supported by Google Play Services; the energy consumption by Google Play has demonstrated to be an additional 12 % daily.

Finally, we have also experimentally evaluated the Cicero latency and promptness to answer user's requests. By considering the relevant aspect of user's activity detection, the ActivityRecognitionAPI has shown performance indicators that depend on the targeted accuracy of detection; for the sake of briefness, here we report that, in the case of detection of a motionless device, latency is on average 550 ms from the starting of the scan and the detected (motionless) activity, with a confidence of 100 %.

---

[8] http://developer.android.com/tools/help/adb.html.

[9] http://developer.android.com/tools/debugging/debugging-devtools.html.

[10] https://developer.qualcomm.com/software/trepn-power-profiler.

7 Conclusion

We presented Cicero, a middleware and tool for developing persuasive mobile apps. Cicero is based on the Action-Behavior Model and assessing user responses to persuasion. We described the design and implementation of Cicero and provided a use case to explain how developers can use it to develop apps within a defined collaboration framework with domain experts. Cicero saves significant development time and waives the requirement that developers need to understand elements of persuasion theory. We presented results of preliminary experiments that characterize Cicero performance and energy use. Cicero software and documentations can be obtained from the Cicero download site[11]. An important future work will provide for a community-based shared resources that document domain experts contributions in the form of short white papers describing positive and negative behaviors related to common or special chronic conditions.

References

1. Lee, D., Helal, S., Sung, Y.S., Anton, S.: Situation-based assess tree for user behavior assessment in persuasive telehealth. IEEE Trans. Hum. Mach. Syst. **45**(5), 624–634 (2015)
2. Lee, D., Helal, S., Sung, Y.: Assessing behavioral responses in persuasive ubiquitous systems. In: Biswas, J., Kobayashi, H., Wong, L., Abdulrazak, B., Mokhtari, M. (eds.) ICOST 2013. LNCS, vol. 7910, pp. 176–186. Springer, Heidelberg (2013)
3. Lee, D., Helal, S.: From activity recognition to situation recognition. In: Biswas, J., Kobayashi, H., Wong, L., Abdulrazak, B., Mokhtari, M. (eds.) ICOST 2013. LNCS, vol. 7910, pp. 245–251. Springer, Heidelberg (2013)
4. Lee, D., Helal, S., Anton, S., De Deugd, S., Smith, A.: Participatory and persuasive tehealth. Gerontology **58**, 269–281 (2012)
5. Lee, D., Helal, S., Johnson, B.D.: An action-based behavior model for persuasive telehealth. In: Lee, Y., Bien, Z., Mokhtari, M., Kim, J.T., Park, M., Kim, J., Lee, H., Khalil, I. (eds.) ICOST 2010. LNCS, vol. 6159, pp. 121–129. Springer, Heidelberg (2010)
6. Riley, W.T., Rivera, D.E., Atienza, A.A., Nilsen, W., Allison, S.M., Mermelstein, R.: Health behavior models in the age of mobile interventions: are our theories up to the task? Transl. Behav. Med. **1**, 53–71 (2011)
7. Fogg, B.J.: A behavior model for persuasive design. In: Proceedings of the Persuasive. ACM, New York (2009)
8. Berdichevsky, D., Neunschwander, E.: Towards an ethics of persuasive technology. Commun. ACM **42**(5), 51–58 (1999)
9. D'Aloia, A.: Persuasive Computing: an Android-based Framework for Developing and Managing Persuasive Applications (2015)
10. Ravindranath, L., Thiagarajan, A., Balakrishnan, H., Madden, S.: Code in the air: simplifying sensing and coordination tasks on smartphones. In: Proceedings of Hot-Mobile. ACM (2012)

---

[11] http://www.icta.ufl.edu/cicero.

11. Kaler, T., Lynch, J.P., Peng, T., Ravindranath, L., Thiagarajan, A., Balakrishnan, H., Madden, S.: Code in the air: simplifying sensing on smartphones. In: Proceedings of SenSys. ACM (2010)
12. Aharony, N., Pan, W., Ip, C., Khayal, I., Pentland, A.: Social fMRI: Investigating and shaping social mechanisms in the real world. Pervasive Mobile Comput. 7(6), 643–659 (2011). ACM
13. Vaka, P., Shen, F., Chandrashekar, M., Lee, Y.: PEMAR: A pervasive middleware for activity recognition with smart phones. In: PerCom Workshops. IEEE (2015)
14. Google Fit SDK: https://developers.google.com/fit/
15. Cardone, G., Cirri, A., Corradi, A., Foschini, L., Montanari, R.: Activity recognition for smart city scenarios: Google play services vs. MoST facilities. In: Computers and Communication (ISCC). IEEE (2014)
16. Zhan, A., Lim, J.H., Terzis, A.: DailyAlert: A generic mobile persuasion toolkit for smartphones. In: PhoneSense. ACM (2011)

Formalization of Computational Human Behavior Models for Contextual Persuasive Technology

Tylar Murray[1,2,3,4](✉), Eric Hekler[1,2,3,4], Donna Spruijt-Metz[1,2,3,4], Daniel E. Rivera[1,2,3,4], and Andrew Raij[1,2,3,4]

[1] University of South Florida, Tampa, USA
tylarmurray@mail.usf.edu
[2] Arizona State University, Tampa, USA
[3] University of Southern California, Los Angeles, USA
[4] University of Central Florida, Orlando, USA

Abstract. In theory, Just-in-Time Adaptive Interventions (JiTAIs) are a persuasive technology which promise to empower personal behavioral goals by optimizing treatments to situational context and user behaviors. This paper outlines open challenges facing the development of JiTAIs and discusses the use of modeling as a common ground between behavioral scientists designing interventions and software engineers building applications. We propose that Computational Human Behavior Modeling (CHBM) has the potential to (1) help create better behavioral theories, (2) enable real-time ideographic intervention optimization, and (3) facilitate more robust data analysis techniques. First, a small set of definitions are presented to clarify ambiguities and mismatches in terminology between these two areas. Next, existing modeling concepts are used to formalize a modeling paradigm designed to fit the needs JiTAI development methodology. Last, potential benefits and open challenges of this modeling paradigm are highlighted through examination of the model-development methodology, run-time user modeling, and model-based data analysis.

Keywords: Persusasive · Just-in-time · Adaptive · JiTAI · Modeling · Computational human behavior modeling

1 Introduction

A recent trend in the area of persuasive technology is the development of mHealth applications which aim to deliver better, smarter, and more effective interventions via mobile and wearable devices. One class of persuasive technologies with this aim is the "Just-In-Time Adaptive Intervention" (or JiTAI) which describes an intervention that adapts to an individual's changing needs and circumstances to deliver tailored support at the time when it is most needed. [12] Thanks to

© Springer International Publishing Switzerland 2016
A. Meschtscherjakov et al. (Eds.): PERSUASIVE 2016, LNCS 9638, pp. 150–161, 2016.
DOI: 10.1007/978-3-319-31510-2_13

great advances in wearable, mobile, and ubiquitous technologies increasingly rich data is now available to characterize the context of the subject for use in JiTAI applications.

Researchers theorize that an intervention which can tailor based on the user and context may be an elegant solution to empower self-management of unhealthy behaviors like substance abuse, overeating, sedentary behavior, and more [11]. These persuasive technologies aim to utilize contextual information — data collected from the subject's surroundings and history — to deliver personalized interventions at the optimal moment in time. Real-time monitoring of data to identify states of special vulnerability to poor behavioral decisions or receptivity to intervention at any given moment is possible [9], but "a major gap exists between the technological capacity to deliver JITAIs and existing health behavior models." [11] Proof-of-concept applications have demonstrated the ability to adapt interventions to users [2,5] and context [3,4], but using current methods the complexity of the behavioral model underlying a JiTAI application grows exponentially as the complexity of the intervention design increases. The needs of a persuasive technology are very different from the needs of extant behavioral research. While the latter places emphasis on the study of the human system's intricacies, the former needs a model which provides generalized insight and specific numerical predictions. Behavioral theories traditionally focus on nomothetic and static insights that do not offer the granularity and specificity to support the full potential of JiTAIs [14]. These methods are sufficient for analysis of traits which do not change much over days or weeks, but data collection and intervention delivery timing is now available to the microsecond for physiological data, behavioral features at the minute-level, and psychological constructs (via EMA [15]).

The current development process for JiTAI-like persuasive technologies requires close collaboration between behavioral scientists and application developers as they struggle to code-ify the model from extant behavioral theories for each individual experiment. The models used by a programmer to describe a *user* and the models used by behavioral scientists to describe a *subject*, have certain key differences which can complicate the process of JiTAI design. In this work we present a hybridization of the two modeling paradigms designed to emphasize the strengths of each approach. As a part of this set of interdisciplinary terms, we introduce the concept of a Computational Human Behavior Model (CHBM) to describe this new class of models which aim to satisfy the demands of persuasive technology. Following definitions, we propose that by formalizing the CHBM underlying persuasive applications, it will be possible to create better behavioral theories, enable real-time ideographic optimization, facilitate more robust data analysis, and reduce application development time. In this section we present a look at how the concept of a CHBM would be applied to address open issues holding back JiTAIs and we highlight the remaining issues which must be addressed to make Just-in-Time Adaptive Interventions a reality.

2   Selected Definitions

This section presents definitions and design considerations relevant to human-behavior modeling from a theory-agnostic standpoint so that different modeling paradigms can be described under a common foundation. This set of definitions draws from both the area of HCI user-modeling and the extant paradigms of human behavior modeling in behavioral science in an attempt to synthesize a pragmatic language for use in the development of persuasive technology by behavioral scientists and application developers alike.

Treatments are defined by M.C. Kaptein [10] as the set of messages or feedback a user receives from a persuasive application. The term treatments seems synonymous with interventions in usage, but a single treatment should be used to unambiguously represent a single instance of user-interaction, whereas a single intervention may represent a set of interactions given as a dose.

Just-in-Time (JiT) is a cross-disciplinary concept defined in the context of behavioral interactions by Nahum-Shani et al. as "the effective provision of timely support, operationalized by offering the type of support needed, precisely when needed, in a way that minimizes waste (i.e., defined as anything that does not benefit the person) and accommodates the real-life setting in which support is needed." [11] Thus, for an intervention to be considered Just-in-Time (JiT), it must attempt to deliver treatment immediately before or after an event associated with the target behavior.

Adaptive interventions must utilize dynamic (time-varying) "information from the person (e.g., changes in psychological distress, response to an intervention, intervention adherence) [...] to make intervention decisions repeatedly in the course of the intervention (e.g., changing the type, dosage, or timing of intervention delivery).' [11] An adaptive intervention is one that responds in real-time to the changing needs of the participant by tailoring the treatment itself based on situational context or the recent behavioral history of a user.

Individualization is defined by Nahum-Shani et al. as the "use of [static] information from the individual to make decisions about when, where and how to intervene." [11] Thus, an intervention is individualized if "relatively stable information from the person (e.g., gender, baseline severity of symptoms) is used to make intervention-related decisions (e.g., to offer intervention package A or B)" [11] For example, a stress-relief intervention regimen may utilize relaxing music treatment based on the subject's favorite songs at study initialization, or a participant's favorite color may be used as the basis for the user interface color palette.

3   Computational Human Behavior Models

The following specification will allow for the formal description of a CHBM, providing a standard approach to describing, designing, and visualizing human behavior models for persuasive applications. A Computational Human Behavior Model (CHBM) is defined here as a mathematical, explicit model which describes how context is transformed into a behavioral outcome through the internal state of the human system. In summary, a Computational Human Behavior Model (CHBM) should have (1) a set of context, state, and behavior variables, (2) a set of computations which define behavior variables as a function of state which is itself a function of context, (3) a logical abstraction which allows researchers to internalize the model's behavior such that they will be better able to estimate control of the human system in general, and (4) guidelines regarding the applicable population and time-scale of the CHBM. The following section details each of these CHBM components, followed by a methodology which makes use of a graph representation to create and describe a particular CHBM.

3.1   Characteristics of a CHBM

User Features: Context, State, Behavior. A distinguishing feature of a CHBM is the separation of the subject definition into environmental *context*, internal *state*, and *behavior* variables. In reality, an individual represents an inseparable component within the larger environment, but this simplification segments out the human system for definition.

In most cases, it is sufficient to define context as a set of selected information from the environment available for inflow into the human system, but contextual information from the environment may be summarized and represented in countless ways. In reality, consider context to be everything that is observed by the senses. Some of this information will alter the internal state of the human system, but some may not. When building a model based on theory alone, modelers should make the selection and summary of contextual constructs to be as generalizable, extensible, and reusable as possible. When utilizing a model to simulate a particular experiment, efforts to connect avaialable data to that which is available during the experiment may be needed, and contextual information not available empirically may need to be simulated. The environmental context influences the human system, which has an internal state represented by a set of internal state variables. In reality, internal state includes all information stored in the chemical and physical arrangement of our bodies. In order to make the model tractable, the mass of information is summarized into a set of meaningful constructs. Information flowing into a CHBM comes from the environment around an individual (the context) as an inflow which is independent of the individual's state in this instant. Similarly, information flowing out of a CHBM (as behaviors) represents actions the individual is taking to impact the environment.

Relationships Between User Features. The relationships between context, state, and behavior variables in a CHBM must be defined computationally. The functional form of these computations is not constrained in this definition, theoretically allowing for the representation of any intervariate relationship. There are numerous benefits to keeping the functional form of these relationships simple and homogenous across variables. Last, a simple formulation is more easily understood, allowing for a straightforward interpretation and abstraction of the model behavior.

Heuristic Interpretation. Statistical models trained on data do qualify as CHBMs in that they can define the relationships between state and context, but typically do not incorporate a logical abstraction of cognition and instead treat the internal state as a *black box*. This abstraction is essential when considering the process of JiTAI design, since the search-space available to a JiTAI designer can only be approached through heuristics guided by an understanding of how the human system will generally behave under given conditions. Though mathematical equations themselves reveal the nature of the system, naming and describing the interpretation of specific constructs or coefficients which play pivotal roles in the model can aid in the process of internalizing model behavior.

Model Metadata. While a CHBM should strive to be as broadly applicable as possible, this inevitably comes at the cost of increased complexity which can make the CHBM's nomothetic abstraction(s) intractable; there is a balance to be struck between a CHBM's inclusivity and the clarity of the abstraction. For this reason, it may be important to specify the circumstances in which a given model is valid. This is not analogous to the issue of over-fitting in machine learning, as the model can remain accurate across the population; the primary reason for limiting the number of variables or the functional complexity of relationships is to preserve the heuristic understanding of the model.

3.2   Creating a CHBM

A network graph is an effective abstraction to describe the relationships (represented by arrows or "edges") between variables (represented by the graph's "nodes") in a CHBM. In this case a directed graph wherein edge arrows represent the flow of information between nodes is used. Thus, a directed graph edge from node A to node B indicates that information flows from node A into node B. This relation can be read as "A influences B", "A informs B", or similar. This choice of notation is in agreement with graphs used in information theory, communications models, and behavioral science. In contrast, some graphing paradigms (such as probabilistic graphical models and software design) prefer to use notation wherein an edge is used to represent dependency.

   While the network graph shows the connectivity of a model, it fails to indicate the meaning of each connection. In the majority of existing applications, the mathematical form of the relationship is implied or else it is neglected completely. The most common analyses assess linear relationships between variables, and thus it is perhaps reasonable to assume that this is the intention of most authors. Assuming this is the case we can return to our simplistic example in Graph 1 and interpret the implied relationship as:

$$B(t) = coeff_{ab}A(t) + const_b \qquad (1)$$

In this formulation $coeff_{ab}$ represents the correlation coefficient which relates A to B, and $const_b$ represents a scalar constant. For nodes with multiple inflow edges, such as node B in the following graph:

$$A => B <= C => D \qquad\qquad (2)$$

Continuing with our assumption that node interrelations act as linear sums, the resulting formulation is simply a sum of the inflows:

$$B(t) = coeff_{ab}A(t) + coeff_{cb}C(t) + const_b \qquad\qquad (3)$$

Using this formulation, the general form of the CHBM is expressed via the network graph alone. The general solution of an CHBM does not require definition of the constants, but a simulation cannot be run until some numerical value is assumed. These constants often have theoretical significance in that they often have meaningful influence upon system behavior. Scaling-coefficients, for instance allow for relative weighting of each inflow. Similarly, the coefficients of a dynamical equation define how quickly variables react to a change "upstream".

This linear, homogeneous-graph representation is useful, but also very limited. One important feature which this formulation does not take into account is the dynamics of the relationship. For instance, the above linear model assumes that there is no delay between variables. This assumption is fine for some applications, but this is a very poor assumption for human behavior models.

Differential equations based on a fluid-flow analogy can be used to describe the relationship between variables as described by Dong et al. [7]. Using the differential formulation our equation for B in Graph 1 becomes:

$$B(t) = coeff_{ab}A(t - \theta_{ab}) - \tau_b\frac{dB}{dt} + const \qquad\qquad (4)$$

Just as before, our general model is not expressed entirely through the graph, and an ideographic example is specified by providing table of coefficient values. Our table is now quite a bit larger, but these coefficients have meaningful definitions which relate to our theory. While this formulation offers a huge improvement over the linear formulation, we can still imagine relationships which it cannot express.

It should be noted at this point that although the linear formulation is too simple to express the dynamics of the differential formulation, the differential formulation is capable of expressing linear relationships. This is accomplished by setting coefficients of dynamical components to 0. One might think, then, that there is some general formula which could express any functional form, and that this form should be used to express the relationships between variables in all CHBM graphs. While such formulations do exist (such as Taylor or Fourier series approximations or even ANN-based relations), this usage tends to make the model difficult to understand and to simulate with. Linear and differential formulations are in such widespread use because of the relative ease with which we can understand and solve them.

Let us now consider the case where a graph-wide assumption is NOT made. That is, we will specify the functional form of each node individually so that each edge on the graph may be linear in form while another may be differential. This has the benefit of allowing for both complex relationships between variables as well as simplistic ones. In this way one could craft a model in which two variables are linearly related and a third is dependent on the variance of another variable (a particularly odd formulation, but one which is relevant to behavioral theory). Unfortunately, this approach also means that a table of formulations must now be included with our graph to show the meaning of each edge in the graph. Consider for example the table below for Graph 2:

Node	Formulation
B	$coeff_{ab}A(t) + coeff_{cb}C(t) + cosnst_b$
D	$coeff_{cd}C(t - \theta_{cd}) - \tau_d\frac{dD}{dt} + const_d$

If a fixed number of functional forms is adhered to, the graph can be made to visually represent these functional forms through the use of different node icon shapes. This approach quickly begins to resemble applications which use flow-based programming. Indeed, they are quite similar in their approach, and the specification of a CHBM is quite similar to the writing of a program.

In conclusion, we propose that an CHBM should be specified using the following rules (1) use a graph-wide formula assumption if possible, else specify formulations for each node individually, (2) when choosing a formulation, consistency between nodes is most important, (3) when choosing a formulation, simplicity and clarity is second only to consistency.

4 Benefits of CHBM-enabled JiTAIs

This section discusses the utility of a CHBM throughout the lifecycle of a JiTAI application. Hypothetical situations are posed to highlight the potential value of CHBM use in the JiTAI development process and show open challenges through establishment of a target user group model, application design, application implementation, data analysis, model personalization, and model iteration.

4.1 *A Priori* CHBMs

Prior to development of a JiTAI, a mental model of the target user group is established. This *a priori* model represents the researcher's understanding of the user group, and the design of the intervention utilizes the model in order to predict user actions. This level of detail to which this model is documented varies greatly between applications, and in some cases the causal descriptive model has little grounding in existing behavioral theory [13]. Nevertheless, a vague description of expected user behaviors and interactions with the persuasive technology still represents a user model. Existing JiTAI-like applications may not have a CHBM, but they always (sometimes informally) imply a CHBM. This section highlights the benefits of defining a CHBM explicitly, rather than relying on implicit behavioral theory.

Model Building. When model-building for a JiTAI, the planned system and underlying model of human behavior becomes very complicated, and user responses may be difficult to predict through thought experiments. Without a concrete framework to describe the model, user behavior becomes oversimplified, giving an even less accurate picture of the complex human system. When a model is under-developed, the application development process will open unaddressed questions and simple assumptions will be made. For instance, delivery of a treatment may be limited to the waking hours or to the weekdays, but this will not be reflected in the described user model. The mismatch between the documented theoretical model and the actually implemented model further muddle the process of study replication and analysis.

In addition to those assumptions knowingly made by application developers, causal descriptive modeling often contains implicit assumptions which are easily overlooked. For instance, the delay between a cause and effect is frequently neglected — that is: how quickly does a participant's behavior respond to an treatment? The process of defining a more detailed a priori model itself can lead to new insights and research questions by eliminating these oversights and forcing critical thinking on the assumptions being made.

Intervention Design. When designing intervention options for a JiTAI application, researchers will consider how a treatment influences the subject in the context of the chosen user model. When using a CHBM, this means quantifying the treatment's effect on user context. For instance, consider an intervention which provides information about the health repercussions of sedentary behavior. Assuming our CHBM uses an adaptation of the Theory of Planned Behavior [1], this intervention targets *behavioral belief* regarding sedentary behavior. Since behavioral belief is part of the internal state and the treatment should be defined as part of the user's context, a context variable should be included in our model to represent external influences on behavioral belief from the environment. After defining the expected effect of a single treatment, the CHBM can then be used to predict a detailed account of user response. The use of simulations such as this in the process of designing controls is well-explored in many other areas, but is nearly unheard of in behavioral science. This is in part due to the prevalence of abstract causal descriptive models and the novelty of CHBMs, but there remain several important issues highlighted below which have not yet been addressed in this space.

Benefits of CHBMs in Persuasive Design:

1. By using a CHBM with dynamical equations, the dynamics of relationships between variables can be explicitly described as a part of the model.
2. The use of an explicit a priori model for intervention design helps researchers formulate testable research questions and experiment designs.
3. The additional pre-study detail removes post-study modeling assumptions that can dilute the underlying behavioral theory or invalidate study results.
4. The process of defining a CHBM itself can lead to new insights and research questions which are almost entirely unaddressed by existing theory.

Open Questions for CHBM-Empowered Persuasive Design:

1. The process of defining a CHBM requires detailed knowledge of both the underlying behavioral theory and the mathematics. Relatively few researchers today possess the necessary skillset.
2. Modeling software exists for other engineering domains, but is not directly applicable to the problem of CHBM development.
3. Software for running simulations to test the function of an *a priori* CHBM is non-existent.
4. Methodologies for creating an *a priori* CHBM are not fully established, and mappings from existing causal descriptive models may be model-dependent.
5. The definition of a treatment's effect on a user is a subjective process. That is: how is one to know what amount of behavioral belief a specific "sedentary activity fact treatment" imparts?
6. In order to get a more realistic look at user responses to an treatments, many simulations with varying parameters set to match the expectations of the researchers should be run and analyzed; this would require a CHBM simulation software suite that does not yet exist.

4.2   CHBMs at Run-Time

In this section methods in which CHBMs may be used in the persuasive technology itself are discussed. Options include model-based intervention optimization, timing, and online ideographic modeling.

A crucial step in the development of a persuasive technology today is to establish a set of *decision rules* based on behavioral theory which codify the circumstances in which a treatment should or should not be delivered. For instance, a treatment might be delivered only during the daytime, right before a meal, only in a particular location, or in response to a behavioral event such as cigarette use. Establishing a set of decision rules for a small number of conditions is feasible for a simple intervention, but as the number of conditions increases the number of rules required increases combinatorially. Even worse, when making use of adaptive interventions this set of rules must be expanded even further to map between all possible contexts and intervention permutations. Relying on simple decision rules loosely guided by existing theory to define the optimization of intervention delivery to control a complex system inevitably leads to under-optimized interventions, over-simplified models, and weakened data. An additional problem with this approach is the use of a binary state (i.e. rule satisfied or not) to optimize delivery over a continuous time. Because of this oversimplification, rules which govern the behavior often become part of the theory underlying the application and are clumsily expressed as decision rules. In contrast, optimization of treatment delivery using a CHBM can be done algorithmically to minimize the area between the desired and observed target behavior.

Because CHBMs are computational in nature, prediction of behavior is possible given information about the user's present and future context. Furthermore, because the behaviors in computational models are quantitative, an application could search available treatment options to find one which produces the ideal amount of a target behavior. Methods for model predictive control are a well studied topic of control systems engineering, but many methods cannot be applied to generic formulations. Without a constrained form to guide optimization, all possible options must be explored with equal feasibility in a brute-force search. With sufficient computational power this is effective for simple problems, but this approach becomes increasingly infeasible as the number of options and the number of future steps to be considered increase. If the functional form describing variable relationships is constrained appropriately, however, mathematical optimizations methods can greatly simplify this problem. Applications of model-predictive control over intervention delivery have been explored for gestational weight gain [8], smoking cessation [16], and fibromyalgia treatment [6] by limiting the functional form of the CHBM specification to a differential equation based on a fluid-flow analogy. In this way, application creators can implement software utilizing the advanced understanding of behavioral science described by the CHBM, without direct knowledge of the underlying behavioral science.

Benefits of CHBMs for Persuasive Applications:

1. Using a CHBM enables the use of optimization algorithms instead of decision rules. This change is needed to apply complex control over target behaviors.
2. CHBMs can be adapted to fit a user's needs at run-time, establishing an idiographic model of each subject from the generalized CHBM.

Open Questions for CHBM-enabled Persuasive Applications:

1. Optimization of intervention delivery can be computationally expensive unless the functional form of modelling is restricted, and it is not yet clear what formulations are most appropriate for behavioral construct relationships.

4.3   CHBMs Post-Study

Another rising challenge for persuasive technology researchers is the increasing complexity of data analysis methods needed to handle large amounts of "in the wild" data. Techniques designed to simplify construct relationships using statistical inferences between distinct groups of measurements cannot address emerging research questions which span the full spectrum of subject demographics, situational context, and time-scale. Contemporary approaches apply data mining and machine learning techniques to fit more advanced models to study data and identify key factors, but findings revealed in these exercises can be difficult to generalize and interpret. By using a model as the hypothesis of an experiment rather than focusing solely on a particular relationship between two variables in specific conditions, research findings can be generalized more easily to practical persuasive applications. Methods for evaluating models, rather than evaluating correlation between two variables should be increasingly focused upon in the analysis of behavioral data. While analysis of correlation between variables looks at the statistical relationship between groups of data points, the evaluation of a model involves comparing the experimental data to the predictions of the model. CHBMs can be used with contextual data to produce a time series of expected behavioral outcomes throughout the study. The simulated "theoretical data" can then be directly compared to the "observed data" to observe how the theory differs from the reality. The process of comparing theoretical predictions to empirical data can be repeated with simulations from alternate theories and a goodness-of-fit metric can be used to evaluate the hypothesis against alternatives. Additionally, unification of existing behavioral models into this common paradigm would enable better collaboration between proponents of different theories.

Benefits of CHBMs Post-Experiment:

1. Analysis of experimental data can shift focus from individual construct relationships to a larger view, evaluating the model as a hypothesis.
2. Comparison between different theories can be informed by a comparison of their respective models using a goodness-of-fit metric against empirical data.
3. The use of CHBMs makes re-use of theory and therefore collaborative improvement on existing theories easier — reversing the existing paradigm which has lead to a dizzying multitude of fragmented theories and sub-theories.

Open Questions for CHBM Post-Experiment Methods:

1. Methods for fitting a model to experimental data require restrictions on the functional form of the relationships between variables, and the optimum functional form is not yet obvious.
2. Methods for evaluating the goodness-of-fit between empirical and simulated data exist, but cutting-edge software for exploring the intricacies of data mismatch may be difficult to apply to this use-case.

5   Conclusion

In this paper we have offered supporting terminology, the CHBM formalization, and a set of open challenges to promote the interdisciplinary discussion needed to push forward the emerging field of JiTAI engineering. The progression of behavioral science towards computational modeling has progressed more slowly than in other scientific domains because of the limited amount of detailed, time-intensive contextual and behavioral measures available. This progression from causal descriptive modeling to causal explanatory modeling and increased mathematical rigor is a natural progression which parallels historical trends in the natural sciences. Now that behavioral and contextual data is becoming accessible, we should expect to see a similar paradigm shift in the behavioral sciences. It is our hope that this formative work towards Computational Human Behavior Modeling and the methods highlighted here act as a jumping-off point for others on the forefront of this impending paradigm shift who can use these methods to unlock the power of context-aware persuasive application driven by CHBMs.

References

1. Ajzen, I.: The theory of planned behavior. Organ. Behav. Hum. Decis. Process. **50**(2), 179–211 (1991)
2. Beck, C., McSweeney, J.C., Richards, K.C., Roberson, P.K., Tsai, P.F., Souder, E.: Challenges in tailored intervention research. Nurs. outlook **58**(2), 104–110 (2010)
3. Brailsford, S.C., Desai, S.M., Viana, J.: Towards the holy grail: combining system dynamics and discrete-event simulation in healthcare. In: Proceedings of the 2010 Winter Simulation Conference (WSC), pp. 2293–2303. IEEE (2010)
4. Collins, L.M., Murphy, S.A., Bierman, K.L.: A conceptual framework for adaptive preventive interventions. Prev. Sci. **5**(3), 185–196 (2004)
5. Dallery, J., Raiff, B.R.: Optimizing behavioral health interventions with single-case designs: from development to dissemination. Transl. Behav. Med. **4**(3), 290–303 (2014)
6. Deshpande, S., Nandola, N.N., Rivera, D.E., Younger, J.W.: Optimized treatment of fibromyalgia using system identification and hybrid model predictive control. Control Eng. Pract. **33**, 161–173 (2014)
7. Dong, Y., Rivera, D.E., Thomas, D.M., Navarro-Barrientos, J.E., Downs, D.S., Savage, J.S., Collins, L.M.: A dynamical systems model for improving gestational weight gain behavioral interventions. In: 2012 American Control Conference (ACC), pp. 4059–4064. IEEE (2012)
8. Dong, Y., Rivera, D.E., Downs, D.S., Savage, J.S., Thomas, D.M., Collins, L.M.: Hybrid model predictive control for optimizing gestational weight gain behavioral interventions. In: 2013 American Control Conference (ACC), pp. 1970–1975. IEEE (2013)
9. Hekler, E.B., Klasnja, P., Traver, V., Hendriks, M.: Realizing effective behavioral management of health: the metamorphosis of behavioral science methods. IEEE Pulse **4**(5), 29–34 (2013)
10. Kaptein, M.C.: Formalizing customization in persuasive technologies. In: MacTavish, T., Basapur, S. (eds.) PERSUASIVE 2015. LNCS, vol. 9072, pp. 27–38. Springer, Heidelberg (2015)
11. Nahum-Shani, I., Hekler, E.B., Spruijt-Metz, D.: Building health behavior models to guide the development of just-in-time adaptive interventions: a pragmatic framework. Health Psychology (2015)
12. Nahum-Shani, I., Smith, S.N., Tewari, A., Witkiewitz, K., Collins, L.M., Spring, B., Murphy, S.: Just in time adaptive interventions (jitais): an organizing framework for ongoing health behavior support. Methodology Center Technical report, pp. 14–126 (2014)
13. Prestwich, A., Sniehotta, F.F., Whittington, C., Dombrowski, S.U., Rogers, L., Michie, S.: Does theory influence the effectiveness of health behavior interventions? Meta-analysis. Health Psychol. **33**(5), 465 (2014)
14. Riley, W.T., Rivera, D.E., Atienza, A.A., Nilsen, W., Allison, S.M., Mermelstein, R.: Health behavior models in the age of mobile interventions: are our theories up to the task? Transl. Behav. Med. **1**(1), 53–71 (2011)
15. Shiffman, S., Stone, A.A., Hufford, M.R.: Ecological momentary assessment. Annu. Rev. Clin. Psychol. **4**, 1–32 (2008)
16. Timms, K.P., Rivera, D.E., Piper, M.E., Collins, L.M.: A hybrid model predictive control strategy for optimizing a smoking cessation intervention. In: 2014 American Control Conference (ACC), pp. 2389–2394. IEEE. (2014)

The Persuasive Potential Questionnaire (PPQ): Challenges, Drawbacks, and Lessons Learned

Alexander Meschtscherjakov[✉], Magdalena Gärtner,
Alexander Mirnig, Christina Rödel, and Manfred Tscheligi

Christian-Doppler-Laboratory "Contextual Interfaces", Center for HCI,
Department of Computer Sciences, University of Salzburg, Salzburg, Austria
{alexander.meschtscherjakov,magdalena.gaertner,
alexander.mirnig,christina.roedel,
manfred.tscheligi}@sbg.ac.at

Abstract. Measuring the potential persuasive effect of non-fully functional prototypes is important in a user-centered design process. A tool for measuring this persuasive potential should be deployable regardless of the persuasive goal, be suited for a generic context, and be targeted at different user groups. In this paper, we make a first step towards such an all-encompassing, quick and easy-to-use tool to measure the potential of persuasive systems: the Persuasive Potential Questionnaire (PPQ). We outline the development stages of the PPQ. A literature analysis led to five dimensions characterizing the persuasive potential of a system. We then formulated 50 items for the PPQ in an iterative generation process and conducted an online survey with 94 participants. Based on a statistical analysis, we propose a first version of the PPQ with 3 dimensions and 15 items. We conclude with a reflection on the identified benefits and drawbacks regarding the current iteration of the PPQ.

Keywords: Methods · Persuasion · Questionnaire

1 Introduction

Measuring the long-term persuasive effect of a system designed to change behaviors can be difficult. It is even more difficult to evaluate the persuasive potential of a persuasive technology, which is not fully developed, and, thus, cannot be incorporated into everyday activities over time. Yet, in early phases of a user-centered design process it may be beneficial to assess the potentials of a proposed persuasive technology even though the system itself is not or only partially implemented at that point.

At the moment, no universally applicable questionnaire to measure both the persuasive potential of not (yet) applicable systems and the persuasive effect of already applicable systems is available. The persuasive research community identified a need for such universal tools, especially to be able to measure and compare the effects of persuasive systems in a generalized way [11]. Of course, some general assessment tools and questionnaires already exist within the community, but overall, these tools either focus on specific strategies (e.g., [8]) or only have validity for one specific system in one specific study context (e.g., [2, 6, 16]). The potential of persuasive systems is often

© Springer International Publishing Switzerland 2016
A. Meschtscherjakov et al. (Eds.): PERSUASIVE 2016, LNCS 9638, pp. 162–175, 2016.
DOI: 10.1007/978-3-319-31510-2_14

determined simply by behavior observation, user self-reporting (e.g., [8]), self-reflection (e.g., [14]), as well as counting (e.g., [3]). Lehto et al. [10] have presented a theoretical model of factors affecting perceived persuasiveness of behavior change support systems based on Oinas-Kukkonen and Harjumaa's Persuasive Systems Design Model (PSD) [12]. They presented a model predicting perceived persuasiveness that may be utilized in various of domains.

If we want to be able to not only measure the potential effect of one system, but also compare different systems regarding their persuasive effects (and their success or lack thereof), a standardized means is necessary. Such a measurement tool should ideally be able to assess persuasive systems regardless of the targeted user group, utilized persuasive strategies, or context in which it is deployed and the complexity of the system itself. A persuasive system might work differently for different user groups, and there exist many persuasive systems to foster the same persuasive goal but employ different strategies, as has been shown (e.g., [9]). Also, the context in which the persuasive system is embedded plays a major role for the success of the system. All of these aspects need to be taken into account when measuring and comparing persuasive systems on a general level.

The overall goal we had in mind was to develop a Persuasive Potential Questionnaire (PPQ) to measure the potential persuasive effect of a system, which is quickly applicable, easy to use for researchers and system users, and open enough regarding the questions it contains to be suitable for all kinds of systems. The PPQ should be:

Item Conservative: The PPQ should be relatively quick and easy to use. A high number of items increase study and evaluation times exponentially. We, therefore, aimed at keeping the item count as low as possible, with a number of 20 items as our first concrete target.

Context Agnostic: Tools and methods that are tailored towards a specific context are often ill-suited to be applied to any other than their originally intended context. The PPQ, therefore, had to be context-agnostic, i.e., either be powerful enough to measure the persuasive effects of a system regardless of the context it is used in *or* be able to accommodate relevant context variables.

User Agnostic: Similar to the previous goal, the PPQ should not depend on or target only one or a number of specific user groups. It needs to be usable either regardless of intended users or be able to accommodate any number of different user groups and their most relevant influence factors.

With these goals in mind, we set out to develop the PPQ in a multi-stage iterative process. We started with an extensive literature analysis and utilized various acceptance, adoption, and persuasion models creating five dimensions characterizing the persuasive potential of a system. In an interdisciplinary item construction workshop, we developed 161 items for these five dimensions. Through a rating process, we selected 50 items to be evaluated in an online questionnaire. The analysis led us to a 3-dimension questionnaire with 15 items. Figure 1 illustrates this process.

In the following we will outline the development stages that led to the present iteration of the PPQ (Sect. 2), present the analysis and results of a first evaluation round

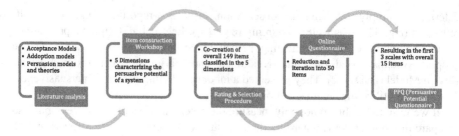

Fig. 1. Development process of the PPQ.

(Sect. 3), discuss challenges, drawbacks, and lessons learned from the development process (Sect. 4), and conclude with an overall summary (Sect. 5).

2 Development of the Questionnaire

2.1 Development of Five Dimensions

Starting point for the questionnaire development was the definition of different dimensions important for a successful persuasive system. As a base, we used the Technology Acceptance model (TAM) by Davis' et al. [5]. This model describes how users come to accept and use a specific technology. In a nutshell, it states that the perceived usefulness of a system and its perceived ease-of use influence the attitude towards using a system, which then again leads to a behavioral intention to use the system, as well as its actual usage. We also used the Unified Theory of Acceptance and Use of Technology (UTAUT) - an extension of the TAM, which states that various factors such as the user's experience and voluntariness, as well as external factors [17], influence the user acceptance and willingness to use a system.

Additionally, our approach was inspired by Lehto and colleagues' [10] structural model for behavior change support systems. Their model consists of eight constructs: primary task support, dialogue support, perceived credibility, design aesthetics, perceived persuasiveness, unobtrusiveness, intention to use, and actual use. They also present measurement items for each of the constructs.

Based on these models three researchers from our department (one psychologist, one communication scientist, and one computer scientist), all researching in the area of persuasive technologies, conducted several informal workshops, which led to five dimensions possibly capable of measuring the persuasive potential of a system.

These five dimensions are:

1. *Persuasion Attitude (PA)*
2. *Perceived Persuasive System Potential (PPSP)*
3. *Perceived Persuasive Individual Potential (PPIP)*
4. *Intention to Use the System (IUS)*, and
5. *Intention to Change Behavior (ICB)*.

The *PA* dimension is intended to measure someone's susceptibility to, and attitude on, persuasive efforts in general. The assumption behind this dimension is that the level of persuadability is different for each individual (see e.g., [4]). We are interested in the general susceptibility towards persuasion and not necessarily towards specific persuasive strategies as highlighted by Kaptein [9]. The *PPSP* dimension is based on the assumption that users of persuasive systems experience the persuasive strategies and efforts a persuasive system is build upon and, therefore, can rate the persuasive potential of the system factually from a user's perspective. This is motivated by Petty and Cacioppo's Elaboration likelihood model (ELM) [13]. Based on cognitive processes via the central route of persuasion, users may assign a general persuasive potential to the system not necessarily suited for them. The *PPIP* dimension, on the other hand, is intended to measure the degree to which participants assess the system's persuasive potential from their personal, subjective perspective. This is also reflected in Lehto et al. [10] construct of "perceived persuasiveness". The *IUS* dimension is defined to measure how willing and motivated users are to keep using the persuasive system from a short- and long-term perspective. This is a crucial factor in many acceptance models (e.g., [5, 17]). Finally, The *ICB* dimension is intended to capture the effectiveness of the persuasive system by capturing the users' true intention to change their behavior as an effect of using the system. This dimension is based on Ajzen's [1] theory of planned behavior. In this model, behavioral intention is an indication of an individual's readiness to perform a certain behavior. Table 1 summarizes the five dimensions and sources used to create them.

Table 1. Five dimensions characterizing the persuasive potential of a system and sources we used to create them.

Dimensions	Sources
D1: Persuasion Attitude (PA)	Busch et al., 2013 [4], Kaptein, 2012 [9], Kaptein et al., 2011 [7]
D2: Perceived Persuasive System Potential (PPSP)	Petty & Cacioppo, 1986 [13]
D3: Perceived Persuasive Individual Potential (PPIP)	Petty & Cacioppo, 1986 [13], Lehto et al., 2012 [10]
D4: Intention to Use the System (IUS)	Davis et al., 1989 [5], Venkatesh et al., 2003 [17], Lehto et al., 2012 [10]
D5: Intention to Change Behavior (ICB)	Ajzen, 1991 [1], Lehto et al., 2012 [10]

2.2 Creation of 50 Items

In a second step, a workshop was conducted in which we made use of Method 635 [15], a more structured variation of the brainstorming technique, to create the items for the pre-defined dimensions. Method 635 was applied as follows: Six human-computer-interaction experts with differing scientific background were instructed to develop items for each of the five aforementioned dimensions, which were to form the basis for the persuasive potential questionnaire (PPQ). To do so, participants were introduced to each dimension and its meaning and then asked to write down three items, i.e. statements, they thought would fit with regard to capturing the meaning of the dimension. After doing so, the three items were passed on to the next participant, who read them and then wrote down another three items. After five rounds of passing along the written notes, item-collection was finished for one dimension. We continued this procedure for all five dimensions. Then, the collected items were presented to all participants to trigger a debate to reconsider, revise or remove the items.

Overall, we collected 149 items; 27 items in the *PA* dimension, 21 items in the *PPSP* dimension, 42 items in the *PPIP* dimension, 24 items in the *IUS* dimension, and 35 items in the *ICB* dimension. The number of items was then further reduced based on the individual rating of three experts in the field of persuasion theory, who evaluated the contribution of every single item to capture the meaning of the corresponding dimension. First, the three experts rated each item individually, then they conducted a separate workshop in which they discussed their ratings, reformulated items were necessary and reduced the number of items to 10 items per dimension, which led to an overall number of 50 items. Finally, the dimensions were renamed, to capture the associated items in a more self-explanatory way.

The PA dimension was renamed to *Susceptibility to Persuasion* (*SP*), the PPSP dimension was renamed to *General Persuasive Potential* of the system (GPP), the PPIP dimension was renamed to *Individual Persuasive Potential* of the system (IPP), and the ICB dimension was renamed to *System Influence on Behavioral Change* (SIBC). The *IUS* dimension remained the same. These tentative items and corresponding dimensions are shown in Table 3 in the Appendix.

2.3   Questionnaire Creation

In order to evaluate the proposed items and to analyze whether items load to the proposed factors, we conducted an online analysis. Items were ordered in a random order and entered into the online questionnaire tool lime survey (www.limesurvey.at). In order to enable study participants to answer the proposed items of the questionnaire we had to describe a potential persuasive system in a fictive scenario.

The scenario introduced the "Healthy Me" application for smartphones (see Fig. 2). Study participants were encouraged to imagine that this application would actively support them in leading a healthier lifestyle. To facilitate the participants' imagination process, the scenario was written in a lively way, so every participant could easily connect with the scenario's content. For example, the "Healthy Me" application was not limited to supporting its users in losing weight, in case this was nothing the participants were interested in, but it was presented as a universally applicable tool, which could support its user in the improvement of every life circumstances, he or she wished for (e.g., weight reduction, quitting smoking, doing more sports, balanced, and healthier nutrition, etc.).

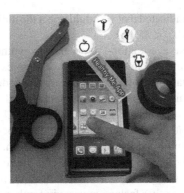

Fig. 2. The picture illustrates the "Healthy Me" Application, the fictional persuasive system, which the scenario of the questionnaire was based on.

Participants were then provided with a concrete scenario. *"Imagine you want to do more sports to increase your personal fitness level. The "Healthy Me" App is supporting you to reach this goal. For example, it suggests to go jogging two to three times a week with a maximum pulse of 150 heartbeats a minute. Additionally, "Healthy Me" recommends to do some strength exercises to buildup some muscles. As you are especially fond of training the upper parts of your body, the app suggests some exercises with dumbbells and floor exercises. After each training session, you record data like duration of training, intensity of training, and frequency of repetitions with the application. "Healthy Me" processes this data to analyze your training program and adapt it to your personal goals. A curve diagram informs you about your progress and steps back over time. Progress is rewarded with cheering up like "You're pretty quick, you did the 5 km in less than 45 min today!" If you are losing sight of your goal, e.g., stopped training for some time, "Healthy Me" encourages you not to give up and defines new interim goals to increase your motivation again."*

After reading the scenario, participants had to rate the questionnaire items on a 7-point Likert scale from *completely disagree* to *completely agree*. A first pre-test with five participants proved the questionnaire to be deployable, so the study was announced through our universities and other email lists. Overall, 94 people participated in the online study. Among participants, five €10 Amazon vouchers were raffled.

3   Analysis

When we developed the questionnaire, we had defined five dimensions, which we considered to be crucially contributing to the persuasive potential of a system. Yet, the actual factorial structure of the dimensions was still to be examined. Further, our aim was the reduction of the 50 existing items to provide a quick and easy-to-use measurement tool. Therefore, we explored the underlying factors of our items by calculating a common-factor analysis. From the results of measures of sampling adequacy, we derived an excellent appropriateness of our data for factor analyses. The Kaiser-Meyer-Olkin measure suggested that the sample was very well factorable (KMO = .907) and the

Bartlett's test of sphericity indicated that we could reject the null hypothesis of an identity matrix ($\chi 2(1225) = 4525.22$, $p < .001$).

Initially, we conducted a common-factor-analysis without presetting a certain number of factors to be extracted. In the settings, we suppressed those factor loadings smaller than .3 and used varimax rotations of the factor-loading matrix. Based on the Kaiser-Guttman-criterion, an 8-factor solution was suggested with eight factors having eigen values above one. In sum, those 8 factors explained 73.85 % of the total variance. The communalities of our items were all above .3, which, besides the high amount of explained total variance, confirmed the factorability of them.

Nevertheless, we noted different problems in this factorial structure. First, the scree plot indicated a maximum number of 3–4 factors. Second, most items loaded on the first four factors, whereas the other factors consisted of only a few items. Third, several items did not show clear primary factor loadings on one factor, indicating a weak and ambiguous definition. Analyzing these problematic items, we detected that almost all of them belonged to our predefined *SP* dimension. Considering these inconsistencies, we examined a three, four, and five factors solution using again varimax rotations of the factor-loading matrix. However, the explained total variance consequently decreased to 59,65 %, 63,66 % and 66,97 %. These solutions resulted in even more ambiguous factor loadings of several items of the susceptibility dimension. We concluded that our original dimension did not represent one personality factor but consisted of many different dimensions, which themselves built separated factors.

Before excluding problematic and redundant items in a next step and conducting factor analyses again, we wanted to investigate the consistency of our original dimensions. We considered this to be an additional decision aid for the following selection of items. Therefore, we conducted several item analyses. Since our questionnaire does not represent a power test, we tested the items only on their internal consistency and not on their difficulty or discrimination power, in order to determine whether the items measured one dimension. Using reliability analysis, we obtained a Cronbach's Alpha of .73 – .95 across the five dimensions, which indicates a very high homogeneity for each dimension. However, the reliability of the *SP* dimension turned out to be lowest in comparison to the others, probably being the consequence of some very low item correlations with the dimension.

We excluded items stepwise, which showed the lowest item-dimension correlations. This resulted in a dimension of four items and an increase of Cronbach's Alpha of the *SP* dimension from .73 to .80. The item reduction across the remaining dimensions was based on content decisions on one hand and statistical decisions derived from the previous factor analyses on the other. Thus, we selected those items of which were, among the others, best verbalized and loaded clearly and highly on one factor. Finally, we again conducted a common factor analysis with the selected items. The loadings of these remaining 15 items showed clear simple-structure solutions with substantial loadings above .5 on one primary factor and negligible secondary loadings on the two other factors.

The first factor includes eight items, which were assigned beforehand to three different dimensions, namely the *SIBC*, the *IUS*, and the *IPP* dimension. Due to the factor analysis, *SIBC* and *IUS* dimensions are now summarized under the *Individual Persuasive Potential* of the system (*IPP*) dimension, meaning the persuasive impact the system has on the single user. The second factor includes three items and is summarized by the *General Persuasive Potential* of the system (*GPP*) dimension, meaning the potentially persuasive impact of the system on any user. Finally, the third factor includes four items and is summarized by the *Susceptibility to Persuasion* by others (*SP*) dimension. This factor represents one personality dimension of the user, which reveals if he/she is easily or hardly influenced by other people which as a consequence may allow to draw conclusions on whether he/she is also easily or hardly persuaded by a system. To prove or falsify this correlation still remains an objective for future iterations of the PPQ questionnaire. Table 2 shows the iterated version of the PPQ.

Table 2. Iterated PPQ questionnaire consisting of 15 items and the three dimensions Susceptibility to Persuasion (SP), General Persuasive Potential of the System (GPP), Individual Persuasive Potential of the System (IPP).

New Dimension	Old Dimension	Item
SP_1	SP_1	What others say brings me to rethink my attitude towards it.
SP_2	SP _2	I do not want to be influenced by others.
SP_3	SP _4	Even my friends have difficulties to influence me.
SP_4	SP _8	No one can tell me what to do.
GPP_1	GPP_1	The system makes people change their behavior.
GPP_2	GPP_2	The system has the potential to influence people.
GPP_3	GPP_5	The system gives the behavior of its users a new direction.
IPP_1	IPP_7	This system is exactly what I need to change my attitude.
IPP_2	IPP_8	Thanks to the system I reach my goals.
IPP_3	IUS_4	I will use this system as often as possible.
IPP_4	IUS_7	I think that I will also use such a system in the future.
IPP_5	IUS_10	I will use this system regularly.
IPP_6	SIBC_2	This system does not cause a change in behavior with me.
IPP_7	SIBC_6	This system causes me to do some things differently.
IPP_8	SIBC_10	With the help of the system, I will behave differently in the future.

3.1 Results of Our Sample

Overall, 94 participants took part in our online-study (70 female, 24 male). They were aged between 15 and 61 years (M = 30.05, SD = 10.60) with most of them (85) having a secondary school qualification or even a university degree. Most of them have not had experiences with a fitness application such as "Healthy Me" before. When analyzing the three dimensions of the PPQ, we found that people in our sample scored rather above average with regard to their susceptibility to be persuaded by others

(M = 3.90, SD = 0.81). They stated a relatively high general persuasive potential of "Healthy Me" (M = 4.48, SD = 1.28). However, the individual persuasive potential of "Healthy Me" was considered to be only average. Thus, we assume that people can distinguish between the general potential of a persuasive system and susceptible they would be themselves. Further, they strengthen our pre-assumption that constructing separate dimensions asking for the general potential of a system and for the actual effect of the system on people's own attitude and behavior is reasonable. In order to check for requirements of the following statistical tests and to make a statement about the generalizability of our data we tested our sample on the assumption of normal distribution. The Kolmogorov-Smirnov tests show that our data are normally distributed.

In a next step, we were interested in whether the individual level of persuadability of people on our *SP* dimension influences their opinion of the general and individual persuasive potential of the tested system. Therefore, we conducted t-tests for independent samples and calculated group comparisons. We made a median split for the *SP* dimension, which served as independent variable, thus comparing people scoring low with people scoring high on that dimension. Dependent variables were the general (*GPP*) and individual (*IPP*) persuasive potential of the system. We found a highly significant difference concerning the individual persuasive potential of the system between people who are sparsely susceptible of persuasion by others and people who are highly susceptible to persuasion by others ($t(92) = 4.11$, $p < .001$). People, who are sparsely susceptible to persuasion by others, show a higher individual persuasive potential by the system than people who are highly susceptible to persuasion by others, meaning that the system has more influence on people, who are less susceptible to social persuasion. Although, this result might seem paradoxical at first sight, a logical explanation for this effect can be that susceptibility of persuasion by others does not necessarily include the same extent of susceptibility of persuasion by systems. Both kinds of persuasion might rather be seen as competing constructs, which exclude each other or are at least not activated at the same time to the same extent. As such, people might either follow advice of other people, such as friends or they have more trust in technological systems but not both.

In order to determine whether *SP* can even serve as a predictor for GPP and IPP, we calculated linear regression analyses with SP as predictor and GPP and IPP as criterion variables. Our results indicate that susceptibility of persuasion by others significantly predicts the general ($b = .54$, $t(92) = 6.20$, $p < .001$) and individual persuasive potential of a system, $b = -.39$, $t(92) = -4.08$, $p < .001$. SP also explained a significant proportion of variance in GPP ($R^2 = .30$, $F(1,92) = 38.45$, $p < .001$) and IPP ($R^2 = .15$, $F(1,92) = 16.61$, $p < .001$) scores. However, the explained proportion of variance, especially concerning IPP, is comparatively small. This indicates that our SP-dimension only covers a small range of factors that contribute to whether the persuasive potential of a system is able to influence the single user or not. We further suggest that even the user's personality and its influence is, to such an extent, diversified that such a narrow personality dimension like ours can impossibly capture the dimensions which actually contribute to the persuasive potential of a system.

Developing a broad and extensive dimension including the different personality aspects would, therefore, be of great relevance in a further iteration of the PPQ.

4 Discussion

This first iteration of the PPQ has confronted us with challenges, drawbacks, and lessons learned. In the following we discuss concrete areas for improvement of the PPQ and findings regarding the potential persuasive effect of a system in general.

4.1 It's all About One's Personality: Traits and Persuadability

The persuasive strength of a system strongly depends on how well the user responds to the persuasive strategies employed. Not all strategies work equally well for everyone, which is why persuasive strategies need to be chosen depending on the targeted demographic and their expected personality spectrum as shown by Kaptein [9]. For the PPQ, we tried to incorporate a person's susceptibility to persuasive strategies in the Susceptibility to Persuasion (SP) dimension. We are aware that this approach reduces the complexity of personality traits in favor of a simple and short questionnaire. But as it turned out, brevity is not quite such a virtue when it comes to assessing personalities. Our personality dimension was too narrow and subsequently inadequate to capture all or most relevant personality factors for the persuasive success of a system. We found that a truly universal questionnaire requires a more broad and detailed personality dimension, containing a much greater number of items than ours had. Of course, this is contrary to the initial goal to keep the item count to a maximum of 20, but it is a necessary modification if we want to achieve the goal of being user agnostic. One can impossibly predict the whole range of potential users of a system, but what one can do is providing a comprehensive personality spectrum, which ultimately serves the same goal of clustering users into persuasion-relevant groups. The immediate next step in this regard is, therefore, the development of a broad and extensive personality dimension for the following iteration(s) of the PPQ.

4.2 Deployment and Validation of the PPQ

Regarding methodology, we have to mention that we used a fictive scenario in the healthcare domain to evaluate the first version of our questionnaire in the online survey. We deliberately formulated this scenario as general as possible. Nonetheless, the scenario might have had an influence on the answers given and therefore the reliability of the PPQ. The natural next step, after further iteration and refinements, is to deploy the questionnaire to evaluate an actually existing system the users can really interact with, but from the same domain. The PPQ is not, however, targeted at only healthcare-related persuasive systems, but *any* system with a persuasive effect. Therefore, the PPQ also needs to be evaluated in a wider number of different contexts in order to show whether it produces adequate data in all of these contexts as well. This is a continuous process, which will accompany the PPQ during its next development and iteration stages. It also is strongly dependent on the community adapting, employing, and criticizing the PPQ in different contexts and with different systems.

4.3   Human- vs. System-Induced Persuasion

Common sense would suggest that a person is either more susceptible to persuasion in general or not. By delineating Individual Persuasive Potential (IPP) from General Persuasive Potential (GPP) and assessing both individually, we found an interesting difference regarding the IPP of a system that contradicts that initial intuition. It appears that people who are highly susceptible to persuasion by others show less persuasive potential by the system than people who are sparsely susceptible to persuasion. This means that for people who are less likely to be influenced by other humans, the better a persuasive technology should work for them. Accordingly, persuasive system strategies cannot mimic human persuasion strategies on-to-one and hope for success, nor can they be measured on the same level. Both system and human persuasion appear to operate on different levels, with different activators and factors that determine success or failure. It is an interesting insight on its own and also brings to light – by means of practical example – the value of a universal assessment tool, which can accommodate such system- and context-independent findings. Nonetheless, these considerations need to be explored thoroughly in the future.

5   Conclusion

In this paper, we presented the development process and first evaluation round of the PPQ, a universal tool to analyze and measure the persuasive potential of a system. The first iteration presented in this paper is already capable of producing usable results but still requires further testing in different contexts, with different user bases and a wide range of systems. So far the PPQ was only applied in one context. Above that, there are still issues that have to be targeted in further iteration such as the effect of the complexity of the system on the persuasive effect, and how we can predict unconscious persuasion [13].

As a next step it would be interesting to compare the results of the PPQ with the actual persuasive effect of a system in order validate that the PPQ actually predicts the persuasive potential. The PPQ will continue to undergo development and iteration, with an appropriate personality and context dimension as the immediate next step. The Persuasion community is encouraged to put the PPQ to the test for different systems, to help speed along this process.

Acknowledgements. The financial support by the Austrian Federal Ministry of Science, Research and Economy and the National Foundation for Research, Technology and Development is gratefully acknowledged (Christian Doppler Laboratory for "Contextual Interfaces").

Appendix

See Table 3

Table 3. The 50 items generated after the workshop. Each of the 5 dimensions is represent-ed with 10 items: Susceptibility to Persuasion (SP), General Persuasive Potential of the System (GPP), Individual Persuasive Potential of the System (IPP), Intention to Use the System (IUS), System Influence on Behavioral Change (SIBC).

Dimension	Item
SP1	What others say brings me to rethink my attitude towards it.
SP2	I do not want to be influenced by others.
SP3	I'm easily influenced.
SP4	Even my friends have difficulties to influence me.
SP5	I often change my attitude.
SP6	I am open to change.
SP7	I find it difficult to change.
SP8	No one can tell me what to do.
SP9	Changes are part of my everyday life
SP10	I have my principles, which are unchangeable.
GPP_1	The system makes people change their behavior.
GPP_2	The system has the potential to influence people.
GPP_3	The system can not change the attitudes of people.
GPP_4	The system is useless for changing my attitudes.
GPP_5	The system gives the behavior of its users a new direction.
GPP_6	The system has almost no influence on behavior.
GPP_7	If you want to change your own behavior, this system is useful.
GPP_8	This system highly encourages a change in behavior.
GPP_9	This system provides little support for a change in behavior.
GPP_10	Few people will behave differently when using the system.
IPP_1	I find it difficult to change my attitude with the help of this system.
IPP_2	My attitude is not affected by the system.
IPP_3	The system has no potential to change my attitude.
IPP_4	This system helps me to change myself.
IPP_5	I think that this system is well suited to make long-term changes to my attitude.
IPP_6	This system shows me the information that I need to change myself.
IPP_7	This system is exactly what I need to change my attitude.
IPP_8	Thanks to the system I reach my goals.
IPP_9	Even if I use the system, I do not change my attitude.
IPP_10	Without the system, I would not change my attitude.
IUS_1	I have no motivation to use this system.
IUS_2	I'll continue to use this system.
IUS_3	I'll never use this system.

(Continued)

Table 3. (*Continued*)

Dimension	Item
IUS_4	I will use this system as often as possible.
IUS_5	I see no point in using such a system again.
IUS_6	Even if I have this system, I will not use it.
IUS_7	I think that I will also use such a system in the future.
IUS_8	I will not utilize this system, although it could help me.
IUS_9	I hope I can possess and use this system.
IUS_10	I will use this system regularly.
SIBC_1	This system persuades me to change my behavior.
SIBC_2	This system does not cause a change in behavior with me.
SIBC_3	I will change my behavior because of this system.
SIBC_4	I think that I will have sustainable behavior change through use of this system.
SIBC_5	This system does not convince me to actively change my personal behavior.
SIBC_6	This system causes me to do some things differently.
SIBC_7	By using this system, I will not change my behavior.
SIBC_8	The functions of this system do not convince me to change my behavior.
SIBC_9	The system is designed so that I would like to change my behavior.
SIBC_10	With the help of the system, I will behave differently in the future.

References

1. Ajzen, I.: The theory of planned behavior. Organ. Behav. Hum. Decis. Process. **50**(2), 179–211 (1991)
2. Anderson, C., et al.: The persuasive power of oral health promotion messages: a theory of planned behavior approach to dental checkups among young adults. Health Commun. **28**(3), 304–313 (2013)
3. Bleich, S.N., et al.: Reduction in purchases of sugar-sweetened beverages among low-income black adolescents after exposure to caloric information. Am. J. Public Health **102**(2), 329–335 (2012)
4. Busch, M., Schrammel, J., Tscheligi, M.: Personalized persuasive technology – development and validation of scales for measuring persuadability. In: Berkovsky, S., Freyne, J. (eds.) PERSUASIVE 2013. LNCS, vol. 7822, pp. 33–38. Springer, Heidelberg (2013)
5. Davis, F.D., Bagozzi, R.P., Warshaw, P.R.: User acceptance of computer technology: a comparison of two theoretical models. Manage. Sci. **35**, 982–1003 (1989)
6. Hendriks, B., et al.: Style congruency and persuasion: a cross-cultural study into the influence of differences in style dimensions on the persuasiveness of business newsletters in Great Britain and the Netherlands. IEEE Trans. Prof. Commun. **55**(2), 122–141 (2012)
7. Kaptein, M., et al.: Means based adaptive persuasive systems. In: Proceedings of the SIGCHI Conference on Human Factors in Computing Systems, pp. 335–344. ACM (2011)
8. Kaptein, M., et al.: Adaptive persuasive systems: a study of tailored persuasive text messages to reduce snacking. ACM Trans. Interact. Intell. Syst. **2**(2), 10 (2012)
9. Kaptein, M.: Personalized persuasion in ambient intelligence. J. Ambient Intell. Smart Environ. **4**(3), 279–280 (2012)

10. Lehto, T., Oinas-Kukkonen, H., Drozd, F.: Factors affecting perceived persuasiveness of a behavior change support system. In: Proceedings of the 33rd International Conference on Information Systems (2012)
11. Meschtscherjakov, A., et al.: Workshop on persuasive technologies in challenging contexts. In: PT 2014: The 9th International Conference on Persuasive Technology (2014)
12. Oinas-Kukkonen, H., Harjumaa, M.: Persuasive systems design: Key issues, process model, and system features. Commun. Assoc. Inf. Syst. **24**(1), 28 (2009)
13. Petty, R.E., Cacioppo, J.T.: The elaboration likelihood model of persuasion, pp. 1–24. Springer, New York (1986)
14. Ramachandran, D., et al.: Mobile-izing health workers in rural India. In: Proceedings of the SIGCHI Conference on Human Factors in Computing Systems. ACM (2010)
15. Rohrbach, B.: Creative by rules—method 635, a new technique for solving problems. Absatzwirtschaft **12**, 73–75 (1969)
16. Thieme, A., et al.: We've bin watching you: designing for reflection and social persuasion to promote sustainable lifestyles. In: Proceedings of the SIGCHI Conference on Human Factors in Computing Systems. ACM (2012)
17. Venkatesh, V., Morris, M. G., Davis, G.B., and Davis, F.D.: User acceptance of information technology: toward a unified view. MIS quarterly, pp. 425–478 (2003)

Persuasive Practices: Learning from Home Security Advisory Services

Mateusz Dolata[1(✉)], Tino Comes[1], Birgit Schenk[2],
and Gerhard Schwabe[1]

[1] Department of Informatics, University of Zurich, Zurich, Switzerland
{dolata, comes, schwabe}@ifi.uzh.ch
[2] University of Applied Science Ludwigsburg, Ludwigsburg, Germany
schenk@hs-ludwigsburg.de

Abstract. Research on persuasive technologies (PT) focuses, primarily, on the design and development of IT for inducing change of individual's behavior and attitude through computer-human and computer-mediated influence. The issue of practices in co-located human-human persuasive encounters remained unattended in the PT community. This study uses the notion of persuasive practices to understand the course of events in face-to-face home security advisory sessions – it specifies and illustrates such practices and discusses their impact on the persuasiveness of the encounter. Furthermore, it presents potential of IT to support such persuasive practices thus opening new research possibilities of PT research.

Keywords: Advisory encounter · Human-Human influence · Practices · F2F

1 Introduction

Persuasive technologies (PT) are engineered to reinforce, change or shape behaviors and attitudes of individuals towards specific areas of their life [21]. Technology can either directly influence an individual's behavior or, alternatively, act as mediator or moderator of social influence [26], i.e., it transfers information on other's opinions or behaviors. In this study, we explore yet another role that technology plays in the context of persuasion: it can facilitate persuasive practices in situations where human influence is exhibited in a face-to-face encounter. There exists a category of such encounters where considering solely the technology – a view that has dominated in PT community so far – does not resemble the complexity of conducted activities and their effect on the persuasive effect. We postulate, that, in such situations, the IT should not be considered as a standalone factor in the success or failure of persuasion efforts – it is not a *machine* that produces persuasiveness. Instead, it becomes a *tool*, which – if embraced in specific practices – can be very effective and support the change of persuadee's attitude and behaviors [3]. Such perspective on PT helps, in particular, in high-touch situations, i.e., where direct influence between humans through practices comes to the fore. Practices are seeable, indigenous actions that participants directly engage in, but do not attend to them in an analytic manner [7, 18]. Still, practices can be object of systematic analytic approach in research [18] – their consideration in the area of PT is a response to the recent call for the practice-turn in human-computer interaction [13].

© Springer International Publishing Switzerland 2016
A. Meschtscherjakov et al. (Eds.): PERSUASIVE 2016, LNCS 9638, pp. 176–188, 2016.
DOI: 10.1007/978-3-319-31510-2_15

In the current study, we focus on the case of home security (HS) advisory services. It is an encounter between (1) a help-seeking homeowner, who wants to make their property more secure (persuadee), and (2) a professional HS advisor (persuader). Even though persuadees often see the need for improving their home's security, they lack ability and motivation to tackle those issues. HS advisory service shall make it easier for them to reach their goal: its goal is to identify most important flaws and pave the way for improvement through mechanical upgrades and security-aware behavior. However, according to a preliminary study, only 20 % of improvements suggested during the advisory sessions are implemented by the homeowners [24]. Given the reportedly successful application of PT in other difficult areas, e.g., preventive healthcare, we propose to include its basic principles in a HS-dedicated *socio-technical persuasive system*, which we define as an information system designed to reinforce, change or shape persuadee's attitudes or behaviors [20]. It consists of a human persuader who engages in *persuasive practices* with use of his tools such as: IT, brochures, notebooks, and exhibits, as well as objects in their surroundings, e.g., windows and doors at persuadee's home. We understand persuasive practices as practices that exhibit the desire to influence the behavior or attitude of conversation partner. We subscribe to very local and timely-limited notion of practices like the one used in conversation analysis [10] or multimodal analysis of encounters [12]. Such practices, normally, involve use of tools and artifacts, which, in turn, shape the practices – the materialistic and social perspective intertwine and form a socio-material view [27]. So far, the socio-material character of IT in persuasive encounters did not attract much attention in research. In particular, the relation between design of PT as a collaborative system and the course of events in persuasive encounters remains unclear. The current study addresses this gap while taking an exploratory mixed-method approach.

To frame the exploration we formulate our research questions as follows:

RQ 1: What persuasive practices emerge in persuasive encounters of HS advisors?

RQ 2: How can we support the persuasive practices of HS advisors by means of IT?

With these research questions in mind, we aim at presenting persuasive practices employed by the advisor with and without an IT tool designed along the basic guidance originating from the field of PT, and we want to show how the application of such IT-enhanced practices improve the persuasive character of the encounters.

2   Related Work

The scenario we address in our research clearly relies on interpersonal, face-to-face persuasion. This mode of influence so far remains outside the core focus of the discourse on PT. We propose to supplement the traditional conversation-based encounter with IT designed, explicitly, to support the persuasion efforts. While it differs from the core PT literature, reconsideration of it informs the design of the proposed tool.

Interpersonal Influence and Persuasive Technologies: Persuasion, being defined as "human communication designed to influence the autonomous judgments and actions of others" [25] as well as "a successful intentional effort at influencing another's mental state through communication in a circumstance in which the persuadee has some measure of freedom" [22], relies on interaction between two actors. Conventionally, the persuader provides arguments [22] and appeals to the deep human drives of the persuadee [4]. The persuadee does or does not undergo changes in their attitudes and behaviors with regard to a topic [4]. This highly interactive nature of persuasion finds acknowledgement in the area of PT where technology is postulated to substitute human and establish a computer-human persuasion scenario [26].

Conventionally, two perspective emerged within PT research of how technology influences the behavior and attitude of an individual: (1) computer-human influence and (2) computer-mediated human-human influence [20]. Persuasive systems belonging to the former category rely on the assumption that technology can act as social agent and, thus, impact the behavior of an individual [26]. In cases where technology acts as mediator (e.g., blogs, forums, and social networks), the individual's behavior or attitude underlies social influence in form of user-generated content mediated by dedicated technology [8, 26]. Recently, a novel technology-dependent mode of persuasion was proposed: computer-moderated influence [26]. Systems belonging to that category transfer information on the behavior of others and influence an individual's behavior or attitude by promoting behavior-based and not content-based social influence [26].

According to the seminal paper of Fogg [6], persuasion is likely to be successful when three interrelated factors are addressed: *motivation* related to the feeling of discomfort and rejection of current state, *ability* describing how simple or difficult it is to reach the target behavior, and *trigger* being a signal, facilitator, or spark that tells people to perform the change at a particular moment [6]. Those factors were developed in the context of computer-human influence, but were applied as design guidelines for computer-mediated influence too [17]. We argue that software developed along those lines, will contribute to the emergence of relevant persuasive practices and thus support persuasion in face-to-face persuasive encounters.

Persuasive Practices: The topic of persuasive practices – as longitudinal gradual changes – was addressed in relation to ubiquitous systems informing users about their behaviors and bringing about change in their attitudes and behaviors [23]. Such systems do well in scenarios with clear goals and clear ways to reach them, such as in the case of WaterBot [1] where the information on used water motivates the user to reduce water wasting or in apps inducing change in the life style [23]. However, in the scenario of HS, the ways of improving things are not straight forward and require involvement of a human actor who can establish understanding for security issues and related topics.

Persuasive practices employed in the traditional service encounters, relying on interpersonal influence, aim at securing the attention of the persuadee and at ensuring the right pre-condition for transferring the message [2]. As discussed in consulting literature, this involves directly addressing the persuadee, posing questions and provocative statements, as well as using various encodings [2]. We expect that an IT tool equipped with dedicated features will impact the way the advisor engages in such practices, thus changing the general impression on the persuasiveness of the HS advisory service.

3   Methodology

Preliminary Studies: This study is a part of a research program on burglary-prevention conducted in collaboration with the responsible authorities, i.e., state police departments from Germany and Switzerland. The preliminary studies focused on shadowing the advisor at real HS advisory sessions, interviews with the involved stakeholders, and formative tests of the proposed technology. It enabled us to better understand how the advisors see their main task and how they behave during advisory sessions. It pointed to persuasion as a central issue in this context.

Technology Design: The tool was designed in a user-centered process according to the requirements collected from stakeholders: advisors requested access to materials they know (schemata, pictures) and wanted an easy-to-carry device; homeowners requested a better understanding of the complex information and more personalization; and authorities requested more standardization of the advisory service. The tool shall improve the persuasive character of the encounter to make the persuadee tackle the security issues. The design was inspired by the persuasion model by Fogg [6]: The tool offers a list of standard needs and fears to give the advisor a possibility to address the emotions and appeal to persuadee's *motivation* (cf. Fig. 1a). It offers multiple ways of visualizing important technical and behavioral information to address persuadee's *ability* (cf. Fig. 1c and d) [5]. A prioritization tool and means to email a PDF with the priorities to the persuadee establishes a *trigger* (cf. Fig. 1b) [5]. We use the tool as a vehicle to observe emerging practices and compare them to the non-IT condition.

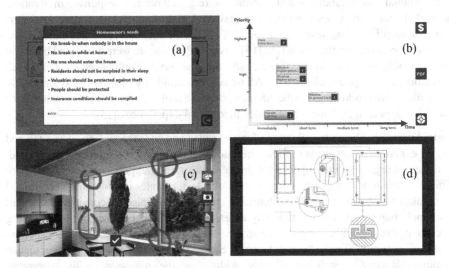

Fig. 1. Exemplary screens included in the HS advisory service support tool (a) Homeowner's needs, (b) Prioritization, (c) Photo taking and annotation, (d) Schemata.

Data Collection: The setting we chose for data collection enables for a natural interaction in a realistic setting. Collecting data from real advisory sessions is nearly impossible because homeowners are reluctant to agree on recordings of their private properties and, in particular, the security flaws thereof. Identification of low-level interactional and conversational practices requires extensive and possibly multimodal data set [10]. We therefore conducted a design experiments [16], thus presuming that introduction of an IT has impact on conversation practices and aiming at their identification.

The overall experiment followed the within-subject design with two conditions: IT and non-IT. It was scenario-driven: each test person was asked to put oneself in a position of a homebuyer who visits two different houses with a home security advisor to receive advice on how to make their future property more secure. No advisor saw the same property twice. We compensate for the order effects while alternating the conditions order. Overall, 20 persuadees and 10 advisors participated in the experiment. Whereas the advisors were policemen who conduct HS encounters on daily basis, the homeowners were a convenience sample acquired through different channels including social media – their age, status, and gender varied, but all of them knew the feelings around buying a new house – they were in a similar situation before. They were not paid for their participation – they were doing it out of interest and received inexpensive gifts after the test. The test was conducted on five days in March 2015 in Mannheim and Frankfurt, Germany, at a pre-fabricated houses fairs. Before the experiment, each advisor participated in a day-long training on the features of the tool and could try it out in role-play exercises. The trainings took part in the same week as the experiments. Additionally, brush-up trainings were conducted on the day of the experiment.

After going through two advisory sessions (IT and non-IT), each persuadee attended a survey and a semi-structured interview built around the topic of interaction quality (e.g., mutual understanding) and persuasion (e.g., emotional response, motivation, ability). In the survey, each participant answered questions related to perceived persuasiveness (PERS) and design aesthetics (DESA) of the encounter on a five-point Likert scale adapted to reflect the HS advice [15]. Overall PERS score were computed based on answers to the such questions as: (1) the *advisory session* (AS) influenced me, (2) the AS was tailored to me personally, (3) the AS makes me rethink my security behavior. DESA score uses on the following: (1) the AS uses attractive tools, (2) the general appearance of the AS is appealing, (3) the AS provides nice visual experiences [15].

Data Analysis: The collected data in form of video and audio recordings was analyzed by an experienced researcher. First, the audio recordings were transcribed. Second, annotations regarding the ongoing actions of advisor and the persuadee were attached. Third, a portion of data (10 random samples of fifteen minutes from various recordings) were taken to identify criteria for interesting episodes – all episodes considered relevant (i.e., including persuasive practices) by at least two researchers either of the following occurred: directly addressing the persuadee with questions including second-person personal pronoun (Engl. "you", Germ. "Sie"), directly addressing the persuadee through directive speech, or directly addressing the persuadee with statements including modal auxiliary verbs (Engl. "you may…", Germ. "Sie mögen…"). Fourth, all episodes extracted from the videos based on the criteria (446 episodes) were clustered based on their similarity in an interactive session involving two researchers. Fourth, abstract descriptions of the clusters were generated based on the transcripts and annotations and put into context of the ongoing action. Moreover, passages from the interviews that related to the particular identified practices were extracted.

Additionally, we applied a mix of statistical tests to identify relation between DESA or PERS values and observed practices. In those tests we treated the observed practices as independent variables with value 1 if a practice was applied in an advisory session and 0 otherwise. We identified practices, that have influence on the dependent variables: DESA and PERS. We run our tests separately for the IT and non-IT conditions – the reported results can be treated as in a between subject study. Following the above, we chose a set of statistical tests appropriate for identification of dependences between nominal independent variables with two or more levels and continuous (interval) dependent variables [11, 14]. We employed the following tests: two-independent-sample t-test, Kruskal-Wallis test, and multiple regression. This approach allowed for formulation of relevant hypotheses and should be treated as indication of possible directions for future research, but not as ultimate evidence for the reported influence or its direction. In particular, our experiment was not designed to detect them and the fact that some of the practices were or were not applied in the particular sessions is more a matter of chance than a consequence of deliberate experiment design. Here, we report on observations with significance coefficient lower or equal to 0.1 (designated by p).

4 Results

In the following, we report on the observations we made across the very extensive data set obtained in the described experiment. First, we show the practices employed by the advisors in the course of their persuasive activities. In particular, we point to the specific practices that are made available by the proposed technology, show how they fit the advisory session, and compare them to corresponding practices in the non-IT condition. Second, we discuss the collected opinions and statistical data that indicate what practices are beneficial or destructive to the overall persuasive character of the encounter.

4.1 Identifying Persuasive Practices in Home Security Advisory Encounters

Thanks to the very extensive preliminary studies in the context of HS advisory services, we could identify three particular goals that advisors follow in their daily work: First, they want to offer help that fits homeowner's needs and situation. Second, they want to provide convincing explanations regarding complicated technical features and behavioral issues. Third, they want to bring the persuadee to tackle the discussed issues – they should contact, e.g., local providers of HS hardware, or change their behaviors. During the analysis of the data, we were able to identify practices in each of the three areas – in the following, we shortly characterize them and provide information on their occurrence across our data set (Tables 1, 2, and 3).

Current Situation and Needs of the Homeowner: According to its definition, persuasion aims at changing, reinforcing or shaping new behaviors and attitudes. This may be ineffective, if the current situation or needs of the persuadee remain hidden. Consequently, that advisors try to approach this topic. If one considers the model proposed by Fogg [6], the work that advisors do while learning to know the homeowner falls into the area of *motivation* – discussing the needs and feelings regarding security makes clear to the persuadee why the encounter takes place and why HS is important.

Table 1. Persuasive practices related to learning and addressing homeowner's needs

Practice and its description
Practice 1 – asking: The advisors introduce the topic of HS mostly by simply asking for the reason of the encounter – after a short introduction they simply pose a question. Often, the answer of the customer is not proceeded by any further discussion. Then, the advisor simply moves to the next point on their agenda, mostly reviewing the security features of doors. Practice 1 occurs with the following frequency: (a) *IT*   5 *times (out of 20)*   (b)   *non-IT*   *11 times (out of 20)* In 3 further non-IT cases, not even a single question was asked regarding the homeowner's HS needs.
Practice 2 – discussing: After receiving an answer, the advisor continues on the topic while paraphrasing the answer and, important, asking further questions to additional information instead of simply moving to the next topic being mostly window's or door's hardware. Practice 2 occurs with the following frequency: (a) *IT*   15 *times (out of 20)*   (b)   *non-IT*   6 *times (out of 20)* We speculate that this frequency results from the fact that the tool includes a screen (Figure 1a) where advisor can choose from a set of standard needs to characterize the current situation of the homeowner. Even though the suggestions in the tool are rather general, the accompanying discussions were more extensive than that.
Practice 3 – recording: While or after listening to the homeowner's HS needs, the advisor takes notes of the needs in the tool by choosing respective fields, but does not show to the client what he chooses or touches – the advisor treats the tool as his private device. In the non-IT setting, the advisors did not make any effort to record the information regarding the homeowner's needs. Practice 3 occurs with the following frequency: (a) *IT*   9 *times (out of 20)*   (b)   *non-IT*   *no comparable practice*
Practice 4 – collaborative recording: As opposite to the previous situation, here the advisor takes care of involving the client into the recording. This happens by sharing the screen with them and by paraphrasing the needs expressed by the client to fit the descriptions in the tool. Advisors leverage this situation to introduce the tool and explain its role in the advisory session. Practice 4 occurs with the following frequency: (a) *IT*   9 *times (out of 20)*   (b)   *non-IT*   *no comparable practice*
Practice 5 – reviewing: The advisor gets back to a particular need or set of needs expressed earlier by the persuadee. This often happens when he presents the final report of the encounter or, in fewer cases, when discusses particular improvement of a security feature. Practice 5 occurs with the following frequency: (a) *IT*   10 *times (out of 20)*   (b)   *non-IT*   0 *times (out of 20)*

Missing Security Features: Persuasion is ineffective if the persuadee does not recognize the attitude or behavior she should change to reach her goals. In our particular case, this includes assembling of new security elements for doors and windows, as well as establishing new routines using those security elements (e.g., locking the windows with a to-be-installed lock mechanism as opposed to simply closing them). The work that the advisors do while teaching the new behaviors falls into the area of *ability* according to Fogg's model [6]. We observe a whole range of practices in this context.

Personalized Recommendation: Given the presented understanding of persuasion, the practices presented above may be ineffective if the persuadee does not know how to approach the set of proposed changes, i.e., what steps to take to reach her goal. In our particular case, a persuadee needs to know what is obligatory and what is optional, what can be done easily (e.g., on changing insecure behaviors), and what requires more

Table 2. Persuasive practices related to presenting security improvements and new routines

Practice and its description
Practice 6 – illustrating through gesture: The advisors explain the flaws of windows and doors directly at the object, while pointing to the particular features (e.g., lock mechanism) and explaining how it may be improved, i.e., how it should look like and be used in the future. This is a practice that seems to be essential to all advisors and is applied at least several times in the IT and non-IT condition.
Practice 7 – taking picture: The advisor takes picture of the particular object or feature via the camera included in the tool. This practice has two different forms: (1) the advisor takes the picture *alone* while the homeowner goes on the side; (2) the advisor tries to keep the homeowner involved by explaining what he does and maintaining the conversation or by incorporating the persuadee in the process of photo taking (encouraging her to look at the picture being taken). Practice 7 occurs with the following frequency: *(a)   alone + IT   17 times (out of 20)*   *(b)   together + IT   3 times (out of 20)*
Practice 8 – annotating picture: The advisor adds specific marking to the previously taken picture in form of rough drawings done by touching the screen – such annotations depict particularly weak or strong points of the object in the picture. Again, this practice is done only by the advisor or in collaborative manner with the persuadee. It can only occur in IT condition. Practice 8 occurs with the following frequency: *(a)   alone + IT   5 times (out of 20)*   *(b)   together + IT   14 times (out of 20)*
Practice 9 – reviewing picture: Advisor reviews the picture and shows it to the homeowner to return to a particular topic from earlier part of the conversation. This typically happens when advisor recapitulates the advisory session, returns to particular object or identifies appropriate solutions to address the issue discussed at the object. This practice occurs only in IT condition; in 18 out of 20 cases.
Practice 10 – adding free text and notes: The advisor adds additional notes or chooses from predefined template notes to denote the problem or the solution related to a particular object. This practice occurs in the IT condition, but can be compared to *Practice 14* from the non-IT case. Nevertheless, *Practice 14* occurs in the late phase of the advisory session, during recapitulation of particular problems and solution. Thanks to the IT, *Practice 10* can occur throughout the service provision – it occurs in 13 out of 20 cases.
Practice 11 – presenting a video: The advisor presents a video illustrating working methods of burglars and how they deal with doors and windows. Advisors introduce the video shortly and then add further explanations or clarifications to the presented material. This practice occurs in 14 out of 20 cases in IT condition.
Practice 12 – presenting a schema: The advisor presents a schema of a technical detail to the persuadee on the IT tool. There are numerous schemas provided in there and they reflect material presented in brochures and other printouts. This practice is the IT-based counterpart of *Practice 13*. It occurs in all 20 IT cases.
Practice 13 – presenting a brochure: The advisor presents a schema of a proposed solution to the persuadee in the brochures and print outs he carries with him. The material includes mostly a technical drawing of the proposed solution. This practice is the paper-based counterpart of *Practice 12*. It occurs in all 20 IT cases.
Practice 14 – annotating a brochure: The advisor adds additional notes and sketches to brochures and print outs. The information he adds to the brochures includes, e.g., information on which window or door it belongs to or what kind of materials can be used in the given context. This practice is the paper-based counterpart of *Practice 11*. It occurs in 10 out of 20 cases – four less than in the IT condition.
Practice 15 – presenting an exhibit: The advisor uses a mechanical example to illustrate how a specific locking mechanism works. In most cases, advisors present difference between mushroom and roller cam in the window fitting while presenting a piece of window hardware. Practice 15 occurs as follows: *(a)   IT   2 times (out of 20)*   *(b)   non-IT   14 times (out of 20)*

effort (e.g., assembly to be done). If the persuadee is clear about all those points, it becomes a *trigger* [6] to tackle the HS issues. The advisors apply particular practices and employ specific materials to support the triggering effect of the advisory encounter.

The identified practices occur across the whole data set and do not show coincidence with the particular advisors or do not result from order effects. However, they are interrelated. Collaboratively visualizing things (like in *Practice 19* and *Practice 4*) imply more extensive discussions (*Practice 17* and *Practice 2*). Some practices are related to the material used and address the visualization of content (*Practices 3, 4, 7–15, 18, 19*), others are conversational practices (*Practices 1, 2, 5, 6, 16, 17*). It is, thou, obvious that this division is not binary – especially the collaborative practices, rely on visualization as a common artifact as a basis for conversation (e.g., *Practice 4, 5, 7, 8, 9, 19*).

Table 3. Persuasive practices related to informing about the next necessary steps

Practice and its description
Practice 16 – mentioning the priorities: In general, the advisors suggest upgrading the mechanical security features (windows and doors) before going for electronics (e.g., alarm system). They provide a list of local craftspeople who are certified to make specific improvements. After making a short utterance about the necessity to contact a respective craftsman, they go over to the next topic. Practice 16 occurs as follows: (a) *IT*   20 *times (out of 20)*   (b)   *non-IT*   17   *times (out of 20)*
Practice 17 – discussing the priorities: After mentioning the general priorities, the advisor discusses them with the homeowner to make sure that they fit her expectations. As opposite to *Practice 16*, here additional questions are asked and the advisor makes sure that the homeowner understood the general tendency in this regard. Practice 17 occurs with the following frequency: (a) *IT*   17 *times (out of 20)*   (b)   *non-IT*   3 *times (out of 20)*
Practice 18 – listing things to be done: The advisor writes down and provides a list of things and issues to be addressed. The list does not give any priority to one or the other problem or solution, but summarizes all topics addressed throughout the provision of the service in a predefined order (door, windows, cellar, etc.). Alternatively, the respective information is written on the brochures or print outs. Practice 18 is characteristic for the non-IT condition and is applied there in 12 cases. In two cases (out of those 12), the advisor places the list between him and the persuadee, such that the notes were made collaboratively.
Practice 19 – prioritizing things to be done: The advisor lists all issues to be addressed and orders them according to the priorities and his personal assessment. This practice is supported by the provided IT and occurs only in the IT condition: the advisor can sort all issues he addressed according to the dimensions of priority and time. In most cases, he encourages the involvement of the persuadee such that the prioritizing has a collaborative character. Practice 19 occurs with the following frequency: (a)   *alone + IT*   6 *times (out of 20)*   (b)   *together + IT*   13   *times (out of 20)*

4.2   Relating Persuasive Practices to the Perceptions of the Persuadee

The above analysis shows that supporting visualization of specific content enables for occurrence of particular conversational and interactional practices. Nevertheless, the effectiveness of the practices cannot be solely related to their occurrence in the advisory encounter. In the following, we discuss the relation between PERS and DESA, as well as the relation between the occurrence of particular practices and those two measures.

Relation DESA – PERS: DESA and PERS stand in relation to each other and both define important aspects of persuadee experience in persuasion regarding health behavior as measured by a general, online survey [15]. Our analysis confirms this for the situation of HS advisory service, by using an onsite survey right after the these sessions. There is a significant and moderate-to-strong correlation between DESA and PERS across all our cases (two-tiled bivariate correlation: Pearson's Coefficient $corr = 0.5, p \leq 0.001$) and, especially, in the non-IT cases ($corr = 0.6, p \leq 0.005$). The coefficient we measure is higher than reported in earlier research (0.43 [15]). Furthermore, we show that DESA is significantly higher in the IT condition than in the non-IT with a large effect size (IT: $\bar{x} = 4.72$; non-IT: $\bar{x} = 3.95$; $t(19) = 3.29, p \leq 0.005$), and, as consequence, PERS is higher in the IT than in the non-IT with a very small effect size (IT: $\bar{x} = 4.71$; non-IT $\bar{x} = 4.58$; $t(19) = 1.05, p \leq 0.1$). We do not observe significant results for other constructs from the model of Lehto et al. [15].

Influence of Practices on PERS and DESA: When asked about the most positive episode across both conditions or about the what increased their understanding, many persuadees point to the visualization potential of the IT – for video: *"I valued the fact, that one could directly show me how a potential burglary can look like"* [H13] and for pictures: *"Schemata made it easy to understand the technical solution – they were* *good in traditional advisory as well as in the modern one – just with the tablet you could directly see it at the object"* [H16]. The visualization potential of modern technologies was emphasized in each interview. In particular, persuadees point to videos and schemata as elements that leverage understanding (*"It was a lot easier to understand the one [advisory session] where I could see the video and pictures"* [H8]), and the practice of recording needs as a way to personalize and individualize the advisory service (*"It was a personalized experience – he addressed my personal situation. One feels respected if their personal situation gets considered. One feels proud"* [H2]).

Asked about their motivation and ability to take next steps on HS, persuadees point to the prioritization practices: *"This was clearer in the IT, because one could see what to do next and what can wait"* [H16]. Some other account for the role of individualized pictures: *"I found the one with tablet more pleasant cause there was a through and individualized discussion towards the end (...). I could take this PDF with the photos of my doors and windows, and go to the craftsman, show this to him and ask for his help"* [H15]. Other persuadees emphasize the role of discussion in general: *"The conversation at the closure, it encouraged me and acts as a reminder of most important things – independent of whether with IT or not"* [H8]. The collaborative character of activities seems to be very central issue for many test participants: *"It helped to understand when we took the picture together. Clack... 'Look, there is your door'."* [H9] and *"So, my advisor, she took the pictures, added markings, made notes with me. And I think, those photos help to remind oneself of what needs to be done"* [H18].

On the one hand, the persuadees refer to particular materials used throughout the advisory sessions: schemata, videos, pictures, etc. On the other hand, they stress the interactional and conversational character of advisory sessions. We explore this issue while providing results of statistical dependence analysis of the PERS and DESA measures and the observed practices. We did not identify any (nearly) significant relation between practices and PERS or DESA for the non-IT condition. All the indications presented below describe solely the IT condition in a between subject mode.

The results of the Kruskal-Wallis test suggest a positive relation between *Practice 2 (discussion of homeowner needs)* and DESA ($H(1) = 2.53, p \leq 0.1$), as well as between *Practice 19-b (prioritizing things to be done – together with IT)* and DESA ($H(1) = 4.24, p \leq 0.05$). We also observe negative relation between *Practice 7-a (taking picture – alone with IT)* and DESA ($H(1) = -3.33, p \leq 0.1$) and between *Practice 7-a* and PERS ($H(1) = -2.46, p \leq 0.1$). Regression analysis, even if it does not produce a general regression equation for DESA or PERS, it still provides indications that confirm two dependencies: the positive relation between *Practice 19-b* and DESA ($B = 1.56, t = 2.91, p = 0.04$), as well as the negative one between *Practice 7-a* and PERS ($B = -0.8, t = -1.8, p \leq 0.1$). Finally, the set of two-independent-sample t-tests suggests the following positive relationships: (1) between presenting the video to the persuadee *(Practice 11)* and PERS ($t(17) = 1.66, p \leq 0.1$), (2) between collaborative annotation of the picture *(Practice 8-b)* and PERS ($t(18) = 1.64, p \leq 0.1$), and (3) between *Practice 19-b* and DESA ($t(17) = 1.66, p \leq 0.1$). In summary, only the relation between *Practice 19-b* and DESA was yielded in all tests, which seems an intuitive and still valuable – collaborative work practices with a shared visualization improve the perceived design aesthetics of the HS session. The other tendencies we observe confirm that practices which have a collaborative character (*discussion, working together with the tool*) may tend to improve perceptions on PERS and DESA, while avoiding engagement in collaborative practices may lead to negative effects in this regard.

5 Discussion and Conclusion

Our analysis shows that advisors employ a whole range of persuasive practices. They differ with regard to use of artifacts (IT, brochures, etc.) and with regard to their collaborative character. Also, some practices address the homeowner's HS needs and the next steps, however the largest variety of practices is employed for addressing the persuadee's *ability* by discussing missing security features. The advisors put by far most effort to support these activities by using brochures, exhibits, and referring to windows and doors. With introduction of IT, new relevant practices emerge, such as: collaborative picture taking or video watching. Practices that improve persuasive character of the encounter involve collaboration and discussion around a shared artifact – according to the interview data and the quantitative analysis of survey responses. Importantly, IT improves design aesthetics (DESA), but has negligible effect on persuasiveness (PERS) as shown by comparison between conditions. Consequently, it is not the technology itself that enhances persuasiveness in HS encounters, but the way it is used makes the difference. In our opinion this is the key for further research in the area of PT for interpersonal interaction where successful persuasion is essential.

Hitherto, the focus of research in PT was on the human-computer influence, as well as computer-mediated and computer-moderated interpersonal influence [26]. The results suggest, that technology designed along the same lines has potential to establish effective practices for face-to-face interpersonal influence – in particular it shows that specific practices can easily emerge and supplement existing practices if appropriate IT is provided. We show that PT can be well applied in situations where a human persuader is needed due to the high complexity of decisions to be taken, as opposite to more classical application scenarios with a clear target state or behavior [1, 23]. This opens a new, fascinating area for PT researchers and shows first directions of research: establishing persuasive practices as work practices between persuader and persuadee.

In the course of generalizing our observations, it is easy to imagine that systems like the one used in current study, can be effortlessly extended in accordance with other design principles borrowed from PT. In the case of HS, this includes information on the improvements done by other people in similar situation and their attitude. We argue that PT community needs to extend its research focus beyond this limit [23] – it is easy to speculate about possible direction of research, e.g., health support apps where computer-mediated or -moderated persuasive systems are linked with advisory services at doctor's office. Through the design and application of the tool presented above, we show that the guidance developed for the computer-human influence [6] is applicable for interpersonal encounters. Our research, also, contributes to the knowledge on IT support in advisory services. So far, research in this area addresses concepts as transparency [19] or education [9], thus addressing the objectivism of such encounters.

However, considering persuasion in this context stresses a different side of those encounters being a meeting of two socially and organizationally linked actors following their goals. The identification of relevant persuasive practices helps the designers to engineer systems inducing those practices and the researcher to identify design elements linked with persuasion and differentiate them from features for facilitation or moderation.

Finally, the set of collaborative practices identified via statistical tests as having potentially strong influence on persuasiveness confirms the importance of practice-based studies for the PT. While following the general description of practices from the consulting literature [2], we are able to identify particular practices specific in the given context and provide a zoom-in analysis [18]. Thereby we confirm the value of such perspective in the PT research and claim, that it is the appropriate way to study effects, especially in human-human influence scenarios. The results do not come without limitations: practices perspective focuses on local, internal validity over the external one. Nevertheless, we show its potential for research in PT to explore human-human influence in IT-supported encounters and claim that the results can be adopted in other scenarios, such as medical advice – doctor who fails to convince a patient via words, could, e.g., employ videos showing negative impact of particular factor on the patient's body. We call for intensification of research oriented at practices resulting from use of PT in real situations and for deepening the understanding of persuasive practices. Alike in general HCI, we call for practice-turn in PT research [13]: What other persuasive practices emerge? Which of them can be supported by PT? How to design appropriate PT?

References

1. Arroyo, E., et al.: Waterbot: exploring feedback and persuasive techniques at the sink. In: Proceedings of International Conference on Human Factors in Computing Systems, pp. 631–639. ACM (2005)
2. Blundel, R.: Effective organisational communication: perspectives, principles, and practices. Financial Times Prentice Hall, Harlow, England; New York (2004)
3. Budde, R., Züllighoven, H.: Software tools in a programming workshop. In: Floyd, C., Züllighoven, H., Budde, R., Keil-Slawik, R. (eds.) Software Development and Reality Construction, pp. 252–268. Springer, Heidelberg (1992)
4. Cialdini, R.B.: Influence: the psychology of persuasion. Collins, New York (2007)
5. Comes, T., Schwabe, G.: From fuzzy exploration to transparent advice: insights into mobile advisory services. In: Hawaii International Conference on System Sciences. Los Alamitos, USA (2016)
6. Fogg, B.J.: A behavior model for persuasive design. In: Proceedings of the 4rd International Conference on Persuasive Technology. ACM (2009)
7. Garfinkel, H.: Studies in Ethnomethodology. Prentice-Hall, Englewood Cliffs (1967)
8. Harjumaa, M., Oinas-Kukkonen, H.: Persuasion theories and IT design. In: de Kort, Y.A., IJsselsteijn, W.A., Midden, C., Eggen, B., Fogg, B.J. (eds.) PERSUASIVE 2007. LNCS, vol. 4744, pp. 311–314. Springer, Heidelberg (2007)
9. Heinrich, P., et al.: Microworlds as the locus of consumer education in financial advisory services. In: Proceedings of the International Conference on Information Systems (2014)

10. Hutchby, I., Wooffitt, R.: Conversation Analysis: Principles, Practices, and Applications. Polity Press, Cambridge (1998)
11. Kanji, G.K.: 100 Statistical Tests. SAGE Pub., London, Thousand Oaks (2006)
12. Kress, G.: Multimodality: A Social Semiotic Approach to Contemporary Communication. Routledge, Abingdon, New York (2009)
13. Kuutti, K., Bannon, L.J.: The turn to practice in HCI: towards a research agenda. In: Proceedings of the Conference Human Factors in Computing Systems, pp. 3543–3552. ACM Press (2014)
14. Leeper, J.D., Hartman, J.: Choosing the Correct Statistical Test (CHS 627: University of Alabama), http://bama.ua.edu/~jleeper/627/choosestat.html
15. Lehto, T. et al.: Factors affecting perceived persuasiveness of a behavior change support system. In: Proceedings of the International Conference on Information Systems (2012)
16. Mettler, T., et al.: On the use of experiments in design science research: a proposition of an evaluation framework. Commun. AIS. **34**(1), 223–240 (2014)
17. Muntean, C.I.: Raising engagement in e-learning through gamification. In: Proceedings of the International Conference on Virtual Learning, pp. 323–329 (2011)
18. Nicolini, D.: Practice Theory, Work, and Organization: An Introduction. Oxford University Press, Oxfor (2012)
19. Nussbaumer, P., et al.: "Enforced" vs. "Casual" transparency – findings from IT-supported financial advisory encounters. ACM Trans. Manag. Inf. Syst. **3**(2), 11:1–11:19 (2012)
20. Oinas-Kukkonen, H., Harjumaa, M.: Persuasive systems design: Key issues, process model, and system features. Commun. Assoc. Inf. Syst. **24**(1), 28 (2009)
21. Oinas-Kukkonen, H., Harjumaa, M.: Towards Deeper Understanding of Persuasion in Software and Information Systems. In: Proceedings of the International Conference on Advances in Human-Computer Interaction. IEEE (2008)
22. O'Keefe, D.J.: Persuasion: Theory & Research. Sage Pub, Thousand Oaks, CA (2002)
23. Rogers, Y.: Moving on from weiser's vision of calm computing: engaging UbiComp experiences. In: Dourish, P., Friday, A. (eds.) UbiComp 2006. LNCS, vol. 4206, pp. 404–421. Springer, Heidelberg (2006)
24. Schwabe, G., et al.: Advancing collaboration engineering: new ThinkLets for dyadic problem solving and an application for mobile advisory services. In: Hawaii International Conference on System Sciences, Los Alamitos, USA (2016)
25. Simons, H.W., Jones, J.: Persuasion in society. Routledge, New York (2011)
26. Stibe, A.: Advancing typology of computer-supported influence: moderation effects in socially influencing systems. In: MacTavish, T., Basapur, S. (eds.) PERSUASIVE 2015. LNCS, vol. 9072, pp. 253–264. Springer, Heidelberg (2015)
27. Suchman, L.A.: Human-machine reconfigurations. Cambridge University Press, Cambridge (2007)

Persuasive Patterns in Q&A Social Networks

Ifeoma Adaji[✉] and Julita Vassileva

University of Saskatchewan, Saskatchewan, Canada
Ita811@mail.usask.ca,jiv@cs.usask.ca

Abstract. Social networks differ in their structure and objectives, hence, the effectiveness of persuasion principles or patterns may vary from one type of network to another. This study aims to identify the persuasive principles that make a typical Q&A network successful. Using Stack Overflow as a case study, we applied the PSD model to evaluate the persuasive principles of the network. Our results show that all but four principles of the PSD model were implemented in Stack Overflow. This study can help social network developers build persuasive Q&A social networks and improve on existing social platforms.

Keywords: Persuasive technology · Social networks · Persuasive systems design

1 Introduction

Online social networks are peculiar in that they have different objectives and operate in different ways, thus making a "one size fits all" model difficult to apply to the various social networks. For instance, the objective of users on Facebook and Stack Overflow differ, and so does the structure of both networks. Hence, the persuasive strategies that will work in Facebook might not work in Stack Overflow. This study aims at identifying the persuasive patterns that make a typical Q&A social network successful. These patterns can help social network developers and stake holders build or improve existing social platforms, and serve as a guide to building a persuasive framework for Q&A social networks.

2 Related Work

2.1 Stack Overflow

Stack Overflow is a Q&A network where users can ask and answer specific IT related questions to gain points and build their reputation. Users do not need to sign up in order to view existing answers to already asked questions. However, in order to ask or answer a question, a user has to sign up. Through active participation, asking good questions and providing good answers, users can gain incentives, such as higher reputation score, badges and privileges. While users can up vote or down vote other users' questions and answers, only the user who asked a question can select the best answer to his/her

© Springer International Publishing Switzerland 2016
A. Meschtscherjakov et al. (Eds.): PERSUASIVE 2016, LNCS 9638, pp. 189–196, 2016.
DOI: 10.1007/978-3-319-31510-2_16

question. Stack Overflow currently has over 4 million registered users and over 9 million questions[1].

2.2 Persuasive Systems Design (PSD) Model

There are currently several frameworks and strategies for designing persuasive systems in different domains. A review carried out by Wiafe and Nakata [1] shows that the frequently applied persuasive frameworks or models include Fogg's functional triad [2] and the transtheoretical model [3]. Despite the popularity of these frameworks, in this study we applied the persuasive systems design model (PSD) [4]. We used this model for two reasons. First, the Fogg's functional triad has been studied extensively over the years and new frameworks have been developed based on his model, the PSD being one of them. Second, as noted by Oinas-Kukkonen and Harjumaa [4], Fogg's framework and principles are too general in terms of designing and evaluating persuasive systems. Though the transtheoretical model is a common framework, it is however mainly used to model health behavior change [3].

PSD is a framework for designing and evaluating persuasive systems. It categorizes and maps the elements of persuasion in a system and also describes the software functionality expected in the end product [4]. The PSD model recommends three phases of development and evaluation: understanding the key issues behind persuasive systems, analyzing the persuasion context and designing of system qualities. In this study, we only evaluated the third stage, designing of system qualities, as we are interested in identifying the persuasive patterns and principles adopted in the design of a system.

3   Research Method and Results

In this study, our focus was on the third phase of the PSD model: design of system qualities. This stage is important as it focuses on the persuasive principles that should be adopted in designing a system to make it more engaging. The principles are categorized into four groups: providing primary task support, dialogue support, system credibility support and social support [4]. We analyzed Stack Overflow and identified the persuasive principles that exist and how they were implemented.

This project is still work in progress. In the next phase of this study, we will validate the different principles identified below, by carrying out a user study with Stack Overflow users to verity if these principles work in practice.

3.1   Primary Task Support

The principles of persuasion in this category assist users of a system in achieving their primary objective. These principles include the following:

---

[1] https://data.stackexchange.com/StackOverflow/revision/325050/420211/count-of-all-users-all-questions-and-all-answers.

Reduction: With the principle of reduction, a system should make complex tasks as easy as possible by reducing them into simpler ones to persuade users to carry out such tasks. For example, a very short registration process for users makes it more likely that users will register since the task of signing up has been reduced to something simpler [5]. Stack Overflow reduces the task of registration by allowing users sign up with their Facebook or Google account, hence eliminating the need for users to fill out a registration form which some could regard as time consuming.

Tunneling: The tunneling principle states that a system should guide users through a process and provide means of persuading them along the way. We could not identify any application of tunneling in Stack Overflow.

Tailoring: A system that allows users to tailor the information or service to their interests or preferences could be more persuasive than one that does not. With the tailoring principle, different user groups should be provided with tailored information for that group. Stack Overflow applies the tailoring principle by letting users specify what subject areas they are interested in and receive notifications when questions are asked in these areas. This is done with the use of tags. Tags are labels or keywords used to classify a question[2]. Users can subscribe to as many tags as they have interest in, and are notified of questions that have those tags. This prevents users from receiving notifications when questions they have no interest in are asked.

Personalization: The principle of personalization states that a system that offers more personalized content is more likely to be persuasive compared to one that does not. In Stack Overflow, when users register for the first time, a profile is created for them. The system uses this profile to personalize their experience. On the profile page, among others, users can change their display name, location, edit what information that other users can see about them, edit the tags they have interest in, and edit what notifications they want to receive. All this information is to ensure the system personalizes the content the user receives. This principle is very similar to tailoring.

Self-monitoring. According to the self-monitoring principle, for a system to be persuasive, users should be able to keep track of their performance or status, as this will support users in attaining their goals. Stack Overflow allows self-monitoring of users' performance. On each user's profile page, they see a summary of their activities on the site. The details of a user's performance include their reputation score, badges they have received, the number of questions they have answered, the number of questions they have asked, any points earned from the questions and answers, number of profile views, how long the user has been a member and the last time the user visited the network. Going by the self-monitoring profile, having access to this information could persuade users to use the system.

Simulation: The simulation principle states that persuasive systems should enable users to see the link between cause and effect. Stack Overflow allows users to observe

---

[2] *Tags in Stack Overflow*, http://stackoverflow.com/tags.

the connection between posts and reputation score. A user's profile page states the number of questions and answers the user has asked and answered and the reputation score earned from those posts. Hence users can see that there is a link between posting questions or answers and their reputation score. This, according to the simulation principle, could persuade users to answer more questions.

Rehearsal: For a system to be persuasive using this principle, the system should provide a means for users to rehearse a target behavior. A typical example is a flying simulator, which student pilots can use to rehearse being certified pilots. We could not identify the use of this principle in Stack Overflow. What we found to be similar to this however, is that unregistered users can view existing questions and answers. They however cannot ask or answer questions. They also do not have a profile so cannot benefit from personalization. Viewing existing questions and answers could give unregistered users a feel of the site and hence persuade them to register.

3.2 Dialogue Support

This category of influence principles uses a feedback system to provide support to users with the aim of bringing them closer to their goal. In Stack Overflow, this goal could include asking a question, answering one, improving one's reputation score or finding questions that could be useful to a user. The dialogue support category includes the following persuasive principles:

Praise: According to the PSD model, a persuasive system should use praise as a means of feedback to users, as praise can make a user more open to persuasion. Praise could be in the form of words, images, symbols or sounds. Stack Overflow uses praise in the form of *up votes*. When a user asks a question and other users find the question valuable, they can vote it up. The number of up votes serve as a feedback to the user who asked the question. The up votes also provide a feedback on the quality of the answers provided to a question. Users can up vote the answers they feel provide the best solution to the question asked. In Stack Overflow, praise is also offered in the form of *favorite question*. Users who think a question is relevant or useful can make it one of their favorite questions. *Accepted answer* is another form of praise in Stack Overflow. The user who asks a question is the one to pick the best answer from the various answers provided. All these forms of praise are displayed beside the question or answer so are visible to all users. They also contribute to the final reputation score of the users who earned them.

Rewards: The rewards principle states that systems that offer rewards to their users could be more persuasive than those that do not. Stack Overflow offers rewards to users in form of privileges and badges. Privileges control what users can do in the network. The higher the privilege, the more actions a user can perform. Privileges are gained by increasing one's reputation score, and reputation score is increased by posting helpful questions and answers[3]. Users with reputation score of over 25,000 for example, are

---

[3] *Privileges in Stack Overflow*, http://stackoverflow.com/help/privileges.

rewarded with the privilege of *access to site analytics* which includes Stack Overflow's internal and Google site analytics.

Badges is another reward offered to users in Stack Overflow. Users receive badges when they are especially helpful[4]. Badges earned by users can be seen on their profile page and on their posts. An example of a badge in Stack Overflow is the Great Question badge. It is rewarded to users who score 100 or more on a question. Scores are computed by the number of up votes a question receives. There are over 40 badges in Stack Overflow and are classified into various categories.

Reminders: The rewards principle asserts that users are expected to achieve their target objective if a system reminds them to do so. Hence, a system that implements a reminder technique could be more persuasive. We could not identify the use of reminders in Stack Overflow.

Suggestion: According to the suggestion principle of the PSD model, systems that offer suggestions to users are more persuasive than systems that do not. Stack Overflow offers suggestions to users in several scenarios, for example, when a user is typing a question. When a user asks a question, the system searches for similar questions that have been asked and answered in the past and suggests such questions to the asker. The asker then has the opportunity to review the suggested questions and decide if they are useful, in which case the user does not go ahead with asking a new question. Another use of suggestion in Stack Overflow is with the use of tags. Tags are labels or keywords used to classify a question. Not all users can create a new tag. *Create tag* is a privilege rewarded only to users when they gain a reputation score of 1,500. However, all users can use existing tags. At the point of typing a new question, the system suggests possible tags that a user can choose for the question.

Similarity: The similarity principle states that systems that remind users of themselves are more likely to be persuasive. In Stack Overflow, we could not identify the use of similarity principle in this context. However, in our future study, one of the questions we will try to answer is "Do users have friends or people they admire who use Stack Overflow, if yes, do they form special networks". This will help us identify how persuasive the similarity principle is.

Liking: This principle asserts that a visually attractive system is likely to be more persuasive. Rating the attractiveness of Stack Overflow is subjective and can only be determined by the users of the system, hence we did not give an opinion of this principle. Validating the persuasiveness of this principle is one of the objectives of the user study that we intend carrying out in the future.

Social Role: The social role principle states that systems that embrace the use of social roles are likely to be more persuasive. Stack Overflow has several social roles which are rewarded to users as they achieve various milestones. For example, when a user attains a reputation score of 10,000, they are awarded the *access to moderator tools* privilege

---

[4] *Badges in Stack Overflow*, http://stackoverflow.com/help/badges.

which enables them access reports, delete inappropriate or duplicate questions and answers, add new tags, create and moderate chat rooms among other functions. Knowing that there are users in such social roles could persuade users to use the system.

3.3 Social Support

This category of principles leverages on social influence to persuade users to use a system. The principles in this category include:

Social Learning: According to the PSD model, a system using the social learning principle should allow users to observe other users performing their target behavior in order to see the outcome of such behavior. In Stack Overflow, users can observe other users performing their target behavior. Since the questions asked by users are public, and so are their comments, votes, favorites, as well as the answers to the questions, their votes and the best answer award, the users can learn from these community actions, both the social norms of posting, answering and providing feedback, and about the subject of the posts.

Social Comparison: This principle asserts that users are more persuaded to perform their target behavior if they can compare their performance to that of others within the system. According to Stack Overflow, reputation is a measure of the confidence the community has in a user[5]. The better the performance of a user, the more reputation score he earns. Users can view the reputation score and other privileges earned by other users within the network by viewing their profile. They can compare their performance with those of others by looking at their profile.

Normative Influence: The principle of normative influence states that a system should take advantage of peer pressure to increase the possibility of persuading a user to adopt a target behavior. According to this principle, a system that can bring users who share the same goals together, is more likely to persuade its users to use the system. In Stack Overflow, users are brought together in chat rooms where they can share knowledge and information. A user with the *communication* privilege can create a chat room and grant talking privileges to other users who can then join in the conversation. Another example of normative influence is the use of the reward system. Users could feel persuaded when their friends earn high reputation or badges in the system.

Social Facilitation: This principle states that a system's users are more likely to be persuaded to use the system if they can discern from the system that other users are carrying out a similar task along with them. In Stack Overflow, an example of the implementation of this principle is the chat room. From Stack Overflow's chat portal[6], users have an overview of active chat rooms including a description of the chat room and the number of active users. If a user clicks on any of the active sessions, he or she

---

[5] *Reputation in Stack Overflow*, http://stackoverflow.com/help/whats-reputation.
[6] *Stack Overflow*, http://chat.stackoverflow.com/?tab=all&sort=people.

can view the details of the chat including the names of the users, the details of their conversation and time stamp. Going by the social facilitation principle, users in the chat room are persuaded to participate because other users are active.

Cooperation: The cooperation principle of the PSD model suggests that for a system to be persuasive, it should take advantage of human beings' natural desire to co-operate. In other words, a system should provide a method of co-operation among users. In Stack Overflow, users are able to co-operate with other users when asking questions. For instance, users can comment on a question in order to improve on it. This kind of co-operation among users is also evident with answers provided on Stack Overflow. It is common for users to comment on answers provided by other users to ask for clarification or to improve an existing answer.

Competition: The competition principle states that for a system to be persuasive, it should take advantage of human beings' natural desire to compete. In other words, a system should provide a method of competition among users. Stack Overflow rewards users who are first to answer a question with a score of ten or more. This type of reward could lead to competition among users who want to receive the *first accepted answer* reward.

Recognition: According to the PSD model, offering public recognition to an individual can increase the possibility of that user being persuaded. In Stack Overflow, a user's reputation score and badges earned form part of the user's display image and are found beside every question, answer or comment posted by the user. Hence, it is easy to see the user with the highest reputation score and rewards from a list of users who answered a question or who posted comments to an answer. This makes recognition of users possible.

4   Conclusion and Future Work

This paper identified the persuasion principles adopted in a typical Q&A social network, Stack Overflow. Using the PSD model, we were able to identify all but four principles of the model namely tunneling, rehearsal, reminders and similarity. Each principle identified promotes engagement of users. This research shows that persuasion in a typical Q&A social network adopts regular observable patterns. Software developers can adopt these principles to develop applications that will possibly succeed.

This study is still work in progress. We were unable to evaluate the *system credibility support* category of the PSD model. This category is based majorly on feedback from users. Evaluation of this category will be carried out in the next phase of the project. In that phase, we will also validate the different principles listed above, by carrying out a user study with Stack Overflow users' data, to show that these principles actually work in practice. For instance, one of the research questions we will answer in the user study is if users are persuaded to answer more questions when they receive a hard to earn badge. The study will show the impact and effect of these persuasive principles on user participation.

References

1. Wiafe, I., Nakata, K.: Bibliographic analysis of persuasive systems: techniques, methods and domains of application. In: Persuasive Technology, vol. 61 (2012)
2. Fogg, B.J.: Persuasive technology: using computers to change what we think and do. Ubiquity **2002**, 5 (2002)
3. Prochaska, J.O., Velicer, W.F.: The transtheoretical model of health behavior change. Am. J. Health Promot. **12**, 38–48 (1997)
4. Oinas-Kukkonen, H., Harjumaa, M.: A systematic framework for designing and evaluating persuasive systems. In: Oinas-Kukkonen, H., Hasle, P., Harjumaa, M., Segerståhl, K., Øhrstrøm, P. (eds.) PERSUASIVE 2008. LNCS, vol. 5033, pp. 164–176. Springer, Heidelberg (2008)
5. Fogg, B.J., Eckles, D.: The behavior chain for online participation: how successful web services structure persuasion. In: de Kort, Y.A., IJsselsteijn, W.A., Midden, C., Eggen, B., Fogg, B.J. (eds.) PERSUASIVE 2007. LNCS, vol. 4744, pp. 199–209. Springer, Heidelberg (2007)

Games and Gamification

Utilizing a Digital Game as a Mediatory Artifact for Social Persuasion to Prevent Speeding

Bernhard Maurer[✉], Magdalena Gärtner, Martin Wuchse,
Alexander Meschtscherjakov, and Manfred Tscheligi

Center for Human-Computer Interaction, Department of Computer Sciences,
University of Salzburg, Salzburg, Austria
{bernhard.maurer,magdalena.gaertner,martin.wuchse,
alexander.meschtscherjakov,manfred.tscheligi}@sbg.ac.at

Abstract. In this paper we present a game-based approach to stop a driver from speeding by means of social persuasion. The approach utilizes a digital game played by a passenger inside the car. The game serves as a mediatory artifact, which translates the speed of the car into in-game events, thus, nudging the passenger to communicate with the driver about his/her driving behavior. As a game we used Tetris, which was coupled to the speed of a virtual vehicle in our driving simulator. We designed four different in-game representations of the real car data and examined, which of these designs is most suitable to trigger an intuitive, understandable linkage between the speeding behavior and the corresponding in-game events in order to enable a prompt intervention of the passenger. We evaluated the four designs in an exploratory user study. Our findings highlight the feasibility of our approach, as even passengers, who were rather uninvolved in the driving task, were successfully encouraged to slow down the driver. Based on our study results, we recommend a hybrid design strategy for the game, between designing for a dynamically increasing in-game challenge to foster passenger engagement based on fun, and simultaneously intervening dynamically in the playability of the game to foster communication with the driver to pave the way for social persuasion in the car.

Keywords: Persuasive game design · Social persuasion · Automotive domain

1 Introduction

Understanding and designing games as socially influencing systems can be an insightful perspective and fruitful opportunity for researchers and designers of persuasive technology, in particular in the automotive domain, because the car is an inherently collaborative and social space that creates social interdependencies between the co-located persons in the car [7]. Yet, the car is also a safety critical environment where incautious driving behaviors such as speeding can result in dangerous, or even fatal incidents, not only affecting the driver but all people in the car. Hence, having a means of persuasion in order to prevent drivers from speeding is an important design challenge for persuasive technologies in the automotive domain.

© Springer International Publishing Switzerland 2016
A. Meschtscherjakov et al. (Eds.): PERSUASIVE 2016, LNCS 9638, pp. 199–210, 2016.
DOI: 10.1007/978-3-319-31510-2_17

Games and play (both digital and physical) have the ability to create a social setting and connect people within the boundaries of this setting. Through collaborative gameplay social couplings are formed by which people communicate and interact with each other for an underlying, common goal [9]. In many games, gameplay is inherently based on combining various social influence principles such as competition, cooperation, recognition, and learning. Thus, interweaving game design and persuasive system design by incorporating these principles into specific game mechanics offers great potential for designers of persuasive technology to generate impact and induce behavior change.

Following this assumption we present an approach that incorporates the real speed of a car in a digital game. With this linkage we are deliberately intervening in the social setting between the driver and a passenger with the aim to utilize the passenger as a resource for social persuasion in order to keep the driver from speeding. Our approach is based on the following scenario: A person is driving a car accompanied by a passenger. The passenger is playing the tile-matching, digital puzzle game Tetris during the car trip. Some features of the game are linked to the actual speed of the car in real time. Thus, when the driver starts speeding, his/her driving style is immediately incorporated in the game. As a consequence the game gets harder to master or even unplayable, and the passenger is alerted that the driver is exceeding the speed limit. By communicating the status of the game to the driver, the passenger consequently persuades the driver to reduce the driving speed – first and foremost, for the safety of the two, but also for keeping up a positive gaming experience.

In terms of interaction design, there are several ways of how to link the car's driving speed to in-game changes. This inlcudes, e.g., directly coupling the game speed with the driving speed (i.e. the faster the driving speed is, the faster the Tetris tiles fall down) or even pausing the game when the car exceeds a certain speed limit. We implemented four different game designs and evaluated their effect in a driving simulator study. We aimed at answering two main research questions:

1. Does a digital game, whose game mechanics are based on real car-data (i.e., speed), serve as a useful mediatory artifact to foster communication as a means of social persuasion in the car to prevent speeding?
2. Which of the four game designs are the most useful and promising ones in order to foster social persuasion in the car?
   i. Which game designs create the most intuitive and easy to understand linkage between the real-world misbehavior of speeding and the in-game consequences/events?
   ii. Which game designs do the passengers prefer and for which reasons?

In the following, we present the theorectical background of our research and describe the development process of the four different game designs we used for our study. To examine our approach and identify the most promising game design(s), we evaluated the designs with 16 participants in an exploratory user study in a car-simulator. We report on the study procedure, the data analysis and discuss the findings of the study with regard to the research questions and future work.

2   Related Work

2.1   Games as Socially Influencing Systems

Digital games are information systems that are highly social and collaborative often incorporating a variety of social influence principles such as social learning, cooperation, or competition. Oinas-Kukkonen et al. [10] highlight the role of social influence as a persuasive strategy by providing a framework with a variety of principles also prevalent in most games (i.e., social learning, social comparison, normative influence, social facilitation, cooperation, competition, recognition). In a similar direction, Bogost argues that the persuasive effect that games create can be understood by seeing them as *procedural rhetorics,* i.e., "the art of persuasion through rule-based representations and interactions" [2].

In our approach, the game uses and embodies the real car speed, thus forming a procedural rhetoric around translating this data related to driving misbehavior into changes within the game (i.e., a rule-based representation of real world data).

2.2   In-Car Technology and Collaboration

Today, cars are pervaded with technology like entertainment systems, or navigation devices. These technologies are often not designed around the social nature and collaborative mechanisms within the car, though. Perterer et al. [7] highlight how the sharing of information (e.g., making it visible for both driver and passenger) can have large impact on the collaborative nature of driving. Previous research has in particular focused on investigating concepts around driver-passenger cooperation e.g., for navigational tasks [3, 4, 7], while Shepherd et al. [8] investigated the influence of the social setting within the car on the driver's behavior itself. They examined a scenario with peers posing as passengers who provide verbal feedback in order to persuade the driver to change his/her driving behavior. Their findings show how effective the influence of peers as passengers can be in risk-related driving scenarios.

Our approach differs from these approaches, though, as we design for the passengers as a means for social persuasion. In providing the passenger with a digital game, which incorporates real-car data, we assign him/her to take the role of a social persuader, who influences the driver. With the game serving as a mediatory artefact in this process, we connect the persuasive powers of digital gaming and social influence in order to change the driver's driving style and keep him/her from the gas pedal.

3   Approach

The motivation for our approach originated from the results of a probing study we conducted to investigate the persuasive potentials of in-car interfaces [5]. This study identified the potential of creating technology driven social spaces within the car for persuasive purposes. Inspired by the design ideas presented in this paper, we developed our approach to use a game to create a social coupling between driver and passenger.

We use and intervene in this coupling based on different embodiments of real car data that are translated into different in-game interventions. The game serves as a mediatory artifact the social coupling is formed around and facilitates social communication as a persuasive means. When the driver starts speeding the game adapts to this problematic behavior, and as a consequence becomes a lot harder to master or even unplayable. This urges the player of the game (i.e., the passenger) to actively communicate with the driver, which potentially results in persuading the driver to stop speeding. In order to make that happen, the passenger, who is playing the game during the ride, is supposed to link the in-game changes to the actual driving behavior. Therefore, one major challenge in the design process was to find a suitable way of translating the problematic, real-world driving behavior of speeding into in-game events and changes in gameplay. This linkage not only had to work on a technical but also on a semantic level for the passenger in order to enable him/her to persuade the driver effectively. Another challenge was to find an accurate balance between maintaining the safety of the driver and passenger, as well as creating a positive gaming experience, which keeps the passenger engaged with the game, hence aware of the driver's behavior.

3.1 Game Design

As a starting point for the different game designs we wanted to explore, we chose the tile-matching game Tetris as it is well known, skill-based and relatively easy to play. As it is also a rather abstract game with little theming, we were able to pursue our approach and adapt the game mechanics according to our design goals (i.e., creating different levels of game interventions) without breaking the aesthetics and recognition value of the game. We used an open-source version of Tetris (www.openprocessing.org/sketch/34481) to develop the prototype and adapt the game towards the different designs. As it would have been an interfering factor for two of our designs (acceleration and deceleration), we decided to remove the possibility for the player to drop the tiles immediately, in contrast to the implementation of the original game. Thus, we ensured that players could not bypass the speed dependent game mechanics, because that would have otherwise made it difficult for them to recognize the linkage between the real-car speed and the in-game changes. In the following the four different game designs we created are described in detail. In each design the car's speed has a different effect on the gameplay. These effects vary in the strength of their consequences on the gameplay. More precisely, the designs are ranked in descending order, from the most severe to the least severe interference regarding the game's playability (see also Fig. 1):

- **Freeze:** The game freezes, when the driver is speeding (i.e., the playing area turns black, tiles are not visible anymore and the game is paused). Playing is no longer possible for the passenger, until the driver reaches accurate driving speed again. The goal of this design was to completely interupt the player in the playing experience.
- **Blocking Input:** The passenger cannot move the tiles to the left or right, or both, or rotate them anymore on a gradual level depending on the severity of the speeding violation (i.e., the faster the driver is driving, the more control elements are blocked). This design aims at removing the player's input capabilities stepwise in order to create a notion of *loss of control* and simultaneously increase the difficulty level.

- **Acceleration:** The speed of the falling tiles is changing according to the actual speed of the car. The faster the driver gets, the faster the tiles fall and the harder the game gets to master. The goal was to gradually increase the challenge for the player up to a point where the game actually becomes unplayable, depending on the severity of the speeding.
- **Deceleration:** This design is similar to the aforementioned design, but this time in reverse manner. The faster the car is driving, the slower the tiles are falling. Our goal with this design was to explore how we could make the game "less fun" for the passenger if the driver is speeding (i.e., making it extremely slow in order to completely remove the challenge aspect of the game as well as the typical expected game progress of tiles falling faster and faster).

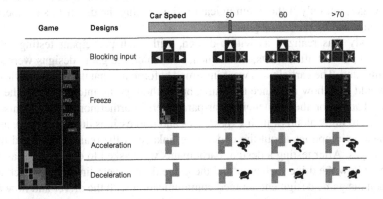

Fig. 1. Schematic of the four different game designs (blocking input, freeze, acceleration, deceleration): Starting with a speed limit of 50 km/h, different changes in the game mechanics and behavior are induced depending on how much the driver exceeds the speed limit.

4 Exploratory User Study

In order to investigate the general potential of our approach to act as a trigger for communication as means of social persuasion, as well as to explore the individual designs, we conducted a user study in the driving simulator (see Fig. 2). We focused on the passenger's role of being a successful persuader by means of the game in order to keep the driver off the gas pedal. Thus, the role of the driver was executed by one of our colleagues.

We conducted our study with 16 participants (9f, 7 m), aged between 22 and 35 years, with a mean age of 30 years, who all took on the role of the passenger in the study. All participants were rather experienced drivers, who held their driving licenses for an average of 11.5 years. The annual mileage travelled by car of all participants averaged out at 7.170 km. Eleven participants declared themselves to be actively playing digital games, whereas five participants don't play digital games at all. The gamers were rather moderate ones regarding the frequency and duration of playing, as the mean gaming frequency was once a week, with one gaming session lasting about 65.5 min on average. All participants were familiar with the game Tetris, and 15 out of 16 participants had already played the game at least once before.

4.1 Study Procedure

At the beginning of the study each participant was asked to sign an informed consent. Then participants were seated next to the driver and introduced to the game and its controls, as well as, the study procedure. To allow for consistent study conditions, we briefed one of our colleagues to take on the role of the driver. He was told to generally stick to the speed limit (50 km/h) but to exceed this limit at certain spots on the track in order to provoke the desired in-game changes. He was allowed to communicate with the passenger, but only if the communication (i.e., asking the driver to stop speeding) was first initiated by the passenger.

The study was realized as within-design, with each participant testing all four designs. To prevent aftereffects, the sequence in which the game designs were tested was permutated. The participants were informed beforehand that the driving style of the driver would somehow influence the game, but without going into details on the exact in-game changes or the influencing car-parameters. Furthermore, participants were encouraged to think aloud of their experiences and impressions during the ride, as well as, to make assumptions about the underlying linkage of the real-car data and the in-game changes. After testing a design, participants were asked to outline their assumptions about how the driver behavior and the game design were linked with each other, how much the game design encouraged communication with the driver and how much fun it was to play. One researcher was present on the backseat of the car to lead through the study and to ask questions after every condition. Another researcher took notes on observations during the ride, as well as on user comments and feedback after the ride. After testing all conditions, participants were asked in a final interview on their opinion on the general approach, as well as, how they would rank the different designs regarding their ability to foster driver-passenger communication as a means of social persuasion.

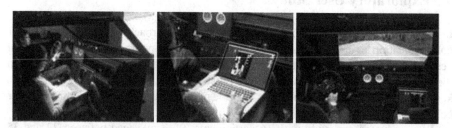

Fig. 2. Picture of the study setup within the car simulator. Passenger is playing Tetris on a laptop while the briefed driver is varying the speed of the car to trigger in-game changes.

4.2   Technical Setup

Our prototype setup used VDrift (vdrift.net) as a simulation software and combined it with Spacebrew (docs.spacebrew.cc) for communication matters between the game (running on a network connected laptop) and the car simulation. Spacebrew, is a websocket-based prototyping framework that was used to connect the game running on a laptop with the car simulation software. The simulation software sent the current speed of the car to the game, which in turn translated the speed into the different in-game changes (based on the aforementioned designs).

5   Results and Findings

5.1   Analysis and Results of Quantitative Data

The quantitative data consisted of participants' answers on which designs were the most intutitive ones regarding the linkage between car speed and in-game changes (multiple answers possible) as well as, the final rankings on which designs were the most fun to play and also which design fostered communication with the driver the most. For a first comparative analysis every rank was associated with a predefined number of points. A first rank was worth 20 points, a second rank 15 points, a third rank 10 points, and a fourth rank 5 points. Every game design received points from 16 participants, which were totaled for the final *fun* and *communication* score. Furthermore, the number of mentions (i.e., how often the specific designs were mentioned to be the most intuitive ones) was counted for each design, and multiplied by 20 for the final linkage score. Finally, each design was assigned an overall score in points, which totaled the scores for fun, communication, and linkage (see Table 1).

Table 1. Rankings of the designs, rated in terms of fun, communication, and best linkage. The overall score combines all three rankings, with a higher score meaning a higher rating.

Condition	Fun	Communication (=based on points)	Best linkage (=nr of mentions)	Overall score
Acceleration	**285**	205	**160**	**650**
Blocking input	150	**235**	120	505
Freeze	155	230	60	445
Deceleration	215	160	40	415

In terms of fun, condition *acceleration* was ranked as being the most fun design by participants, followed by condition *deceleration*. We think that this is due to the fact that the design of condition *acceleration* was based on increasing the challenge for the players, and for many players in-game challenge is directly related to the fun-level of a game. Further, we assume that condition *deceleration* was ranked second highest, because it represented the least severe interventions in terms of playability of the game (i.e., the game only got slower). The conditions *blocking input* and *freeze* were clearly ranked last in terms of fun. A reason for this could be, that both of them strongly interfere with the playability of the game. Additionally, the *blocking input* design, which was ranked last, was experienced to be the most frustrating one.

In turn, the conditions *blocking input* and *freeze* triggered driver-passenger communication the most, whereas condition *acceleration* and *deceleration* were ranked as being the last in terms of communication. We conclude that the more severe the interference in the playability and the higher the experienced frustration level were the more the driver and passenger communicated with each other.

Regarding the linkage of the car speed and the in-game changes, design *acceleration* was rated best, which was presumably a result of the direct mapping between the in-game speed and car speed and corresponded to the general expectations of Tetris tiles falling faster as the game progresses. That is also, why we reason, that the reverse design implementation *deceleration* was experienced to be the least intuitive one. We assume, that *blocking input* was ranked second, due to the stepwise removal of input controls which was linked to a stepwise rise in car speed. Condition *freeze* on the other hand was designed to be binary (i.e., the game was either on or off), which could have made it slightly more difficult for participants to establish a reasonable connection between the speeding and the in-game changes.

Condition *accelerate* and *blocking input* received the best overall scores with all three rankings combined. Based on this result, we argue that a potential real world implementation of our approach should follow a hybrid strategy between designing around increasing the challenge for the player (to foster engagement based on fun) and intervening drastically in the players' game experience e.g., by stepwise removing the player's input capabilities (to foster driver-passenger communication). Such a hybrid design could dynamically adapt the in-game changes based on the severity of real world driving misbehavior and change in-game embodiments accordingly (i.e., the more the driver is speeding the more drastic the in-game interventions could get).

5.2   Analysis and Results of Qualitative Data

The qualitative data consisted of data and notes based on the observations during the study and questions asked at the end of the game sessions. The data was analyzed according to the basics of qualitative content analysis [6].

In general, participants thought our approach was fun and that it was feasible in terms of providing them with a means to stop the driver from speeding. One participant stated: "The game is an indirect way of keeping more eyes on the road, and it encouraged me to tell the driver to slow down". A point of critique was that the mappings of car data and in-game changes were not dynamic, meaning that the game did not adapt to differently skilled players, or players that became better at the game over time. Thus, the balance between creating enough challenge for the player to have an engaging gaming experience but at the same time creating in-game situations that to some extent force the player to give verbal feedback to the driver, is a design challenge for future work. Participants liked the designs that increased the challenge better than those that punished the player. Participants also suggested to create game designs around rewarding the passenger-driver couple for positive driving behavior, rather than punishing the passenger for the driver's neagtive behavior.

In the following, the "common themes" and similarities among the different designs that emerged during the study are described:

Challenge (condition *accelerate* and *decelerate*)**:** At a certain point, the game became boring or unplayable for the participants in these conditions. Thus, the initiated communication with the driver was based on the game getting too easy or too difficult. Some players also felt the need to get better at the game. However, perceived challenge of the game was a matter of individual player skills. This shows, that for a real world implementation of our approach, the mappings between real world misbehavior and in-game changes would need to be dynamic to the current driving scenario and the player's skills and/or game progression in order to enable more long term engagement in the game, hence awareness for the driving style.

Frustration/Punishment/Loss of control (*condition blocking input* and *freeze*)**:** The communication between driver and player was often a direct result of the player being interrupted in the flow of gameplay. The discrepancy between seeing the visuals of the game, but not having adequate control (*condition blocking tiles*) over the game, felt punishing and frustrating for the players. This frustration and loss of control was reported to lead to an increased amount of communication and feedback from player to driver. Attempts to slow down the driver like "Your speeding is breaking my game!" or "I can't play this way, drive slower!" illustrate that the interventions of *condition blocking input* and *condition freeze* were not perceived as being fun for the player, although on the other hand fostered immediate intervention of the passenger.

Commands/Agreements/Common Goal: The commands and feedback from the players were very precise and clearly targeted at slowing down the driver in order to make the game playable and fun to play again. This, in turn, also led to a negotiation process between the driver and passenger regarding the "ideal speed" as a common goal in order to have the best gaming experience but also stick to the speed limit. One participant stated "I achieve more within the game if the driver is sticking to the speedlimit" which illustrates the interconnectedness and common goal between the two of them.

Changing Visual Attention: Some participants were very aware of the speedometer in the central dashboard of the car simulator. They constantly switched their visual attention between the game and the speedometer to compare the car speed and the in-game changes, whereas others were completely focused on the game itself without actually looking at the surroundings. Nevertheless, all types of passengers – the active and the rather passive ones – were aware of the driver's behavior and interfered, when the driver was speeding, which proves our approach to be a viable means of involving even an inattentive passenger in the driving situation.

Social connection: Regardless of the game design, the better the passengers understood how and why the in-game changes were related to the driving behavior, the more interaction between them and the driver emerged. Some participants stated that they felt like "playing together co-operatively" and said that the more dependent they were towards the driver, the more they communicated and wanted to persuade him to stick to the speed limit. One participant concluded: "I like the idea, of influencing someone's behavior, like the driving style, by communicating with each other, which in turn influences the game, and hence, my gaming experience, and so on." This mutual influence loop described by the participant exemplarily illustrates the potential of our approach to deploy gaming technologies in the car, which unfold their persuasive effects based on social influence.

6 Discussion

Our approach proved to be feasible in presenting a game that acts as a mediatory artifact to trigger social persuasion. The different game designs involved the front-seat passenger into the driving experience even when focused on playing the game. This resulted in increased amounts of communication between the front-seat passenger and the driver. Hence, our approach allows to involve co-located passengers in the driving task based on creating a social coupling between them and fostering embodied communication through a shared resource and task (i.e., the game).

Dynamic Mappings: In a real world implementation of our prototype, the mappings between in-game changes and driving behavior would have to be dynamic in terms of presenting the right challenge to the player at the right time to be applicable in a real car setting. As perceived challenge is a matter of individual player skills and preferences, a future iteration of our game prototype could start at a level that suits these factors (i.e., being aware of the player's skill level and game progression).

A major challenge will be to find a balance between safety (i.e., preventing unsafe driving behavior) and a positive gaming experience. For instance, if the players are getting better, they can handle the speed of the falling tiles better but should nevertheless encourage the driver to stop speeding. Hence, the better the player gets, the more the driver could speed, which would be an undesired side effect. As real world settings are much more complex, a future implementation of a game in the real car would need more "intelligence" to react to the ever changing surroundings and traffic situations as well as the player's skill level and game progression, in order to present the right in-game consequence at the right time. If in a future iteration of our approach this level of intelligence in the game is reached, the game itself as well as the mappings between in-game changes and real world driving behavior could also be much more complex thus, being closer to real world scenarios. In that sense, new designs around multiple disadvantageous driving behavior (e.g., tailgating, insufficient lane keeping, etc.) could be incorporated in one game.

Balance of In-game Interventions (Frustration vs. Persuasion): Regarding the in-game interventions, the biggest design challenge would be to find the right level between presenting an appropriate challenge to the player, but also encouraging him/her to actually influence the driver. In our study, we found that intervening in the input and control capabilities of the player, as well as pulling the player out of the game by pausing and interrupting the experience (conditions *blocking input* and *freeze*), create frustration and punishment for the player. These designs provoked more and immediate communication between driver and passenger, though. On the other hand the designs that worked with continous effects (condition *accelerate* and *decelerate*) were ranked as being more fun. However, these designs were not ranked as high in terms of fostering driver-passenger communication, thus, proved to be harder to achieve the desired persuasive effect of keeping the driver from the gas pedal through social influence of the passenger. Finding the right balance between creating an understandable link between in-game and real world, while presenting the right level of challenge and at the same time also increasing communication based on in-game consequences, is an enormous design challenge. Based on our study results, we argue for a *hybrid design strategy* based on creating a game that, depending on the severity of speeding, also adapts the severity of in-game interventions as needed. This would in turn be an ideal compromise between passenger-game engagement and increased communication between driver and passenger. Based on the results and observations, we conclude that intervening in a player's input capabilities or taking her/him out of the game itself (condition freeze), can result in immediate frustration, however also fostering communication rapidly. Thus, we argue that designs based on such input interventions are more likely to be applicable for short term settings where a player is only playing over a short period of time. On the other hand, designs around the mentioned challenge aspect have the potential to create long term engagement, but are a bigger design challenge.

Our approach presents an opportunity to let a person currently focused on gameplay, simultaneously take part in the driving situation. Creating a shared embodied resource, i.e., the game itself, in order to foster communication and social interdependence as a persuasive strategy, proofed to be feasible. This notion is supported by the theory of embodied simulation [1] which describes how humans create meaning by continuously constructing mental models of the currently perceived scene, which in our case is mirroring the experience of the driver based on the current game scene. Different in-game embodiments can facilitate this mirroring process and create a "window" for the player to mirror the behavior of the driver to interfere if necessary.

Limitations and Future Work. A persuasive approach in a safety critical environment like the car that focuses on verbal feedback and increased communication, also has some conflict potential for the passengers (e.g., increased distraction for the driver). In future iterations of our prototype this challenge of potentially increased driver distraction through increased verbal activities has to be mitigated (e.g., by allowing the driver to take over control and disable the connection of the real-car data and the in-game events at some point). In our future work we plan to iterate our designs based on the study findings and create a game that incorporates the mentioned *dynamic mappings* in order to investigate our approach in a real car scenario.

7 Conclusion

We presented an approach that utilizes a digital in-car game, which translates real-world misbehavior (i.e., speeding) into in-game interventions. We designed different levels of in-game interventions and investigated their potentials of acting as a communication trigger for social persuasion, as well as their impact on fun and engagement. Our approach fostered communication between driver and front-seat passenger by using different in-game embodiments of car data to create a connection between the real- and the game world. Thus, the approach proved to be effective in terms of positive short-term effects on the speeding behavior of car drivers.

Our study findings illustrate how using a game as a facilitator for social persuasion and mediatory artifact in a safety critical scenario can be implemented. The respective game should be dynamic to player skills and preferences as well as dynamic to the current driving situation and environment (i.e., a hybrid design strategy with dynamic mappings between in-game changes and driving behavior based on the severity of speeding). Based on our findings we argue, that there is great potential in using contextual data for creating new interactive persuasive systems that are designed around social couplings in the car.

Acknowledgements. The financial support by the Austrian Federal Ministry of Science, Research and Economy and the National Foundation for Research, Technology and Development is gratefully acknowledged (Christian Doppler Laboratory for Contextual Interfaces).

References

1. Bergen, B.K.: Louder than Words: the New Science of How the Mind Makes Meaning. Basic Books, New York (2012)
2. Bogost, I.: Persuasive Games: the Expressive Power of Videogames. MIT Press, Cambridge (2007)
3. Brunnberg, L., Juhlin, O.: Motion and spatiality in a gaming situation–enhancing mobile computer games with the highway experience. In: Proceedings of Interact 2003 (2003)
4. Forlizzi, J., Barley, W.C., Seder, T.: Where should i turn: moving from individual to collaborative navigation strategies to inform the interaction design of future navigation systems. In: Proceedings of CHI 2010. ACM (2010)
5. Gärtner, M., Meschtscherjakov, A., Maurer, B., Wilfinger, D., Tscheligi, M.: Dad, stop crashing my car!: Making use of probing to inspire the design of future in-car interfaces. In Proceedings of AUI 2014. ACM (2014)
6. Mayring, P.: Qualitative content analysis. In: Flick, U., von Kardoff, E., Steinke, I. (eds.) A Companion to Qualitative Research. Sage, London (2004)
7. Perterer, N., Sundström, P., Meschtscherjakov, A., Wilfinger, D., Tscheligi, M.: Come drive with me: an ethnographic study of driver-passenger pairs to inform future in-car assistance. In: Proceedings of the CSCW. ACM (2013)
8. Shepherd, J.L., Lane, D.J., Tapscott, R.L., Gentile, D.A.: Susceptible to social influence: risky "Driving" in response to peer pressure. J. Appl. Soc. Psychol. **41**(4), 773–797 (2011)
9. Sjöblom, B.: Gaming as a situated collaborative practice. Human IT: J. Inf. Technol. Stud. Hum. Sci. **9**(3), 128–165 (2013)
10. Oinas-Kukkonen, H., Harjumaa, M.: Persuasive systems design: key issues, process model, and system features. Commun. Assoc. Inf. Syst. **24**(1), 28 (2009)

Smile Catcher: Can Game Design Lead to Positive Social Interactions?

Niaja Farve[✉] and Pattie Maes

MIT Media Lab, Massachusetts Institute of Technology, Cambridge, MA 02139, USA
nfarve@mit.edu,pattie@media.mit.edu

Abstract. Our hectic and increasingly digital lives can have a negative effect on our health and well-being. Some authors have argued that we socialize less frequently with other people in person and that people feel increasingly lonely [1]. Loneliness has been shown to significantly affect health and wellbeing in a negative way. To combat this, we designed a game, Smile Catcher, which encourages players to engage in in-person, social interactions and get others to smile. Participants wear a device that takes regular pictures of what is in front of them and the system analyzes the pictures captured to detect the number of smiles. The game was evaluated with a two-week study that sought to determine if game design can increase positive social interactions and thereby people's well-being. Our results show that users increased their frequency of positive interactions as a result of playing our game.

Contribution Statement: This paper describes a unique game that improves well-being by encouraging positive social interactions.

Keywords: Happiness · Well-being · Gamification

1 Introduction

Research has shown for years that having a healthy social life is good for well-being and can double life expectancy [2]. Smile Catcher is a multi-user real world game that encourages players to catch as many smiles as possible in a single day or session. The motivation for the game is to have players interact with other people in a positive way, which hopefully results in an overall increase in their well-being and happiness. To play, users only need to wear a Narrative Clip [3] or Google Glass that can take pictures at regular intervals of whatever is in front of the user. At the end of the day, the players upload their images to be analyzed. The simple implementation of the game allows users to play with only minor changes in their apparel and daily behavior. While other projects have tried to log smiles or even force smiles, not many projects have tried to combine the two in a mobile game for players to enjoy.

© Springer International Publishing Switzerland 2016
A. Meschtscherjakov et al. (Eds.): PERSUASIVE 2016, LNCS 9638, pp. 211–218, 2016.
DOI: 10.1007/978-3-319-31510-2_18

2   Previous Work

Previous research has shown that smiles directly correlate to happiness and can even incite happiness in a person [4]. This has resulted in several projects that attempt to measure or force users to smile. All of the projects discussed below primarily focus on inducing smiles in the user. In contrast, the Smile Catcher project encourages the user to induce a smile in another person, which means that they benefit not only from producing a positive affect, but also possibly from emotional contagion [5] and a strengthening of social connections.

2.1   Mood Meter

The mood meter [6] was a MIT project that displayed mood that was measured in terms of the number of people smiling in a particular location. Camera systems were placed in several areas around MIT's campus. These systems were then used to detect smiles in community members as they frequented these areas. The data collected was used to try to raise awareness of how smiles can positively effect an environment. In contrast with our system, the mood meter captured smiles but did not actively encourage users to smile.

2.2   HappinessCounter

The HappinessCounter [7] was a project that attempted to force smiles through the use of an electronic magnet system attached to a fridge. To open the fridge, the user had to smile. This project was intended for users that lived alone and had limited human inter-action. While the HappinessCounter forced smiles and logged smiles, the applications were limited to static locations. Smiles occurring in areas away from the system were not logged. In contrast with our system, the HappinessCounter did not involve any human interactions and dealt with contrived smiles.

2.3   Emotional Flowers

Emotional Flowers [8] is a game that also utilizes the player's emotion. A user can play with several people in their social circle. A webcam on each player's computer monitors his or her facial expression. Facial expressions classified as happy or surprised allow their personal flower to grow and change its color. Negative emotions result in their flowers shrinking. Players attempt to competitively grow the most flowers. Emotional Flowers also utilizes gamification to encourage happiness, however it does not encourage positive interactions among players in the game. Besides competing against each other, there was no advantage to interacting socially. The short interval at which a smile would be captured resulted in players forcing smiles several times an hour. This resulted in players quickly becoming tired of having to smile at such frequent time periods.

3   Game Implementation

The hypothesis of our study is that we can improve people's mood and increase their number of positive social interactions by making a game of catching smiles they encounter in their day. For our study, players utilized Narrative Clips to play Smile Catcher. Game implementation consisted of three parts: image capture, image processing and feedback. A session is typically played over the course of the day; however the game can last indefinitely.

On the Narrative Clip, a game or session does not need to be started as images are taken automatically every 30 s. Proper capture depended on correct placement of the camera and the moment being captured by the camera. Placement of the camera differed per person and took some trial and error.

To process the images captured by the Narrative Clip, players use an online application to upload images. Each image is processed using the Face++ [9] API. The images were analyzed for faces and subsequently smiles. If a smile is present, the image is saved for the player to review. Other images are not saved as the player already has the image saved on their personal hard drive and on the Narrative Clip server. The web application saves their daily counter of smiles and shows trends.

At the end of the day, players are given a score calculated from the day or game counter (if multiple days). The score is used to help the player gauge the happiness they have created over a period of time. This score can be sent to others to incite a long-term competition. Hopefully, this score will become as important as how many steps were taken or how many calories were consumed during a day.

4   Methodology

4.1   Participants and Methods

Our game was evaluated using a two-week study with thirty-three participants. Participant's ages ranged from 19 to 67 (14 males and 19 females). The participants were recruited from a database of willing study participants. Each were told they would be required to wear the Narrative Clip for two weeks and would upload the images at the end of each day. So that their first week could be used as a baseline, they were not told the intention of the study. The only criterion for participation was daily access to a computer with reliable Internet.

A participant was considered to have successfully completed the study if they fully participated throughout the two weeks. Twenty participants successfully completed the study. Full participation consisted of uploading all of the images captured at the end of each day. Successful participants uploaded at least 100 images each day; ten participants did not upload a sufficient number of images (less than 100 over the two week period). Three participants lost their tracker and therefore were unable to participate for the full two weeks.

4.2   Study Procedures

Prior to starting the study, each participant attended a thirty minute orientation session where they were given the Narrative Clip, shown how it worked and given an overview of the website they would be using throughout the duration of the study. Each participant was given suggestions for how to avoid privacy issues. They were permitted to remove the device if an individual felt uncomfortable or they were in a private environment.

Each night, participants visited the website to upload their images. The first week of the study the website was called Life Logger and did not mention anything about smiles. Participants were asked several questions in regards to their mood (see Fig. 1). Once they completed the quick survey, they would gain access to a form to upload their images. During the first week, this was the final step needed to be successfully complete the daily requirements.

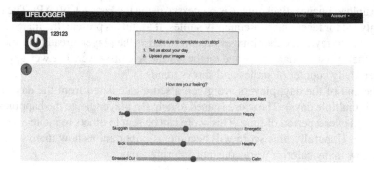

Fig. 1. Baseline week upload page

At the start of the second week of the study the website name changed to be called Smile Catcher. A smile goal was visible at the top of the website as well as a tracker

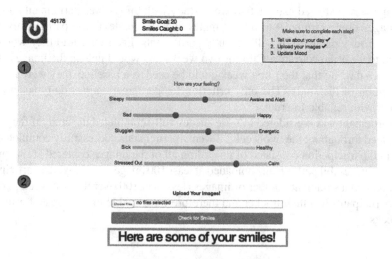

Fig. 2. Week 2 upload page

that reflected any past smiles caught. This goal was the same for all participants and set by averaging daily smile totals from test participants. Participants once again had to report on their day before uploading their images. After uploading, the users were able to review five randomly selected smiles caught in previous days and were once more asked about their mood. After completing the survey, they were shown graphs illustrating any trends in the number of smiles they caught. Participants were not rewarded for reaching their smile goals (Figs. 2 and 3).

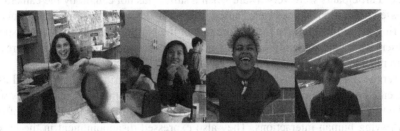

Fig. 3. Smiles caught by participants

At the conclusion of the study each participant attended a thirty-minute closing session. During this time they returned the Narrative Clips, completed a post survey and were asked about their experience playing the game.

5   Results

We analyzed the total count of smiles caught to determine if participants had more positive social interactions during the study. The first week of the study was treated as baseline. When introducing a new device to users, a novelty effect may occur [10]. Our participants were not initially aware of the purpose of the study. If a novelty effect were present, any peak over the baseline week would further confirm that we were able to influence social behavior.

Evaluating the smiles caught by the twenty successful participants, we were able to find, with significance ($p < .05$), that participants caught more smiles during the second week of the study. Users caught an average of 6.25 smiles during the baseline week and 10.85 smiles during the following week. Those that caught more smiles in the second week increased the number of smiles caught by 9 images on average, while other participants caught an average of 3.57 less smiles in the second week.

During the closing session most participants were able to report on smiles that were caught or missed. Participants developed tactics to increase their chances of catching smiles. Several participants noted making efforts to engage with strangers in an attempt to gain more smiles. Other participants chose to smile more at individuals hoping they would reciprocate the gesture.

While users were able to mentally recall smiles in their day, this did not have any significant effect on their self-reported mood. This may be due to participants only submitting their mood at the end of the day. Pervious work has shown that recall of mood can be inaccurate [11]. Our participants may have more accurately submitted their current mood and not an accurate measure of the day's mood. While there were no apparent trends between number of smiles and the mood data collected at the end of the day, 13 participants commented on how the number of smiles they caught affected them either positively or negatively.

Not catching smiles was disappointing to many participants; this may be due to limitations of the system. Due to the nature of the Clip, it was easy for smiles to be missed. Participants were very aware when a smile was not caught by the camera and expressed frustration. Misses were caused by error in detection software and simply not capturing the moment due to the capture rate of the Narrative Clip. This demonstrated that users were independently searching their images for smiles and that they were also able to mentally log smiles during the day.

Users found other trends in the images they captured during the day. Several users commented on the majority of their images being of their computer screens. They were shocked by the amount of time they spent in front of a computer and the lack of time spent having human interactions. They also expressed disappointment in the lack of smiles they caught during the study.

Three participants enjoyed the process of capturing their day and the introspection it provided that they decided to purchase their own devices so they could continue after the study ended (Fig. 4).

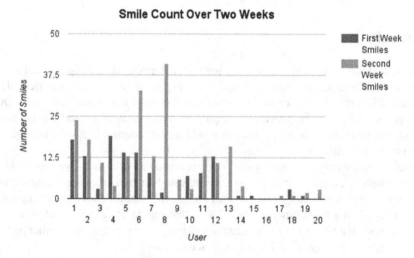

Fig. 4. Total smiles caught by week

6   Discussion

6.1   User Feedback

Through user feedback we were able to identify several areas where the game could be improved. It was clear that for long-term adoption accuracy of the game and ease of use would need to be improved. Accuracy can be improved in further iterations by utilizing a more accurate API to analyze images. Newer versions of the narrative clip have the ability to change the image capture frequency. Increasing the capture rate decreases the chance that a smile would be missed. Outside of the study we would like participants to be able to play without having to upload their images. However, there is currently no open API to develop directly with the Narrative Clip.

Women also expressed frustration in trying to find an effective location to wear the clip. Most examples given by the company highlight men and clothing typically worn by men on a regular basis. Women tend to not have a flat surface on their chest that the clip could be easily pinned.

6.2 System Limitations

Using a computer vision algorithm to determine smiles allows for errors in detection and false positives. Several participants used public transportation daily. Advertising used on public transportation often uses images of happy people. If this were in the participant's field of view, it would result in several "catches". However these catches accounted for less than 10 % of all smiles caught and only three participants caught smiles of this nature. We allowed these to be counted toward the overall total, as emotional contagion is effective in print materials [12].

6.3 Future Work

While we were able to influence the number of smiles caught by participants, it would also be interesting to see how their interactions have changed. Do they have more social interactions overall? Do they target the same people when they try to get their smiles? Other goals could be provided to users to challenge who they target to get smiles.

7 Conclusion

Through a two-week study we were able to show that gamification could be used to persuade users to attempt to have more positive social interactions in their day-to-day lives. By simply tracking the smiles users witnessed during the day and giving a goal, users significantly changed their behavior. We expected users to attempt to target people in their social circles when attempting to catch smiles. However, many users reported engaging with people outside their social circles. We also expected users to be aware of the positive moments in their day. This proved to be the case, but users were also made aware of their lack of social interactions. By simply asking users to catch smiles, they became more cognizant of the smiles in their day-to-day actions. This ability to positively recall memories can be linked to an increase in overall mood and gratitude [13] and therefore an improvement in well-being.

Overall, we were able to positively persuade study participants of all ages to change how they will interact with individuals inside and outside of their social networks through the use of very simple mechanisms. While game design was used to encourage behavior change, participants were not rewarded for completing their goals. We hope this self-motivation will lend to long-term change. As there is no end to the game, users simply monitor their progress.

References

1. Coget, J.-F., Yamauchi, Y., Suman, M.: The internet, social networks and loneliness. It Soc. **1**(1), 180 (2002)
2. Holt-Lunstad, J., Smith, T.B., Bradley Layton, J.: Social relationships and mortality risk: a meta-analytic review. PLoS Med. **7**(7), 859 (2010)
3. Narrative Clip - The Wearable Camera For Moments That Matter. Narrative. Web. 23 March 2015. http://getnarrative.com
4. James, W.: The principles of psychology, vol. 2
5. Hatfield, E., Cacioppo, J.T., Rapson, R.L.: Emotional Contagion. Cambridge University Press, Cambridge (1994)
6. Hernandez, J., Hoque, M., Drevo, W., Picard, R.: Mood meter: counting smiles in the wild. In: UbiComp 2012, pp. 301–310. ACM Press (2012). Dover Publications, New York (1950)
7. Tsujita, H., Rekimoto, J.: HappinessCounter: smile-encouraging appliance to increase positive mood. In: Alt-Chi: Emotions, Ethics and Civics, CHI 2011 (2011)
8. Using emotion in games: Emotional flowers. In: Proceedings of the International Conference on Advances in Computer Entertainment Technology
9. Face++- Leading Face Recognition on Cloud. Face++. Web, 23 November 2015. http://www.faceplusplus.com
10. Kormi-Nouri, R., Nilsson, L.-G., Ohta, N.: The novelty effect: support for the novelty-encoding hypothesis. Scand. J. Psychol. **46**(2), 133–143 (2005)
11. Thomas, D.L., Diener, E.: Memory accuracy in the recall of emotions. J. Pers. Soc. Psychol. **59**(2), 291–297 (1990). doi:10.1037/0022-3514.59.2.291
12. Small, D.A., Verrochi, N.M.: The face of need: facial emotion expression on charity advertisements. J. Mark. Res. **46**(6), 777–787 (2009)
13. Watkins, P.C., Grimm, D.L., Kolts, R.: Counting your blessings: positive memories among grateful persons. Curr. Psychol. **23**(1), 52–67 (2004)

More than Sex: The Role of Femininity and Masculinity in the Design of Personalized Persuasive Games

Marc Busch[1(✉)], Elke Mattheiss[1], Michaela Reisinger[1], Rita Orji[2],
Peter Fröhlich[1], and Manfred Tscheligi[1,3]

[1] AIT Austrian Institute of Technology, Vienna, Austria
{Marc.Busch,Elke.Mattheiss,Michaela.Reisinger,
Peter.Froehlich,Manfred.Tscheligi}@ait.ac.at
[2] McGill University, Montreal, Canada
rita.orji@mail.mcgill.ca
[3] University of Salzburg, Salzburg, Austria
Manfred.Tscheligi@sbg.ac.at

Abstract. The goal of persuasive games is to change behavior and attitudes in a desirable manner, e.g., to promote physical activity. Research has shown that personalized persuasive approaches are more successful than one-size-fits-all approaches. As a means for personalization, sex has been investigated with results showing that women are overall more persuadable than men. We argue that considering only a dichotomous sex-type categorization may not be able to fully capture the differences in the persuasiveness of persuasion strategies. To that end we apply a dimensional approach of capturing gender identity – femininity and masculinity. We investigate the relationship between masculinity, femininity, sex and the persuasiveness of ten persuasion strategies in an online study (n = 592). Results show that femininity is significantly associated with seven of the ten strategies, while sex does only show differences for two strategies, suggesting gender identity could be a reliable variable for personalizing persuasive games.

Keywords: Persuasive games · Personalization · Gender identity · Sex · Femininity · Masculinity

1 Introduction

Persuasive games (PGs) are games that aim at changing human behavior and underlying attitudes [1]. PGs have been used for achieving several behavioral outcomes, such as promoting healthy eating [2] and physical activity [3]. PGs designed in a way that take individual differences into account are more effective than using a "one-size-fits-all" approach [4]. One way of tailoring persuasive technologies (PTs) to individual differences is to design for individual susceptibility to certain persuasion strategies, which is called persuadability [5]. Another popular approach is to tailor PTs based on gender or sex [6].

However, research and design based on gender or sex differences are inherently biased, as recent studies [7] show that sex/gender differences (e.g., in spatial abilities) may be more a product of society and education than of biological differences. Although

© Springer International Publishing Switzerland 2016
A. Meschtscherjakov et al. (Eds.): PERSUASIVE 2016, LNCS 9638, pp. 219–229, 2016.
DOI: 10.1007/978-3-319-31510-2_19

sex and gender are often used interchangeably, the world health organization differentiates the two terms[1]. While sex refers to "biological and physiological characteristics that define men and women", gender refers to "socially constructed roles, behaviors, activities, and attributes that a given society considers appropriate for men and women". This differentiation shows a clear need to depart from a dichotomous classification of women and men and to establish more enduring differentiable characteristics. In this paper, we will use the term sex to refer to the dichotomous categorization of men and women, and the term gender identity, when we refer to a multi-dimensional construct that includes fine-grained notions on masculinity and femininity.

While sex has been investigated in the area of persuasive games [6, 8, 9], there has been – to the best of our knowledge – no previous work investigating whether there are significant relationships between factors of gender identity (such as the degree of femininity and masculinity of people) and the persuasiveness of selected strategies. If such relationships exist, gender identity could meaningfully contribute to the understanding and the personalization of persuasive games.

We selected the same persuasion strategies that have been investigated by Orji et al. in the context of a persuasive game to foster healthy eating [8, 9] and let 592 participants evaluate the persuasiveness of these strategies in an online study. We assessed participants' sex as well as femininity and masculinity by using a short version of these scales that are included in Bem's Sex Role Inventory [10], a self-assessment questionnaire designed to assess the degree of femininity and masculinity of a person. We hypothesized that the more fine-grained notion of femininity and masculinity can provide a better understanding of the persuasiveness of persuasion strategies than biological sex recorded as female or male alone. Our results show that femininity and masculinity affect the persuasiveness of more strategies than sex does and that sex differences might not be a reliable predictor of persuasiveness of persuasion strategies or are strongly depending on the target behavior. We investigated very similar relationships as Orji et al. [8, 9], but have different results.

Our contribution is twofold: First, in opposite to self-reported biological sex, we introduce femininity and masculinity into the domain of persuasive games, and second, we show that accounting for femininity and masculinity can meaningfully inform personalized persuasive game design. The rest of the paper is organized as follows: We start with a review of related work in the area of sex and gender studies and how they account for differences in the effectiveness of PTs and PGs. We describe our online study procedure and the results. We contrast our results to the results of Orji et al. [8, 9] and give an outlook into the future of personalized persuasive game design based on gender identity.

2   Previous Work

Sex and gender are complex constructs that encompass a number of sub dimensions: measurements of sex can include assessment of bodily characteristics, fetal testosterone

---

[1] http://apps.who.int/gender/whatisgender/en/index.html.

markers, chromosomal or hormonal status. Many studies have investigated how and when to measure sex, and what levels of assessment could support defining differences between participants and groups of participants. Gender identity refers to the personal conception of oneself – a conception that is culturally derived. This often refers to masculine and feminine personality traits [e.g., 11, 12], though some employ a broader definition of gender identity, which includes those gendered personality traits as one factor (multifactorial gender identity theory).

Only few authors explicitly discuss routine sex/gender items and different operationalizations of sex and gender in questionnaires [e.g., 13]. Sex and gender are usually assessed through single item measures, within which participants are asked to indicate their sex/gender by checking "male" or "female" (or, sometimes used for the latter, "masculine" or "feminine") and which results in a dichotomous variable. A strong connection between sex and gender is often presumed – so extensively, that they are used synonymously, or one is consciously used to account for the other.

Since items like "are you male/female?" can be associated with "biological sex" (i.e. concepts the individual holds thereof) as well as gender (identity), they are hardly unambiguous. It has also been noted that male/female are neither exclusive nor exhaustive categories, which would also be necessary to use them as nominally scaled data [13]. Using psychometric scales to assess gender identity on the other hand is much less common. Of these scales, the Bem Sex Role Inventory (BSRI) [10] and its shortened versions, e.g., the Gender Traits Index (GTI) [14] are most frequently used. For an overview of other scales for the assessment of gender see Döring [13]. Originally, the BSRI has three subscales (femininity, masculinity and androgyny) and consists of 60 items. Identification with these attributes categorizes individuals across four categories: feminine, masculine, androgynous and undifferentiated. In this research we did not want to assign people to categories (similar to assigning them to sex categories), instead we wanted to understand the finer grained notion of gender identity regarding masculinity and femininity in relation to persuasion strategies. To achieve this, we adopted a shorter version of the BSRI with ten items of the femininity and masculinity scales each that had the highest item-scale correlations [15].

Sex/Gender have been shown to influence interests and behavior [2, 16]. Both constructs also play a role within persuasion pathways – persuasiveness can be moderated by gender similarity of human as well as non-human interaction partners [17, 18], and message pathway preferences differ according to sex/gender [19–21]. Gender (no details on assessment given) and age can impact the effectiveness of gain- or loss-framed messages promoting physical activity, with gender furthermore acting as moderating factor in promoting physical activity [22].

In the last years, personalization of PTs and PGs has been in the focus of research [23]: For example Kaptein et al. [24] showed that in the health promotion domain, tailored messages were more successful in persuading people to perform more physical activity or to eat more healthy. Investigating the persuasiveness of selected persuasion strategies from Fogg [25] and Oinas-Kukkonen and Harjumaa [26], Orji et al. [8] found that females evaluate the strategies cooperation, customization, personalization, praise and simulation as significantly more persuasive. Investigating sex differences in the strategies by Cialdini [27], Orji et al. [6] found that females evaluate the strategies reciprocity, commitment and consensus as significantly more persuasive. Regarding a model of persuasiveness, Drozd [28] found that the relationships between several variables in that model (e.g., unobtrusiveness of technology and intention to use) was the same for women and men.

We aim to combine and advance these different research streams: we apply an existing method from gender studies (scales from BSRI) to explore gender identity as a possible new meaningful factor for the personalization of PGs.

3 Method

To answer the research question whether femininity and masculinity as measured through a short version of the BSRI can contribute more to the understanding of persuasiveness of persuasion strategies than sex alone, we conducted an online study with 592 participants. A link to the online study was distributed to a database consisting of people volunteering to participate in research studies.

3.1 Procedure of the Online Study

The procedure of the online study was as follows: After a short introduction into the goal of the study (the design of videogames for promoting physical activity), participants saw the persuasion strategies, which were presented as storyboards. Storyboards are considered to be a useful tool in product design to communicate concepts in a visually appealing way [29] and they have also been successfully used in prior work in the area of persuasive technology [8, 9]. In this regard, storyboards have been used to operationalize the persuasion strategies and to empirically compare the persuasiveness of these strategies to ultimately decide which persuasion strategies should be implemented in real systems. We chose the same persuasion strategies as Orji et al. [8, 9], which were taken from Fogg [25] and Oinas-Kukkonen and Harjumaa [26], but investigated all of them separately (e.g., to be able to have results for these strategies separately, we did not investigate competition and comparison in one storyboard). Each of the ten persuasion strategies that we investigated in this study was operationalized in one storyboard. Every participant saw each persuasion strategy one by one in a random order.

After each storyboard, participants had to answer the following three questions on a 7-step Likert-type scale ranging from *Totally Disagree* to *Totally Agree*:

- *This approach is fun.*
- *This approach would help me to be more aware of my physical activity.*
- *This approach would motivate me to do more physical activity.*

From the three items, one persuasiveness score per persuasion strategy was calculated. Next, gender identity was assessed with a short version of the BSRI containing 20 adjectives (e.g., "strong"). There are ten adjectives that are more associated with women and ten adjectives that are more associated with men. On a 7-step Likert-type scale, participants were asked to decide how much each adjective applied to them. From these ratings, we calculated an overall score for masculinity and one for femininity for each participant.

We report Cronbach's Alpha as a measure for internal consistency of the scales used in this study: Femininity has an Alpha of .83, masculinity has .86 and the mean Alpha of the persuasiveness scales is .93. These values are satisfying for internal consistency, which allows us to calculate and interpret overall scores from the single items.

At the end, participants were asked basic demographic variables such as biological sex and age as well as interest in video games.

3.2 Storyboard Development

In the following section, we describe how we designed the storyboards used in this study. Although the design of the storyboards was inspired by Orji et al. [8, 9], the storyboards in this study were modified as follows: The gamer shown in the storyboards of Orji et al. [8, 9] was always female. Instead of showing a person which can be identified as either female or male, we used a sketch/outline of a hand to account for potential biases. To ensure internal validity of this study, we checked the following quality criteria in the (message) design of the storyboards:

- The storyboards should only vary in the persuasion strategies, not in the level of detail, design fidelity or other factors.
- The storyboards should clearly represent one and only one strategy.
- The storyboards should comprehensively relay the persuasion message.

We evaluated and iteratively refined the persuasion strategies in two subsequent expert interviews with HCI experts in a research organization. Initial interviews conducted with five experts led to a first design iteration, further interviews with two different experts led to a second design iteration. An example for a storyboard representing the persuasion strategy reward is depicted in Fig. 1.

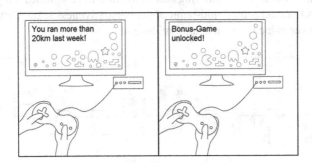

Fig. 1. Storyboard representing the persuasion strategy *Reward*

Graphically, all ten storyboards looked the same. What differed was the text on the left and on the right picture. This is a list with all texts of all ten storyboards:

- **Customization**: Indicate, how your results regarding running should be displayed in the game – Settings: o Speed/o Distance/o Burned calories.
- **Personalization**: Enter some information about you: Age, Weight – Your training plan will be personalized accordingly.

- **Praise**: You managed to run more than 20 km in the last week – Very good! That is quite a lot!
- **Self-Monitoring**: You ran 21 km in the last week – You improved: the week before it was 19 km.
- **Simulation**: The number of km that you ran has increased from week to week – A sneak peek into the future: if you continue with your progress, you will run 30 km per week in two months.
- **Suggestion**: To improve your running performance, here is a tip – Try to walk some distances occasionally during running. Doing that, you manage longer distances.
- **Comparison**: You ran 21 km in the last week – Alex ran 23 km.
- **Competition**: In the next week you can enter a competition against Alex – Will you manage to run more km than Alex?
- **Cooperation**: In the next week Alex' and your results will be added – Can you manage to run over 75 km together?

4 Sample and Results

Sample. The sample (n = 592) indicated a medium interest in video games (M = 3.77; SD = 2.17). Participants' age ranged from 14 to 80 (M = 35.14; SD = 14.06) and 272 (46 %) assessed themselves as female.

Distribution of Persuasion Strategies. To get an overall view on how persuasive the single persuasion strategies were rated, Fig. 2 presents notched boxplots. The notch represents the 95 % confidence interval of the median and allows estimating significant differences between the strategies regarding their persuasiveness. Customization, personalization, reward, self-monitoring and simulation have significant higher persuasiveness values than the neutral mid-point of the persuasiveness scale. Comparison has a significant lower value than the neutral mid-point.

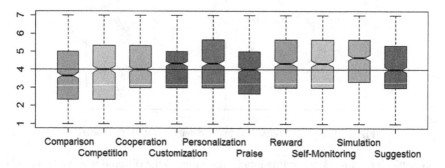

Fig. 2. Evaluation of the *persuasiveness* (y-axis) of the ten persuasion strategies (x-axis) on a Likert-type scale ranging from 1 to 7 (higher numbers indicate a higher persuasiveness; the black line at 4 indicates the neutral mid-point).

Distribution of Masculinity and Femininity and Influence of Sex. Masculinity (M = 4.92; SD = .91) and femininity (M = 4.89; SD = .85) are similarly distributed.

Femininity and masculinity show a medium correlation of .16. According to two-sample t-tests, self-reported sex has a significant influence on femininity, $t(585) = 5.81$, $p < .001$, $d = .46$, with women describing themselves as more feminine ($M = 5.13$; $SD = .77$) as men ($M = 4.75$; $SD = .87$). Self-reported sex has not a significant influence on masculinity, $t(567) = -1.58$, $p = .12$, $d = .13$, however men described themselves slightly more masculine ($M = 4.94$; $SD = .89$) than women ($M = 4.82$; $SD = .92$).

Table 1. Influence of femininity, masculinity and sex on persuasion strategies (it is indicated in bold when a gender identity factor has a significant influence on persuasiveness of a strategy).

Strategy	Regression Statistic	Influence of femininity/masculinity
Customization	$R^2=.01^a$, $F(3,584)=3.27$, $p<.05$	**Femininity ($\beta=.19$, $p<.05$)** Masculinity ($\beta=-.05$, $p=.53$) Sex ($\beta=-.19$, $p=.16$)
Personalization	$R^2=.01$, $F(3,584)=3.34$, $p<.05$	**Femininity ($\beta=.22$, $p<.01$)** Masculinity ($\beta=.00$, $p=.97$) Sex ($\beta=-.15$, $p=.28$)
Praise	$R^2=.01$, $F(3,584)=5.52$, $p<.05$	**Femininity ($\beta=.24$, $p<.01$)** Masculinity ($\beta=-.04$, $p=.62$) Sex ($\beta=-.12$, $p=.41$)
Reward	$R^2=.01$, $F(3,584)=3.47$, $p<.05$	**Femininity ($\beta=.26$, $p<.01$)** Masculinity ($\beta=-.05$, $p=.54$) Sex ($\beta=-.27$, $p=.07$)
Self-Monitoring	$R^2=.00$, $F(3,584)=2.08$, $p=.10$	**Femininity ($\beta=.20$, $p<.05$)** Masculinity ($\beta=-.06$, $p=.45$) Sex ($\beta=-.05$, $p=.74$)
Simulation	$R^2=.01$, $F(3,584)=2.67$, $p<.05$	**Femininity ($\beta=.22$, $p<.01$)** Masculinity ($\beta=.01$, $p=.88$) Sex ($\beta=-.05$, $p=.70$)
Suggestion	$R^2=.00$, $F(3,584)=1.91$, $p=.13$	**Femininity ($\beta=.18$, $p<.05$)** Masculinity ($\beta=-.02$, $p=.76$) Sex ($\beta=-.04$, $p=.76$)
Comparison	$R^2=.02$, $F(3,584)=6.774$, $p=.00$	Femininity ($\beta=.15$, $p=.07$) Masculinity ($\beta=.06$, $p=.47$) **Sex ($\beta=.60$, $p=<.001$)**
Competition	$R^2=.03$, $F(3,584)=7.101$, $p=.00$	**Femininity ($\beta=.20$, $p<.001$)** Masculinity ($\beta=.08$, $p=.31$) **Sex ($\beta=.59$, $p<.001$)**
Cooperation	$R^2=.00$, $F(3,584)=1.607$, $p=.19$	Femininity ($\beta=.15$, $p=.07$) Masculinity ($\beta=-.05$, $p=.51$) Sex ($\beta=-.24$, $p=.10$)

[a] Adjusted R^2

Influence of Femininity, Masculinity and Sex on Persuasion Strategies. To answer our main research question – whether femininity and masculinity can contribute more to the understanding of the persuasiveness of persuasion strategies than sex– we calculated multiple regressions. We chose not to perform multivariate analyses, as we had no hypotheses about the interdependencies of the persuasion strategies, but only about the influence of the predictor variables (femininity, masculinity, sex) on the outcome variable (persuasiveness of a persuasion strategy). The results are displayed in Table 1. In eight out of ten strategies, femininity has a significant positive influence on the subjective persuasiveness. The more feminine a person describes him-/herself, the more persuasive he/she rates the persuasion strategies customization, personalization, praise, reward, self-monitoring, simulation and suggestion and competition. Regarding the influence of sex: Men rate the strategies comparison (men: M = 3.99, SD = 1.64; women: M = 3.44, SD = 1.71) and competition (Men: M = 4.09, SD = 1.65; Women: M = 3.57, SD = 1.77) as significantly more persuasive than women.

5   Summary and Discussion

Persuasive games (PGs) can be successful tools in changing behavior and attitudes towards specific desirable goals. For several years now, researchers and designers have aimed at defining and discovering methods for personalizing PGs, as personalized PGs has been shown to be more effective in motivating behavior change than one-size-fits-all approaches. To add to and extend existing work on tailoring persuasive technology to individual characteristics including sex and gender, we explored whether femininity and masculinity (as a dimensional construct) can be a useful and more predictive characteristic for tailoring persuasion strategies than sex alone.

To that end, we conducted a large-scale study with 592 participants to evaluate the persuasiveness of 10 commonly employed strategies in PG design. Participants did a self-assessment on both femininity and masculinity scales (short version of BSRI). Our results show that femininity and masculinity can indeed provide more insight into the persuasiveness of persuasion strategies than sex alone: In our study, men find comparison and competition significantly more persuasive than women. This finding reflects a common male tendency in our society, which is reproduced in our results. However, considering the gender identity factors masculinity and femininity, our results show that participants (regardless of sex) who self-assessed as more feminine find the strategies customization, personalization, praise, reward, self-monitoring, simulation, suggestion and competition more persuasive. Masculinity does not have a significant effect on the perceived persuasiveness. Overall, gender identity factors femininity and masculinity mediates the perceived persuasiveness of more strategies than sex.

We have a finding that might appear counterintuitive: Men find competition significantly more persuasive than women while femininity (but not masculinity) is positively associated with the persuasiveness of competition. However, we argue that this finding shows that sex and gender identity – although related – are not the same construct, they reflect different factors and cannot be used interchangeably.

Since the study by Orji et al. [8, 9] investigated the same persuasion principles as we did, we expected similar results. However, our results stand partly in contrast to their study, where women rated the persuasiveness of cooperation, customization, personalization, praise and simulation significantly higher than men (which is reflected in our finding on the effect of femininity), while for comparison and competition no sex effects were shown. Also, Orji et al. [6] showed that for the Cialdini persuasion principles [27], women are in general more susceptible to persuasion than men. There are several explanations for such different results: Their operationalization of the persuasion strategies differed slightly (e.g., they investigated competition and comparison in one storyboard). Furthermore, while Orji's et al. study [8, 9] was targeted at promoting healthy eating, the current study was targeted at promoting physical activity. Although both target behaviors referred to healthy living and lifestyle, the nutrition topic could be more appealing to women, while the physical activity topic could be more appealing to men, which could in turn have influenced the perceived persuasiveness of persuasion strategies in these topics. This leads to an important conclusion: The application domain in which the technology is applied is an important determining factor of its effectiveness. Furthermore, also potential predictors of the effectiveness of persuasive technology (e.g., sex, gender identity) are mediated by the behavior that should be changed.

In a broader sense, the influence of sex (and gender) on the persuasiveness of persuasion strategies could depend on contextual and situational factors. Under this consideration it is not only necessary to personalize PTs and PGs – assuming that a strategy that persuades a person might not persuade another person - but also to contextualize them, assuming that a strategy that persuades in a specific context or situation might not persuade in another specific context or situation.

Surprisingly, sex was only significantly associated with femininity, not with masculinity. This could be attributed to the instrument with which femininity and masculinity was measured: although the Bem Sex Role Inventory (BSRI) [10] is one of the most widely used inventories to assess gender identity, it is possible that other (psychometric) operationalization methods of gender identity might produce other results, which is a limitation of this study.

6 Conclusion and Future Work

This paper presents the first exploratory study on gender identity, sex and persuasion strategies for persuasive games (PGs). Our results have the following implications for the personalization of PGs: The sex of the target audience, but also how feminine they describe themselves, can influence the effectiveness of persuasion strategies. Taking into consideration that different sexes and gender identities might perceive persuasion strategies differently depending on target behavior (e.g., healthy eating, physical activity), strategies should be selected with care and on the basis of empirical data: When promoting physical activity through PGs, strategies comparison and competition are more persuasive for men than women; strategies customization, personalization, praise, reward, self-monitoring, simulation, suggestion and competition are more persuasive the more the target audience describes themselves as feminine.

To understand the underlying mechanisms of these effects future work has to critically explore the interactions between societal images of men and women and how this affects their perception of PGs. We have to investigate if and to which extent the findings in this and related studies [9] can be generalized to other domains (e.g., personal transportation, security) and target behaviors. Additionally, the stability of the findings needs investigation: Long-term studies under realistic conditions will shed more light on the interrelations between gender identity, sex and persuasiveness of PGs.

Acknowledgements. This research has partly been funded by the Austrian Research Promotion Agency under contract no. 844845 (GEMPLAY).

References

1. Bogost, I.: Persuasive Games: The Expressive Power of Videogames. MIT Press, Cambridge (2007)
2. Orji, R., Vassileva, J., Mandryk, R.L.: Modeling gender differences in healthy eating determinants for persuasive intervention design. In: Berkovsky, S., Freyne, J. (eds.) Persuasive 2013. LNCS, vol. 4128, pp. 161–173. Springer, Heidelberg (2013)
3. Berkovsky, S., Freyne, J., Coombe, M.: Physical activity motivating games. ACM Trans. Comput. Interact. **19**, 1–41 (2012)
4. Orji, R., Mandryk, R.L., Vassileva, J., Gerling, K.M.: Tailoring persuasive health games to gamer type. In: Proceedings of the SIGCHI Conference on Human Factors in Computing Systems - CHI 2013, pp. 2467–2476. ACM Press, New York (2013)
5. Kaptein, M.C.: Personalized persuasion in ambient intelligence. J. Ambient Intell. Smart Environ. **4**, 279–280 (2012)
6. Orji, R., Mandryk, R.L., Vassileva, J.: Gender, age, and responsiveness to Cialdini's persuasion strategies. In: MacTavish, T., Basapur, S. (eds.) PERSUASIVE 2015. LNCS, vol. 9072, pp. 147–159. Springer, Heidelberg (2015)
7. Hoffman, M., Gneezy, U., List, J.A.: Nurture affects gender differences in spatial abilities. Proc. Natl. Acad. Sci. **108**, 14786–14788 (2011)
8. Orji, R.: Exploring the persuasiveness of behavior change support strategies and possible gender differences. In: Öörni, A., Kelders, S., van Gemert-Pijnen, L., Oinas-Kukkonen, H. (eds.) Second International Workshop on Behavior Change Support Systems, CEUR, vol. 1153, pp. 41–57 (2014)
9. Orji, R., Mandryk, R.L., Vassileva, J.: Gender and persuasive technology: examining the persuasiveness of persuasive strategies by gender groups. In: Gamberini, L., Spagnolli, A., Chittaro, L., Zamboni, L. (eds.) Persuasive 2014, Adjunct Proceedings, pp. 48–52. University of Padova, Padova (2014)
10. Bem, S.L.: Bem Sex-Role Inventory: Professional Manual. Consulting Psychologists Press, Palo Alto (1981)
11. Palan, K.M.: Gender identity in consumer behavior research: a literature review and research agenda. Acad. Mark. Sci. Rev. **2001**, 1–24 (2001)
12. Tate, C.: The "problem of number" revisited: the relative contributions of psychosocial, experiential, and evolutionary factors to the desired number of sexual partners. Sex Roles **64**, 644–657 (2011)
13. Döring, N.: Zur Operationalisierung von Geschlecht im Fragebogen: Probleme und Lösungsansätze aus Sicht von Mess-, Umfrage-, Gender- und Queer-Theorie. Gend. – Zeitschrift für Geschlecht, Kult. und Gesellschaft. vol. 5, pp. 94–113 (2013)

14. Barak, B., Stern, B.: Sex-linked trait indexes among baby-boomers and pre-boomers: a research note. Adv. Consum. Res. **13**, 204–210 (1986)
15. Schneider-Düker, M., Kohler, A.: Die Erfassung von Geschlechtsrollen: Ergebnisse zur deutschen Neukonstruktion des Bem Sex-Role Inventory. Diagnostica **34**, 256–270 (1988)
16. Vilela, A.M., Nelson, M.R.: Testing the selectivity hypothesis in cause-related marketing among generation Y: [when] does gender matter for short- and long-term persuasion? J. Mark. Commun. 1–18 (2013)
17. Siegel, M., Breazeal, C., Norton, M.I.: Persuasive robotics: the influence of robot gender on human behavior. In: IROS 2009, IEEE/RSJ International Conference on Intelligent Robots and Systems, pp. 2563–2568. IEEE Press, New York (2009)
18. Mellor, S., Barclay, L.A., Bulger, C.A., Kath, L.M.: Augmenting the effect of verbal persuasion on self-efficacy to serve as a steward: gender similarity in a union environment. J. Occup. Organ. Psychol. **79**, 121–129 (2006)
19. Guadagno, R.E., Cialdini, R.B.: Persuade him by email, but see her in person: online persuasion revisited. Comput. Human Behav. **23**, 999–1015 (2007)
20. Vossen, S., Ham, J., Midden, C.: Social influence of a persuasive agent: the role of agent embodiment and evaluative feedback. In: Persuasive 2009, pp. 46–52. ACM Press, New York (2009)
21. Ruijten, P.A.M., Midden, C.J.H., Ham, J.: Lonely and susceptible: the influence of social exclusion and gender on persuasion by an artificial agent. Int. J. Hum. Comput. Interact. **31**, 832–842 (2015)
22. Li, K.-K., Cheng, S.-T., Fung, H.H.: Effects of message framing on self-report and accelerometer-assessed physical activity across age and gender groups. J. Sport Exerc. Psychol. **36**, 40–51 (2014)
23. Kaptein, M., Markopoulos, P., de Ruyter, B., Aarts, E.: Personalizing persuasive technologies: explicit and implicit personalization using persuasion profiles. Int. J. Hum. Comput. Stud. **77**, 38–51 (2015)
24. Kaptein, M., Lacroix, J., Saini, P.: Individual differences in persuadability in the health promotion domain. In: Ploug, T., Hasle, P., Oinas-Kukkonen, H. (eds.) PERSUASIVE 2010. LNCS, vol. 6137, pp. 94–105. Springer, Heidelberg (2010)
25. Fogg, B.J.: Persuasive Technology - Using Computers to Change What We Think and Do. Morgan Kaufmann Publishers, San Francisco (2002)
26. Oinas-Kukkonen, H., Harjumaa, M.: A systematic framework for designing and evaluating persuasive systems. In: Oinas-Kukkonen, H., Hasle, P., Harjumaa, M., Segerståhl, K., Øhrstrøm, P. (eds.) PERSUASIVE 2008. LNCS, vol. 5033, pp. 164–176. Springer, Heidelberg (2008)
27. Cialdini, R.B.: Harnessing the science of persuasion. Harv. Bus. Rev. **79**, 72–81 (2001)
28. Drozd, F., Lehto, T., Oinas-Kukkonen, H.: Exploring perceived persuasiveness of a behavior change support system: a structural model. In: Bang, M., Ragnemalm, E.L. (eds.) PERSUASIVE 2012. LNCS, vol. 7284, pp. 157–168. Springer, Heidelberg (2012)
29. van der Lelie, C.: The value of storyboards in the product design process. Pers. Ubiquit. Comput. **10**, 159–162 (2006)

A Gamified Solution to Brief Interventions for Nightlife Well-Being

L. Gamberini[1]([⊠]), A. Spagnolli[1], M. Nucci[1], G. DeGiuli[2], C. Villa[2],
V. Monarca[2], A. Privitera[1], L. Zamboni[2], and S. Leclerq[2,3]

[1] HtLab, Department of General Psychology, University of Padua, Padova, Italy
luciano.gamberini@unipd.it
[2] Psicologi Senza Frontiere Onlus, Padova, Italy
[3] ABD - Energy Control, Barcelona, Spain

Abstract. This paper addresses a specific type of intervention for health and wellbeing, i.e., brief interventions during nightlife events, aimed at improving partygoers' awareness of the risks related to the consumption of psychoactive substances. It is argued that a gamified modality would help overcome some limiting contextual constraints while preserving the seriousness of the intervention purpose. To support this last point, the paper describes two studies (N = 227, N = 81 respectively). The first study was conducted in the field; it was found that after a game session, users' self-reported awareness of nightlife risks increased significantly from pre-session scores. In addition, users evaluated the intervention as credible in terms of its accuracy, novelty, and contextual appropriateness. The second study showed, under controlled laboratory conditions, that the number of correct answers about substance consumption consequences, substance characteristics, and risk prevention choices improved after the game session. Together, these studies suggest that using gamification as an attractor would not compromise the serious goals of this intervention modality.

Keywords: Well-being intervention · Risk awareness · Nightlife · Serious games

1 Introduction

Substance consumption is so common in recreational venues such as clubs, festivals, raves, or parties [9] that the terms "club drugs" has emerged to identify a set of substances commonly associated with raves and parties. A recently survey in nine cities across Europe reported that only 9.8 % of the interviewees were nonusers [6]. Practices such as binge drinking [17] or polydrug abuse [31] are not restricted to deviant groups but are diffuse in the young population, supported by specific cultures and lifestyles [18]. The abuse or misuse of recreational drugs can generate serious health problems, jeopardize relationships, and lower performance in activities such as driving [5]. Interventions range from prevention programs addressing the community, law enforcement, and alcohol sellers to interventions carried out in nightlife settings. The latter are brief [23] and devoted to sensitizing to the need for acquiring better information or changing habits. They generally employ leaflets and infocards [3]. On the

© Springer International Publishing Switzerland 2016
A. Meschtscherjakov et al. (Eds.): PERSUASIVE 2016, LNCS 9638, pp. 230–241, 2016.
DOI: 10.1007/978-3-319-31510-2_20

one hand, organizing brief interventions in nightlife settings allows people to reach consumers of recreational drugs where they are likely to perform risk behaviors. On the other hand, this context makes the intervention difficult because it might seem inconsistent with the situational cultures and values and because the hectic environment hampers sustained attention. We built on the opportunities offered by digital technology to overcome some of the contextual constraints and developed a multiplayer digital quiz projected on a large screen to deliver prevention information during such interventions. Whereas noise, crowd, and dominant mood during these events can deter serious information-seeking about prevention behavior, these features might turn into assets if the intervention takes place via a game.

Digital environments for health treatment designed as full-fledged games or that include game elements such as scores, competition among players, roleplaying, chance, rules, goals, levels, rewards, and narratives [8] have added persuasive value [15]. They exploit fun and entertainment to increase the users' motivation to undertake and commit with the intervention, and emphasize the progression of challenges and achievements that boosts the users' self-efficacy by overcoming a progressive set of challenges [e.g., 20]. In addition, they can appeal to classes of users that are particularly attracted or accustomed to digital technology. The World Health Organization acknowledges that the "widespread appeal of computer and videogame playing among children and adults creates a unique opportunity to deliver health education during leisure time" [21, p. 27].

A few examples of interventions directed to young adults to prevent drug abuse and supported by serious games are in the literature. "Reach Out Central" [4] and "Climate" [35] are school-based interventions, which require a different stylistic register and level of explicitness than interventions at parties, are often longer than one session, and do not focus on nightlife and its specificities. "Spot the Triggers Challenge," [24, North] targets alcohol and drug abuse and aims at addiction treatment through a structured program requiring multiple sessions. Closer to our purpose are Happy Farm [13] and VideoDope [12]; the first relies on an interactive storytelling paradigm, which is too complex for nightlife interventions; the latter is limited in scope, being focused on substance effects on driving.

Compared with the existing computer-based solutions to deliver prevention information in this domain, our gamified intervention has a unique combination of characteristics: it is a brief intervention specifically targeting nightlife events, targets a large set of nightlife behaviors, and is especially designed for use in nightlife settings (e.g., multiplayer interface, easy rationale, party aesthetics). Although serious games [2] can be used for health information in general [7, 27, 32, 33], we believe a crucial point in gamified applications is proving that they do not spoil the serious purpose of the intervention, in each context in which they are applied. In this paper, we report two studies with the purpose of assessing whether this was the case with our solution. We will start by describing the game and then report the two validation studies.

2 Game

The intervention presented here represents the gamification of a typical nightlife intervention, which is usually brief [23], with an information area in a relaxed zone of the party, and expert operators—most often peer operators—available to hand out prevention material and provide information. In our intervention, information and advice reside in a digital database and their provision occurs through quiz questions. This is then a serious game [2], in that it exploits for serious purposes the motivational characteristics of a game to provide serious prevention information. The full version of the game contains 4,032 questions in five different languages (English, Italian, German, French, and Spanish), including 1,193 multiple choice and 2,839 true/false questions. We categorized questions according to the 11 risk areas[1] and 13 topics[2].

The game logic includes a set of steps: a training video showing the use of the remote control and the basic rationale of the game (Fig. 1); avatar selection; the set of quiz questions and related explanations; and a player's ranking screen. Questions are randomly selected from the database. Players can select their answer via the controller; after a predefined time, the correct answer is displayed with an explanation and the players' scores are updated and displayed. Players can modify and set some features before each intervention: the language, difficulty level, number of participants, and time to answer each question.

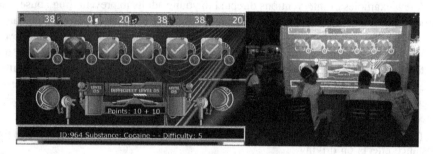

Fig. 1. (a, b). A screenshot from the game interface, where the scores of the players are shown along with the correctness of the last response provided and the difficulty level of the last quiz question (a, left); an image from one field intervention (b, right).

The base system is composed of several modules, each dealing with a different aspect of the game.

---

[1] Alcohol, Cannabis, Ecstasy and Methamphetamines, Hallucinogenic Substances, Ketamine, GHB-GBL, Popper and other Solvents, Cocaine, Heroin, Friendship & Sexuality-Mix.

[2] Desired Effects, Not Desirable Acute Psycho Effects, Not Desirable Long-Term Psycho Effects, Not Desirable Physical/Medical Effects, Legal Issues, Historical-Political-Geographical Issues, Curiosities-Myths and Legends, Woman Specificities & Pregnancy, Driving, Sex & Sexually Transmitted Diseases, Other Indirect Risks, Violence-Bullies-Micro Interethnic Conflicts, First Aid and Precautions.

The data management module contains the quiz questions and the data collected by players' data (ID, date, avatar, scores, and response time). The scoring system module is responsible for storing and correctly calculating the scores depending on the answers selected by the player and on the question category. The event triggering module receives messages from the controller's handler and interacts with the game logic. The controller handler collects inputs from up to six players' controllers and converts them into messages to the base system. It also contains a console for starting the game and an anti-piracy system for preventing the improper use of the software.

Technically, the base system was developed with Web application technology, using the Ruby on Rails framework for development and SQLite as a database for storing all data involved (questions, scoring system, user data collection, and level data). This technology permits easy delivery of the game to the most used platforms and the Web. The controller handler is written in is written in C#, using a .NET framework. The data management module is a SQLite Database. Game controller support in Web platforms is at an early stage of development and not yet implemented in all browsers. For this reason, we designed and developed this module as a separate piece of software, in C# using Microsoft DirectInput Library. It runs on Microsoft Windows. We created audio content using Ableton Live8. We tested the game for usability before the studies described here.

2.1 Additional Design Strategies to Improve Persuasion

We benefited from the specific persuasive characteristic of a game to attract users, but put great emphasis during design into ensuring that the game was credible and contextually appropriate, which are preconditions to persuasion [11, 26].

Credibility required accurate information and institutional or scientific sources for the questions. We built the database by collecting and examining scientific publications and prevention material produced by reliable sources. Experts double-checked each piece of information and turned the pieces into questions in various formats (e.g., multiple choice, true/false, and numeric entry). A component of credibility is the perception that the information is unbiased [e.g., 14]. Indeed, in the specific context of nightlife interventions and health communication, International guidelines [9, 30, 35] stress the need that the recipient perceives the intervention as consonant with his/her prior experience. Thus, our conceptual approach is not to question users' repertoire of values framing certain risky behaviors, which are well rooted in their culture [16, 19], but to appeal to alternative values still consistent with their goals during their nights and parties: well-being and friendship. To be *contextually appropriate*, the game appearance was curated so as to fit the aesthetics of nightlife events. Two professional designers developed graphics, avatars, and music especially for the game, close to those from nightlife parties. The soundtrack changed according to the category of the question; for instance, the music had a fast pace for exciting substances, a reggae rhythm for marijuana, and a soft melody for sexuality. For outdoor interventions (such as during summer music festivals), a gazebo was equipped with an information desk and projection wall and decorated according to party-like aesthetics.

In addition, the game used illustrated narratives (Fig. 2), which increase recall in health communication [22, 29] and allowed some tailoring (selection of topic categories, kind of substance addressed in the questions, questions' difficulty, and time to respond before each intervention), which increases persuasiveness [11].

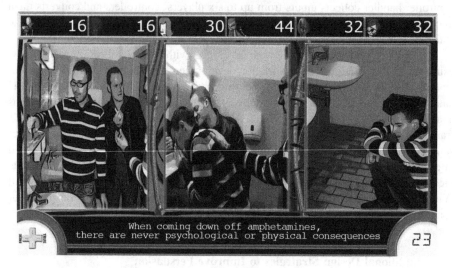

Fig. 2. An instance of an illustrated narrative accompanying a question, here in the form of a statement, which players had to determine was true or false.

The whole design process was participatory [1], which maximizes the probability that the design fit the context of use and the target users' perspective and was in line with the recommendation for persuasive technologies to build upon users' own motivation or goal [25]. This entailed a brainstorming session with 21 European peer operators and experienced nightlife operators; five workshops with peer operators, experienced operators and minors with legal issues related to drug consumption. Each workshop involved 8–10 participants to produce narratives about the risky situations, from initial brainstorming to shooting the scenes; experts participating in the European network Newnet (www.safernightlife.org) to localize the questions.

3 Study 1: Risk Awareness and User Experience

The first validation study reported here was conducted in the field. This forced us to keep the validation instrument as short as possible to avoid dropouts. We hypothesize that after using the game, users' awareness of nightlife risks increased significantly compared with the pre-session scores (H1). We also hypothesized that the scores of the user experience items were positive and significantly higher than the central value of the response scale (H2). We ran analyses with SPSS.

3.1 Method

Setting. The intervention was carried out within two events in Italy. The former took place during the summer; our intervention took place along three days on 4–7 July 2013 and was located beside a park where a dance party was organized with famous radio deejays targeting young adults. Since the event was outdoors, we projected game images onto a wall of a specially designed gazebo. Players could sit in a row of chairs in front of it. The second event was a techno music event with a program consisting of several concerts. We carried out the intervention during three concerts in 2013, on October 5, October 31, and November 23. In this case, the event was indoors and our intervention took place in a space (the "chill-out" zone), where attendees could find less noise, seating, and information. All interventions took place in agreement with the event organizers.

Questionnaire. This intervention used a brief questionnaire, since long, articulated questionnaires were not possible in these conditions. It was a paper-and-pencil questionnaire with pre- and post-session parts. The pre-session questionnaire contained demographic items asking the participants' age, gender, education, and nationality, as well as two statements assessing risk awareness, which could be answered on a 6-degree Likert scale where 6 meant "full agreement" (Table 1). The post-session questionnaire included the same two statements as the pre-session questionnaire in addition to 10 statements (Table 2) investigating whether the intervention was appreciated and was considered appropriate, relevant, and useful. In particular, items 1, 2, 5, and 6 (Cronbach's $\alpha = 0.62$) addressed enjoyment, namely the emotional engagement with the game [28]; items 3 and 4 (Cronbach's $\alpha = 0.77$) take inspiration from the Technology Acceptance Model, where acceptance is measured in terms of intention of using a certain technology and is affected by the extent to which important others would think that the system is worth being used [34]. Items 8, 10, 11, and 12 (Cronbach's $\alpha = 0.73$) measured distinct components of credibility [10, 14]: Items 8 and 10 measured the perceived novelty of the information given in the game; item 12 checked the perceived accuracy of the information; and item 11 investigated the contextual appropriateness of the intervention to the context of use, an important dimension for nightlife interventions in general [9, 30, 35]. All questions were in Italian.

Participants and procedure. The sample consisted of 227 participants (77 women, 150 men, age: $M = 24.69$, $SD = 6.78$). Participants were event attendees who voluntarily approached the intervention area. After signing an informed consent form, participants were shown how to interact with the game. Then, the sessions started. The game included 9 questions and up to 6 players per session. After completing the session, they were administered the post-session questionnaire.

3.2 Results

Let's consider first the items administered twice, the pre- and post-sessions (Table 1). We compared the scores obtained before and after the game with a Wilcoxon test for paired samples, finding the difference significant in both cases ($Z = -3.16$; $p < 0.05$; $r = -0.210$ and $Z = -2.103$; $p < 0.05$; $r = -0.14$).

Table 1. Median, mean value, and standard deviation of the awareness items in the pre- and post-session questionnaires

	Pre	Mdn	M	SD	Post	Mdn	M	SD
7. I am aware that with the proper company I can avoid some risks.		5	4.75	1.46		5	5.05	1.28
9. I am aware of the risks one can run during a night out.		5	4.65	1.58		5	4.87	1.45

For the other user experience items (Table 2), we compared the scores obtained with the central value of the scale (3.5) with the nonparametric signed rank Wilcoxon test with a single sample. The underlying dimension is assumed to vary on a continuum. This justifies comparison with a central point even if this point is not provided in the response scale. The results are shown in Table 2, which indicates that all scores are positive and significantly different from the central value of the scale.

Table 2. Mean value, standard deviation, and result of Wilcoxon signed rank test for each item of the questionnaire. * = $P < 0.001$

Item	M	SD	V
1. I liked playing the game	4.98	1.25	23936.5*
2. Had I played alone, I'd have less fun	4.40	1.89	18676*
3. I'd like to use this game again in the future	4.33	1.49	20122.5*
4. I would recommend my friends to play	4.65	1.38	22148*
5. I liked the remote control used in the game	4.20	1.56	18679.5*
6. The game is attractive	4.61	1.34	22157.5*
7. I am aware that with the proper company I can avoid some risks	4.87	1.45	22659*
8. While playing, I felt the wish to get better informed about substances	3.94	1.60	16701*
9. I am aware of the risks one can run during a night out	5.10	1.19	23865.5*
10. By playing I learned something new about substances	4.57	1.56	21039.5*
11. I think that a videogame is a good way to provide information during a night out	4.93	1.28	23733*
12. Although brief, the information provided by the game is accurate	4.85	1.26	23513*

4 Study 2: Knowledge Increase

The goal of the second study was to test whether a game session was able to increase users' short-term knowledge about substance consumption risks and coping skills. This is in line with the goals of a so-called "brief intervention" in general [23] and in this domain in particular, which does not aim at long-term effects or providing articulated information. We therefore assessed the players' knowledge before and after the game session. We hypothesized that the number of correct answers to test questions increased after the game session (H1), whereas no variation was observed in the control questions unrelated to the game material (H2). This study does not test long-term knowledge improvements.

4.1   Method

From the database of the game, we selected 40 quiz items for the study. They were items that, during previous interventions, received the highest percentage of wrong answers and varied to cover different kinds of substances (alcohol, amphetamines, cannabis, ketamine, cocaine and other stimulants, ecstasy, heroin and methamphetamines, GHB-GBL, popper and others solvents, and hallucinogens) and effects (first aid, sexually transmitted diseases, urban legends, medical effects, pregnancy, history, and short- and long-terms effects). We used these 40 items as follows (Table 3):

- 20 items made up the pre- and post-test questions, assessing users' knowledge, and also appeared in the game, where the user could see the correct answer and learn its explanation;
- 5 items informed pre- and post-session questions but not the game, so players could not learn the correct answer from the game;
- 15 were distracting questions with no related pre- and post-test.

Table 3. Study 2 design

	Pre-game	Game	Post-game
20 test questions	x	x	x
5 control questions	x	-	x
15 distracting questions	-	x	-

A game session consisted of 35 questions, 20 test, and 15 distracting; their order was randomized automatically by the game system. Before and after each session the participant was asked 25 questions, i.e., 20 test questions and 5 control. Each test and control question was asked twice, once before the game session, and once after the game session. They were multiple choice, with one correct response option only. The order of response options changed between pre- and post-game session.

Participants and procedure. The sample consisted of 81 participants (51 men, 30 women), aged 23.36 on average (SD = 2.02). We recruited university students by asking people encountered on campus, and offered no compensation for participating. The game sessions were multiplayer, as this is the modality in the field interventions. Four participated in each. A session started by welcoming the participants and having them read and sign the informed consent form. Afterwards, we collected background data (gender, age, nationality, mother tongue, education, and familiarity with videogames), the 25-item, we administered the pre-session questionnaire, followed by the game sessions. After the game session, we collected the 25-item post-session questionnaire. During the game, participants could talk but not make shared decisions or affect each other's responses in other ways. They were reminded that game ranked their individual performance so they were actually competing with each other. The whole procedure took 45–50 min to complete.

4.2   Results

We have run analyses with SPSS. Regarding the percentage of correct answers pre- and post-game session, the Wilcoxon test shows that the latter is higher than the former (Mdn = 90 vs. 60), $Z = -7.785$, $p < 0.05$, $r = -0.865$ (Fig. 3).

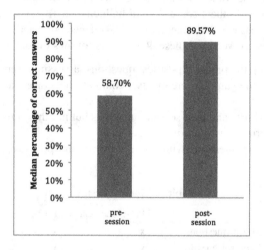

Fig. 3. The median percentage of correct answers before and after the game session.

Regarding the five control questions, we analyzed their variation before and after the session and found it very low: only 18.52 % of them varied after the session, suggesting that it was the specific content acquired during the game to modify the answers in the test questions. Finally, actual performance in the game is not related to the percentage of correct answers before or after the session, $F (3, 77) = 0.62$, $p = .60$. showing that test performance at the test questions improved also if the performance at the game was bad, thanks to the explanation provided during the game (and offering a learning opportunity).

5   General Discussion and Conclusions

The two validation studies gave encouraging results. The strength of the first study was to test the game reception in the field. The reasons for carrying out the second study in the lab were twofold. First, its controlled design needed a limited number of questions;

had the test taken place in the field, the large screen of the game would have shown the same quiz questions over and over, spoiling the sample after just a few sessions. Second, the scientific purposes of the study demanded it follow a pre-defined, rigid structure, difficult to maintain under the shifting circumstances of a field intervention. Nonetheless, none of these requirements are necessary for field intervention or an effective learning experience. In addition, during field interventions, participants volunteer because of their interest in the topic and the information acquired has immediate relevance, both preconditions for effective learning. A higher motivation would increase their ability to retain the information learnt in a field intervention, compensating for the lower ability to sustain attention due to noise and physical state.

Together, the first and second studies prove that gamified intervention is able to reach its goals, in terms of user experience and learning, in addition to its powerful attraction by default. These results encourage more testing and adoption of (carefully designed) serious games in brief field interventions.

Acknowledgments. The European Commission, via the Nightlife, Empowerment and Well-being Implementation (NEW-IP, n. 29299) project, supported this work. The authors would also like to thank Leonardo Montecchi, the Rimini Municipality, Giuseppe di Pino (Municipality of Venice) and S.E.R.T in Faenza for their support. The funding body did not affect the authors' decisions about the study design, collection, analysis and interpretation of data, the writing of the report, or the decision to submit the article for publication.

References

1. Bødker, S., Grønbæk, K.: Cooperative prototyping: users and designers in mutual activity. Int. J. Man Mach. Stud. **34**(3), 453–478 (1991)
2. Bogost, I.: Persuasive Games: The Expressive Power of Videogames. MIT Press, Cambridge (2007)
3. Bolier, L., Voorham, L., Monshouwer, K., Hasselt, N.V., Bellis, M.: Alcohol and drug prevention in nightlife settings: a review of experimental studies. Subst. Use Misuse **46**(13), 1569–1591 (2011)
4. Burns, J.M., Webb, M., Durkin, L.A., Hickie, I.B.: Reach out central: a serious game designed to engage young men to improve mental health and wellbeing. Med. J. Aust. **192** (11), S27 (2010)
5. Calafat, A., Blay, N., Juan, M., Adrover, D., Bellis, M.A., Hughes, K., et al.: Traffic risk behaviors at nightlife: drinking, taking drugs, driving, and use of public transport by young people. J. Traffic Inj. Prev. **10**, 162–169 (2009)
6. Calafat, A., Fernàndez, C., Juan, M., Becona, E.: Weekend nightlife recreational habits: prominent intrapersonal "risk factors" for drug use? Subst. Use Misuse **42**, 1443–1454 (2007)
7. Connolly, T., Boyle, E., MacArthur, E., Hainey, T., Boyle, J.: A systematic literature review of empirical evidence on computer games and serious games. Comput. Educ. **59**(2), 661–686 (2012)
8. Deterding, S., Dixon, D., Khaled, R., Nacke, L.: From game design elements to gamefulness: defining "gamification". In: Proceedings of the 15th International Academic MindTrek Conference: Envisioning Future Media Environments, pp. 9–15. ACM, New York, NY (2011)

9. European Monitoring Centre for Drugs and Drug Addiction: Responding to drug use and related problems in recreational settings. Document n. TDXA12003ENN (2012). http://www.emcdda.europa.eu/attachements.cfm/att_184673_EN_Recreational_settings_WEB.pdf

10. Flanagin, A.J., Metzger, M.J.: The role of site features, user attributes, and information verification behaviors on the perceived credibility of web-based information. New Media Soc. 9(2), 319–342 (2007)

11. Fogg, B.J.: Persuasive Technology: Using Computers to Change What We Think and Do. Morgan Kaufmann Publishers, San Francisco (2003)

12. Gamberini, L., Breda, L., Grassi, A.: VIDEODOPE: applying persuasive technology to improve awareness of drugs abuse effects. In: Shumaker, R. (ed.) HCII 2007 and ICVR 2007. LNCS, vol. 4563, pp. 633–641. Springer, Heidelberg (2007)

13. Gamberini, L., Marchetti, F., Martino, F., Spagnolli, A.: Designing a serious game for young users: the case of happy farm. Annu. Rev. Cybertherapy Telemedicine 7, 77–81 (2009)

14. Gaziano, C., McGrath, K.: Measuring the concept of credibility. J. Q. 63, 451 (1986)

15. Hamari, J., Koivisto, J.: "Working out for likes": an empirical study on social influence in exercise gamification. Comput. Hum. Behav. 50, 333–347 (2015)

16. Hunt, G., Moloney, M., Evans, K.: Youth, Drugs, and Nightlife: Pleasures, Risks, and Identity. Routledge, London (2010)

17. Hunt, G., Moloney, M., Fazio, A.: "A cool little buzz": alcohol intoxication in the dance club scene. Subst. Use Misuse 49(8), 968–981 (2014)

18. Kelly, B.C.: Conceptions of risk in the lives of ectasy-using youth. In: Sanders, B. (ed.) Drug, Clubs and Young People—Sociological and Public Health Perspectives, pp. 50–66. Ashgate Publishing, Hampshire (2006)

19. Kelly, B.C., LeClair, A., Parsons, J.T.: Methamphetamine use in club subcultures. Subst. Use Misuse 48(14), 1541–1552 (2013)

20. Kraft, P., Drozd, F., Olsen, E.: ePsychology: designing theory-based health promotion interventions. Commun. Assoc. Inf. Syst. 24, 399–426 (2009)

21. Lieberman, D.: Management of chronic pediatric diseases with interactive health games: theory and research findings. J. Ambul. Care Manag. 24(1), 26–38 (2001)

22. Miller-Day, M., Hecht, M.L.: Narrative means to preventative ends: a narrative engagement framework for designing prevention interventions. Health Commun. 28, 657–670 (2013)

23. Moyer, A., Finney, J.W.: Brief interventions for alcohol problems: factors that facilitate implementation. Alcohol Res. Health 28(1), 44–50 (2004)

24. North, L., Robinson, C., Haffegee, A., Sharkey, P.M., Hwang, F.: Using virtual environments for trigger identification in addiction treatment. In: Proceedings of the 9th International Conference on Disability, Virtual Reality & Associated Technologies, pp. 345–353. Laval, France, 10–12 September 2012

25. Oinas-Kukkonen, H.: A foundation for the study of behavior change support systems. Pers. Ubiquit. Comput. 17(6), 1223–1235 (2013)

26. Oinas-Kukkonen, H., Harjumaa, M.: Persuasive systems design: key issues, process model, and system features. Commun. Assoc. Inf. Syst. 24(1), 28 (2009)

27. Papastergiou, M.: Exploring the potential of computer and video games for health and physical education: a literature review. Comput. Educ. 53(3), 603–622 (2009)

28. Phillips, R.S., Horstman, T., Vye, N., Bransford, J.: Engagement and games for learning expanding definitions and methodologies. Simul. Gaming 45(4–5), 548–568 (2014)

29. Quintero, G., Peterson, J., Young, B.: An exploratory study of socio-cultural factors contributing to prescription drug misuse among college students. J. Drug Issues 22, 903–926 (2006)

30. Roberts, G., McCall, D., Stevens, Lavigne, A., Anderson, J., Paglia, A., Bollenbach. S., et al.: Preventing substance use problems among young people: a compendium of best practices. Report n. Cat. No. H39-580/2001E, Produced by Canadian Centre on Substance Abuse   (2001).   http://www.hc-sc.gc.ca/hc-ps/alt_formats/hecs-sesc/pdf/pubs/adp-apd/prevent/young-jeune-eng.pdf

31. Schensul, J.J., Convey, M., Burkholder, G.: Challenges in measuring concurrency, agency and intentionality in polydrug research. Addict. Behav. **30**(3), 571–574 (2005)

32. Seaborn, K., Fels, D.J.: Gamification in theory and action: a survey. Int. J. Hum.-Comput. Stud. **74**(2015), 14–31 (2015)

33. Stewart, J., Bleumers, L., Van Looy, J., Mariln, I., Schurmans, D., Willaert, K., De Grove, F., Jacobs, A., Misuraca, G.: The potential of digital games for empowerment and social inclusion of groups at risk of social and economic exclusion: evidence and opportunity for policy. EU JRC Institute for Prospective Technological Studies, Scientific and Policy Reports, 2013 (2013)

34. Venkatesh, V., Davis, F.D.: A theoretical extension of the technology acceptance model: four longitudinal field studies. Manag. Sci. **46**(2), 186–204 (2000)

35. Vogl, L.E., Teesson, M., Newton, N.C., Andrews, G.: Developing a school-based drug prevention program to overcome barriers to effective program implementation: the CLIMATE schools: alcohol module. Open J. Prev. Med. **2**(3), 410–422 (2012)

Long-Term Effects of Computerized Simulations in Protracted Conflicts: The Case of Global Conflicts

Ronit Kampf[✉]

Tel Aviv University, Tel Aviv, Israel
ronit.kampf@gmail.com

Abstract. This article presents an experimental study examining the short term and long term effects of Global Conflicts on attitude change towards the Israeli-Palestinian conflict. Global Conflicts is a role-playing computer game simulating this conflict. 180 undergraduate students from Israel and Palestine participating in the study were divided into game intervention and no-game controls. The participants were required to fill in questionnaires measuring attitudes regarding the conflict immediately before and after the game intervention and 12 months following this intervention. Results suggested that participants who played the game, unlike those who did not play it, shifted towards a more impartial perspective, being able to look at the conflict from both Israeli and Palestinian points of view immediately after the game intervention, and retained this perspective even one year after participation in this intervention, despite the serious clashes between Israel and the Palestinians that occurred during this time.

Keywords: Games for change · Israeli-Palestinian conflict · Attitude change · Conflict resolution · Long term effects · Computerized simulations

1 Introduction

This article investigates the effectiveness of a computer based peace game called Global Conflicts that simulates the Israeli-Palestinian situation, in order to see whether this game enhances the taking of an impartial perspective regarding the conflict (i.e., being able to look at the conflict from both Israeli and Palestinian points of view) and if this learning outcome is retained 12 months following the game intervention. The study compares the short term and long term learning outcomes of Israeli-Jewish and Palestinian undergraduate students playing the game with those not playing it in order to examine whether this game-based intervention actually works.

Global Conflicts is an award-winning educational game developed in 2010 by Serious Games Interactive in Denmark (http://globalconflicts.eu/). The game illustrating the tensions between Israeli and Palestinian sides in a checkpoint scenario. The player is represented by the avatar of a Western reporter who arrives in Jerusalem. Her task is to write for one of the following newspapers: Israeli, Palestinian, or Western. The player is expected to produce a news report geared to the audience of one of these newspapers, based on the interviews she conducts with various Israeli and Palestinian characters at the checkpoint in the Palestinian territories.

© Springer International Publishing Switzerland 2016
A. Meschtscherjakov et al. (Eds.): PERSUASIVE 2016, LNCS 9638, pp. 242–247, 2016.
DOI: 10.1007/978-3-319-31510-2_21

Previous studies have already shown that Israeli and Palestinian young people (like those participating in this study) know almost nothing about what transpires on the other side of the Israeli-Palestinian divide, except for the stereotypic and ethnocentric images constructed by key socialization agents (e.g., the media) and daily incidents [e.g., 1]. Moreover, since these young people have never actually experienced a state of peace they may not regard it as a significant value for which a price should be paid [e.g., 2].

Interestingly, studies have indicated the positive short term learning effects of computerized simulations like Global Conflicts [e.g., 3, 4], but no empirical research, to my knowledge, have been conducted to evaluate the long term effects of game-based interventions in intractable conflicts like the Israeli-Palestinian situation. In general, the number of studies on the long-term effects of peace workshops in such protracted conflicts is extremely limited [e.g., 2, 5].

Previous studies have suggested that peace games like Global Conflicts may be successful as tools for learning about the "other" for youth on the Israeli-Palestinian divide, for a few key considerations. First, Global Conflicts may induce more immersion and can therefore be more enjoyable, boosting players' engagement and motivation [e.g., 6, 7]. Second, Global Conflicts focuses on the hardships of both Israeli soldiers and Palestinian civilians at a checkpoint in the Palestinian territories, an experience which may produce empathy and identification with both sides [e.g., 8]. Finally, in Global Conflicts, a player assumes the role of a more distant party to the conflict who is obliged to look at the situation from both perspectives and act according to norms of balance and objectivity (i.e., a Western journalist). Therefore, the player may be less prone towards the tendency to interpret, favor, and recall information in a way that confirms her own beliefs while giving disproportionately less attention to information that contradicts it [e.g., 9]. As a result, the player may find it easier to look at the conflict through the lenses of both sides [e.g., 10, 11].

2 Research Hypotheses

H1: Participants will hold ethnocentric attitudes before the game intervention.
H2: Participants playing the game will become more impartial toward the conflict immediately after the game intervention, while those who do not play it will retain ethnocentric attitudes toward the conflict during this time.
H3: Participants playing the game will retain impartial attitudes toward the conflict even one year after participation in the game intervention, while those who do not play it will retain ethnocentric attitudes toward the conflict during the same period.

3 Methodology

3.1 Participants

100 Israeli-Jewish participants were from the Departments of Communication and Political Science at Tel Aviv University and 80 Palestinian students were from the Department of Political Science at Al-Quds University.

60 Israeli-Jewish students and 45 Palestinian students played the game (experimental group), while 40 Israeli-Jewish students and 35 Palestinian students did not play it (control group). The experimental and control groups did not differ in key characteristics that could provide alternative explanation for the results (Table 1).

Table 1. Characteristics of the experimental and control groups

	Age	Male	Political attitudes		Religiosity		Playing a digital game in the last six months	Political interest	
			1	10	1	10		1	4
			Left	Right	Religious	Secular		Not at all	Very much
	M(SD)		M(SD)		M(SD)			M(SD)	
Global Conflicts	23.1 (1.25)	36 %	6.12 (2.45)		6.7(1.17)		45 %	3.5 (0.47)	
No Game	22.9 (1.23)	34 %	5.87 (2.29)		6.45(1.12)		48 %	3.46 (0.65)	

3.2 Design and Procedure

The experimental condition took three hours including four parts. First, participants were introduced to the Global Conflicts game and played a short demo (not related to the Israeli-Palestinian conflict). Second, they filled in a short questionnaire. Third, the participants were randomly divided to play a Western journalist representing either an Israeli or a Palestinian newspaper in the game. Finally, the participants again filled in a short questionnaire.

The control condition took three hours including three parts. First, participants filled in a short questionnaire. They were then given a lecture about digital natives (not related to the conflict). Finally, they again filled in a short questionnaire.

Both participants who played the game and those who did not play it were told that they would be contacted by email a year later to answer a short questionnaire and they will receive credit for their participation. The experimental group was told that the questionnaire would examine what they remembered from the game and the control group was told that the questionnaire would examine what they remembered from the lecture about digital natives in order to learn about the effectiveness of the two classes.

3.3 Measures

The attitude measure examined the 'rightness' of each side on key issues in the conflict including water, refugees, borders, settlements, Jerusalem, and security, using the following scale: 1. Palestinians are absolutely right, 2. Palestinians are somewhat right, 3. Both sides are equally right, 4. Israelis are somewhat right, and 5. Israelis are absolutely right. After conducting a factor analysis, the average of answers given on the six key issues was used as a measure of attitude change about key issues in the conflict before and after playing the game. This measure has already been used in previous studies conducted with computerized simulations of the Israeli-Palestinian conflict [3, 4, 12–14], and is based on a questionnaire developed by conflict resolution scholars from Israel and Palestine [e.g., 2].

3.4 Statistical Procedures

A Repeated Measures ANOVA was used to test the research hypotheses, investigating the effects of playing the game (yes or no) and nationality (Israeli-Jewish or Palestinian) on attitude values at three separate time points: immediately before and after the game intervention and 12 months following this intervention. The important point with this study design is that the same participants are measured three times on the same dependent variable, so this test can detect any overall differences between related means.

4 Results

The interaction between time, playing the game and nationality was significant, suggesting that Israeli-Jewish and Palestinian participants playing the game and those who did not play it differed in attitude change regarding key issues in the conflict ($F(3, 176) = 71.03$, $p < .0001$, $\eta^2 = .36$).

Table 2. Nationality and game-playing effects on attitudes toward the conflict

	Pre-game intervention M:SD	Post-game intervention M:SD	12 months following game intervention M:SD
Israeli-Jews			
Game	3.92:.59***	2.91:.31***	2.93:.26***
No Game	3.71:.53***	3.62:.53***	3.52:.47***
Palestinians			
Game	1.07:.09***	1.44:.34***	1.58:.36***
No Game	1.06:.12***	1.07:.11***	1.14:.16***

***$p < .0001$

Before the game intervention, Israeli-Jewish participants playing the game held a pro-Israeli view, while Palestinian participants playing the game held a pro-Palestinian view (i.e., ethnocentric attitudes). Similarly, Israeli-Jewish participants who didn't play the game held a pro-Israeli view during this time, while Palestinian participants who didn't play the game held a pro-Palestinian view (Table 2). Therefore, hypothesis 1 is confirmed.

Immediately after the game intervention, Israeli-Jewish and Palestinian participants playing the game got closer to thinking that both Israelis and Palestinians are equally right regarding key issues in the conflict (i.e., an impartial perspective). In contrast, Israeli-Jews and Palestinians who did not play the game retained ethnocentric attitudes toward the conflict during this time (Table 2). Therefore, hypothesis 2 is confirmed.

12 months following the game intervention, Israeli-Jewish and Palestinian participants playing the game retained impartial perspective regarding the conflict. In contrast, Israeli-Jewish and Palestinian participants who did not play the game retained ethnocentric perspective regarding the conflict during this time (Table 2). Therefore, hypothesis 3 is confirmed.

5 Discussion and Conclusions

By using the Global Conflicts game, which is a simulation of the Israeli-Palestinian conflict, this study assessed whether participants could develop an impartial perspective and whether this learning outcome persisted 12 months after the game intervention. Results suggested that participants held ethnocentric attitudes toward the conflict before the game intervention. In addition, participants playing the game developed more impartial attitudes toward the conflict immediately after the game intervention, while those who didn't play it retained ethnocentric attitudes toward the conflict during the same time. Finally, participants playing the game retained impartial attitudes even 12 months following the game intervention, while those who didn't play it retained ethnocentric attitudes toward the conflict during this time.

The results are promising in terms of showing that computer based peace games can be used not only for teaching purposes in courses related to conflict and peace studies, but also as part of peace building trainings. The results indicate that such games are not only useful in teaching a more complex view of the conflict to direct parties to the conflict with strong and ethnocentric attitudes on the issues, but also in engendering attitude change especially in the form of taking a more impartial perspective and being able to look at the conflict from both sides points of view, even one year following the game intervention, despite the serious clashes between Israel and the Palestinians that occurred during this time.

This study has a few limitations that should be addressed in future research. First, the study focused on Political Science students who may be more interested in politics and therefore most likely do not represent the general public. In addition, it is unclear whether participants would have enjoyed the game and changed their attitudes to an equal degree, if no incentive had been presented at the end. Finally, it remains unclear to what extent the change in attitude is caused by the information the students were exposed to, and to what degree the change is caused by the game-aspect of Global Conflicts.

Further research can isolate different dimensions of computerized simulations like Global Conflicts to understand how such games achieve their short term and long term effects in the shadow of intractable conflicts such as the Israeli-Palestinian situation. It could have also been interesting to examine the impact of Global Conflicts compared with another format presenting the same information (e.g., a lecture, a written text, a presentation or videos of others playing the game) in order to examine specifically whether the game- aspect of Global Conflicts adds more than other formats to the change in attitude.

References

1. Wolfsfeld, G., Frosh, P., Awabdy, M.: Covering death in conflicts: coverage of the Second Intifada on Israeli and Palestinian television. J. Peace Res. **45**, 401–417 (2008)
2. Rosen, I., Salomon, G.: Durability of peace education effects in the shadow of conflict. Soc. Psychol. Educ. **14**, 135–147 (2011)
3. Cuhadar, E., Kampf, R.: A cross-national inquiry into the Israeli-Palestinian and Guatemalan scenarios in global conflicts. Negot. Confl. Manage. Res. **8**(4), 243–260 (2015)
4. Kampf, R., Cuhadar, E.: Do computer games enhance learning about conflicts? A cross-national inquiry into proximate and distant scenarios in global conflicts. Comput. Hum. Behav. **52**, 541–549 (2015)
5. Schroeder, J., Risen, J.L.: Befriending the enemy: outgroup friendship longitudinally predicts intergroup attitudes in a coexistence program for Israelis and Palestinians. Group Process. Intergroup Relat. **4**(5), 1–22 (2014)
6. Fu, F.L., Su, R.S., Yu, S.C.: EGameFlow: a scale to measure learners enjoyment of e-Learning games. Comput. Educ. **52**(1), 101–112 (2009)
7. Kiili, K.: Digital game-based learning: towards an experiential game model. Internet High. Educ. **8**(1), 13–24 (2005)
8. Gross, K.: Framing persuasive appeals: episodic and thematic framing, emotional response, and policy opinion. Polit. Psychol. **29**(2), 169–192 (2008)
9. Stanovich, K.E., West, R.F., Toplak, M.E.: Myside bias, rational thinking, and intelligence. Curr. Dir. Psychol. Sci. **22**(4), 259–264 (2013)
10. Halperin, E., Pliskin, R., Saguy, T., Liebrman, V., Gross, J.J.: Emotion regulation and the cultivation of political tolerance: searching for a new track for intervention. J. Confl. Resolut. **58**(6), 1100–1138 (2014)
11. Halperin, E., Porat, R., Tamir, M., Gross, J.J.: Can emotion regulation change political attitudes in intractable conflicts? From the laboratory to the field. Psychol. Sci. **24**(2), 106–111 (2013)
12. Kampf, R., Cuhadar, E.: Learning about the Israeli-Palestinian conflict and negotiations through simulations: the case of peacemaker. Int. Stud. Perspect. **15**(4), 509–524 (2014)
13. Kampf, R.: Playing singly, playing in dyads in a computerized simulation of the Israeli-Palestinian conflict. Comput. Hum. Behav. **32**, 9–14 (2014)
14. Kampf, R.: Computerized Simulations of the Israeli-Palestinian Conflict and Attitude Change. eLearning Pap. **43** (2015)

Interventions for Behavior Change

Understanding Changes in the Motivation of Stroke Patients Undergoing Rehabilitation in Hospital

Michelle Pickrell[1(✉)], Bert Bongers[1], and Elise van den Hoven[1,2,3]

[1] Faculty of Design, Architecture and Building, University of Technology Sydney,
Sydney, Australia
Michelle.Pickrell@student.uts.edu.au, Bert.Bongers@uts.edu.au
[2] Department of Industrial Design, Eindhoven University of Technology,
Eindhoven, The Netherlands
[3] Duncan of Jordanstone College of Art and Design, University of Dundee, Dundee, UK
Elise.vandenHoven@uts.edu.au

Abstract. Stroke patient motivation can fluctuate during rehabilitation due to a range of factors. This study reports on qualitative research, consisting of observations of stroke patients undergoing rehabilitation and interviews with patients about the changes in motivation they identified during their time completing rehabilitation in the hospital. We found a range of positive and negative factors which affect motivation. Positive factors include improvements in patient movement and support from other patients and family members. Negative factors include pain and psychological issues such as changes in mood. From this fieldwork, a set of design guidelines has been developed to act as a platform for researchers and designers developing equipment for the rehabilitation of stroke patients.

Keywords: Rehabilitation · Stroke · Healthcare · Feedback · Design research

1 Introduction

Rehabilitation following stroke can be a time intensive process with patients having to commit to multiple repetitions of specific exercises [1]. Interactive equipment could be used to help patients with their rehabilitation by offering feedback about their limb movements and balance. Currently however, there are few interactive technologies available to patients who are completing their rehabilitation in the hospital.

The research goals for this project are:

1. To understand the patients' perspective of the differences between high and low motivation towards completing their daily rehabilitation exercises
2. To understand the patient perception of the reasons for changes in motivation

This paper focuses on the best ways of encouraging patients to be motivated during stroke rehabilitation. The aim of this paper is to support designers who are creating interactive rehabilitation equipment for patients undergoing rehabilitation, both in the

© Springer International Publishing Switzerland 2016
A. Meschtscherjakov et al. (Eds.): PERSUASIVE 2016, LNCS 9638, pp. 251–262, 2016.
DOI: 10.1007/978-3-319-31510-2_22

ward and home environments. 'Motivation', for the purpose of this study, is defined as the reason or reasons a person acts in a particular way.

2 Background

To support this research, the topics of stroke, stroke rehabilitation and persuasive technology are important. It is also important to understand motivation as it is the main focus of this research. These topics are discussed in this section, together with the existing work that focuses on the use of interactive equipment to motivate patients.

2.1 Motivation

The level of motivation a stroke patient has will influence the outcome of their rehabilitation [2]. Knowing the direct relationship between motivation and success, we can work to design appropriate equipment to motivate patients. This paper focuses on the theories of motivation, including goal- setting theory and self-efficacy theory.

Goal setting has been proven to have a positive effect on patient motivation [3]. It is however, important that patients have input into the goal creation process so that they feel a sense of ownership over their goals [4]. It is also important that goals are small and achievable, with goals that are relevant to the patient's interests and hobbies being the most successful [3].

Self-efficacy theory is a central concept of Bandura's Social Cognitive Theory and focuses on the relationship between an individual's degree of confidence to complete a task and their ability to do so [5]. As stroke patients have to re-learn how to complete basic tasks such as walking or standing up, confidence in their ability to do this learning is important. Existing research into self-efficacy in stroke patients, which focuses on the subject of falls, shows that there is a relationship between self-efficacy and a patient's rehabilitation success over time [5]. Some patients, however, do not feel the same motivation to get better. This can result from factors such as having family members that can help with activities of daily living when they return home. Another factor is age. Younger patients often feel more of a need to get better as they have their life ahead of them, whereas older patients are not always motivated in the same way [3].

2.2 Persuasive Technology

The Persuasive Technology field of research focuses on the use of technology to change behaviour. Persuasive technology research often focuses on motivation, in particular around the topic of exercise [6–8]. Existing research identifies a number of strategies that can be used when designing for motivation. Firstly, setting goals that are relevant to the user and making them public to the community so the person feels an obligation to their community [9]. Secondly, ensuring the technology channel used is relevant to the target market [10]. Finally, a strategy that focuses on stroke rehabilitation is to provide both immediate and long term feedback to patients [8].

In the context of stroke rehabilitation, interactive technology could support the time-poor physiotherapists and play an important role in persuading patients to exercise [11]. As BJ Fogg points out, in some cases computers can have a number of distinct advantages over humans when it comes to persuasion, as they are persistent and can use many modalities for example, text, audio and sensory feedback [12]. Together with these factors, interactive technology can have a positive role as it can be motivating and stimulating [13, 14].

2.3   Stroke and Stroke Rehabilitation

An understanding of stroke and stroke rehabilitation is important to the context of this research. A stroke results from an interruption to the blood supply to the brain. This can be caused by either a blockage or bleeding from a blood vessel [15]. The damage caused by a stroke is due to the brain not receiving enough oxygenated blood and as a result the affected brain cells cannot survive. The physical and cognitive effects of a stroke are dependent on the size and location of the stroke in the brain. In most cases of stroke, one side of a patient's body will be affected. Some other effects of stroke include memory loss, speech difficulties, changes in vision and behavioural changes [16].

Following a stroke, patients undergo rehabilitation that includes extensive interaction between a patient and their therapist [17]. However, patients are often dealing with a range of different factors that result from their stroke. Such factors include depression and lack of motivation, as well as their coming to terms with the massive physical change that has just happened in their lives [18]. Patients have differing success with motivation with 31% of patients who have motor deficiencies resulting from their stroke not completing the exercises their physiotherapist has prescribed [19].

Stroke rehabilitation often consists of repetitive, simple exercises such as sitting down and standing up or walking up and down stairs. The repetitive nature of these exercises can result in patients becoming bored [20]. The objects used in the rehabilitation ward tend to be everyday objects such as styrofoam cups, popsicle sticks and wooden blocks. Whilst these are objects that patients are familiar with, they don't offer the patient much feedback about the way they are completing movements.

Some gaming technologies have been introduced into the rehabilitation ward such as the Nintendo Wii and the Microsoft Xbox Kinect, however as these are designed for able-bodied people, they often do not give patients appropriate and beneficial feedback for their condition [20, 21].

2.4   Related Work

The changes in motivation of stroke patients who are completing rehabilitation have been explored by studying relevant publications, particularly in the healthcare domain. As well as healthcare, this section presents a review of motivation related human computer interaction (HCI) studies and persuasive technology studies.

From the clinical perspective, there are few recent studies that focus on understanding the motivation of stroke patients when undergoing rehabilitation. The few studies that do focus on the topic of motivation, report on clinical implications, focusing on the clinician's interaction with the patient as opposed to design outcomes that focus on equipment and technology. Important aspects of motivation, however, are identified, including a patient's understanding of the reasons for rehabilitation and understanding the role of nurses and physiotherapists as well as understanding what their own role is in the rehabilitation process [3, 18].

In the field of HCI, there are some equipment designs that have been created to support motivation within the hospital. One such design is the stepping tiles used by patients to measure the number of stepping repetitions they complete during their rehabilitation session. This includes a simple interface, which can be easily interpreted by patients, as well as rich and varied feedback, similar to video games [20].

Persuasive technology research focuses on motivation in a range of different contexts including motivation for exercise, [7] healthy eating [7, 22] and helping people live more sustainably [23]. A number of tools have been identified within this field to aid with motivation, including triggers, goal setting, comparison between subjects, asking users to pledge a commitment and finally giving subjects useful feedback at the right time [10, 22, 23].

3   Study Design

As a result of previous work on a set of sensor floor tiles and a sensor sleeve, we identified the importance of using design to help patients with motivation during stroke rehabilitation [24]. This previous work demonstrated the positive effect on motivation of showing patients the incremental improvements they have made. The results of this work identified the need to conduct a study that specifically focuses on motivation by observing and interviewing patients who have been undergoing rehabilitation for an extended period of time. This section outlines the study design for this project.

3.1   Participants and Recruitment

The six participants in the study were inpatients at the Bankstown-Lidcombe hospital in Sydney. All had suffered from a stroke and had been completing rehabilitation for over four weeks. The patients ranged in age between 64 and 89 years of age. Four of the patients were male and two were female. The physiotherapists at the hospital identified suitable patients and the researcher started observation. After the period of observation, if the patient was willing to participate in the interview, the researcher would obtain informed consent. All interview data was later anonymised to comply with ethics guidelines.

After patients had given consent, they were screened using the Mini Mental State examination. This is a 30-point questionnaire used to assess cognitive ability and screen for cognitive impairment [25], including situational questions, memory-based questions and completing simple tasks such as folding a piece of paper and placing it on the floor. Healthy individuals score 30. Patients who scored at least 23 out of 30 were accepted for the study.

3.2   Observations and Interviews

Observations of the six patients completing various rehabilitation exercises in the rehabilitation gymnasium were conducted. In particular the researcher was focusing on the willingness of the patients to exercise, their relationship with the physiotherapists and their interactions with other patients. This allowed the researcher to understand each patient's level of motivation and the differences between how they acted and how they talked about motivation. When observing the patient, the researcher observed from the other side of the gymnasium and did not interact with the patients.

This approach was taken to reduce any bias on the results as patients may act differently or try harder when they know they are being observed. During the rehabilitation sessions, family members and friends of the patients were often present in the gym, so the researcher was able to fit in with other plain clothed people. At the time of observation, the patients did not know the researcher. The researcher did not introduce herself and the patients did not know what the researcher's interests were.

After the observations were finished, the patients were introduced to the researcher and a one-on-one interview was conducted. All interviews took place in the patient's room or in the physiotherapy gym at the Bankstown-Lidcombe Hospital. All interviews explored the rehabilitation exercises that are prescribed by the physiotherapists at the Stroke and Aged care rehabilitation gymnasium.

The interviews were structured in three sections. Firstly the patient was asked about their stroke and the rehabilitation they were completing at the time. Secondly, the patients was asked about their understanding and definition of motivation to ensure there was a shared understanding. The patient was then asked to map their motivation over the weeks they were completing rehabilitation on a scale between high motivation and low motivation. This graph was then explored in detail with patients to explore high and low motivation from their perspective. Finally the patient was asked about which exercises they identified as being least and most motivating.

4   Results

This section presents the combined results from the observations and interviews. Affinity diagramming was used to extract themes from the interviews and observations.

4.1   Changes in Motivation

Most patients commented that they had ups and downs in their motivation towards completing their rehabilitation. During the interviews patients were asked to map their level of motivation on a scale between low motivation and high motivation during their time in the rehabilitation ward. The results presented in Fig. 1 were self-reported during the interview.

The graphs created by each patient showed that motivation went through ups and downs as they completed their rehabilitation over a period of 4 weeks. In several cases patients became slightly less motivated in the first week of exercise. Patients commented that this was due to the fact that they had not completed exercise of this intensity for years. The graph shows that most patients felt as though they were highly motivated, whilst one patient, who was dealing with a lot of pain, explained that their motivation towards rehabilitation was low due to the pain associated with completing their exercises.

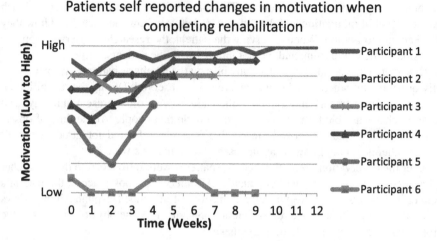

Fig. 1. Changes in patient motivation while completing rehabilitation

The patients who showed signs of being engaged and interested by their rehabilitation exercises were often observed to align that level of interest with motivation when they graphed it on their chart. For four of the six patients this also directly aligned with the number of repetitions they were able to do in any one session.

4.2 Progress and Improvement Aids with Motivation

Patients commented on the links they identified between their motivation and their progress and improvement. Patients also commented that changes in their ability made them feel better, "When there are changes with my legs and my arms then that makes me feel good" (Participant 4). Patients also commented that it is important to them to clearly understand if and when they have improved. As one patient commented when talking about the benefits they saw when getting feedback, "In the arm class, at the start, I had a bottle that only had a little bit of water in it. Now I have one that is nearly full. I know I have achieved something" (Participant 2).

Goal setting (as discussed in Sect. 2.1) is another factor that aids with motivation. The goal of the majority of patients is to get home and live unassisted. This was described by all patients as being their main motivator. As one patient commented, "Sometimes I wish I didn't have to do the exercises, but I have been pushing myself because if I don't push myself I'm not going to get out of here and that is my motivation" (Participant 3).

4.3 Attitude and Understanding of the Reasons for Completing Exercises

Lifestyle and the patient's attitude towards exercise before their stroke are other factors affecting motivation. During the interviews all patients commented on their level and frequency of exercise pre-stroke. There was a close link between a patient's attitude to exercise before and after their stroke. One patient who exercised frequently and felt they had a good understanding of the benefits of exercise commented, "I always want to go to the rehab gym, I know that it will make me better if I do more and more exercise" (Participant 1). On the other hand, patients who had not done much exercise before their stroke commented on how it was the most exercise they had done in years and that they did not see the point in it. "It just makes my muscles hurt, I don't see why I need to do it if it's just making me feel worse" (Participant 5).

Patients commented that they were not always sure why they were asked to complete certain exercises. It was observed that the reasons for completing exercises that used more mundane equipment such as pegs, buckets and balls were not always as clear as the more obvious exercises such as sit to stand and walking up and down a staircase of four steps. One patient commented, "I rather do the 'exercises' than the silly ones with pegs. I prefer to do the ones that help my ability" (Participant 3).

Accepting the fact that the stroke had happened was another topic frequently mentioned in the interviews. Patients talked about the importance of accepting the change that has happened to them before being able to move forward and complete their rehabilitation. As one patient commented, "You have to accept what has happened. When I first got here I was still sad and shocked that this had happened to me. But now I have accepted what the physiotherapists need me to do to get better. There are no days that I don't feel like getting up and exercising" (Participant 4). In some cases, patients felt they did not understand enough about their stroke and what had happened.

4.4 Physical Pain and Psychological Factors Hinder Motivation

Pain was a common theme throughout the interviews. Patients talked about the pain they faced both as a result of the effects of their stroke as well as the pain of doing intensive exercise which they had not done for long periods of time. One patient commented, "I am angry every day because I am in so much pain because of the arthritis in my right knee. It is ten times worse since I had my stroke" (Participant 6). Other patients commented on the immediate pain that resulted from them completing intensive exercise, "You have to be careful not to exercise too much, otherwise you get too sore and can't exercise the next day" (Participant 3).

Temporary psychological factors such as mood can also affect patient motivation. Mood is usually temporary and can be caused by frustration, being overwhelmed or sad [26]. One patient commented, "I have low motivation sometimes because of what has happened (the stroke). It is very overwhelming" (Participant 4).

4.5 Social Factors

Social factors such as having other patients and family around are another factor affecting motivation. Patients commented that the people around them; other patients, physiotherapists and family are very motivating. One patient commented, "I am becoming more motivated as I am getting more used to the people in the ward. When I look around I see that you have to appreciate all the small improvements that people make. They tell me I am improving which gets me more motivated" (Participant 5). Another patient commented "For me, seeing my family is a big thing, so I don't ever lack motivation to go down to the gym because I want to show my family how much I have improved" (Participant 1).

It was also observed that patients take a motivational role in each other's rehabilitation. In the rehabilitation ward, patients will often cheer each other on and encourage each other to complete more repetitions of an exercise. This camaraderie was observed to be particularly strong amongst patients who shared a ward as they had already formed a friendship outside of the gymnasium.

The presence of family members was also observed to be particularly motivating for patients when completing their rehabilitation. Patient's spouses and children would often visit the gymnasium when the patients were completing their exercise. Where possible, family members were encouraged by the physiotherapists to support the patients by completing the rehabilitation exercises with them. Patients would often complete more repetitions of an exercise when their family members were completing them as well.

5   Discussion

In this section we will discuss the results of the study in relation to the research goals.

Research goal 1 - To understand the patients' perspective of the differences between high and low motivation towards completing their daily rehabilitation exercises

Overall, it was found that patients were able to indicate their perceived levels of motivation when completing rehabilitation. Patients identified the causes of low motivation as being physical factors such as pain, as well as psychological factors such as their mood. The causes of higher levels of motivation include improvement in the patient's range of movement and control over their movement, as well as external factors such as the community of patients, family and friends in the rehabilitation gymnasium. Whilst there are factors that affect motivation, most patients accepted that they needed to complete their rehabilitation regardless of whether they felt motivated to or not. This was because these patients had an understanding that the amount of rehabilitation they completed would directly affect their rehabilitation outcomes.

Maclean et al. [3] also discusses the differences between high and low motivation patients. In line with our research, Maclean identifies the patient's desire to leave hospital as a major goal and motivator. In line with our findings that patients did not understand the reason that they need to complete particular exercises, Maclean also identifies the importance of patients understanding the context and possible outcomes which will result from completing different exercises. The Knowledge Attitude Behaviour (KAB) model is used in the persuasive technology domain to explain the importance of knowledge for motivation, both "awareness" and "how-to" information [22]. In the context of stroke rehabilitation, this could translate to both "awareness" of why a patient needs to do an exercise as well as the "how to" instructional information.

Existing literature [3] also identifies the concept that motivation is a personality factor and that some people are motivated and some are not. This was not something that we found in our study. It was clear that patients are motivated by activities other than exercise, so instead of being a personality factor motivation was related to what a patient was passionate about and interested in.

In general, our study found that patients who had a good relationship with exercise before their stroke were more likely to be motivated to complete their rehabilitation exercises. In addition, situational factors such as mood, affected patients day to day and resulted in fluctuating changes in motivation.

Research goal 2 - To understand the patient perception of the reasons for changes in motivation

During the interviews, patients commented that their changes in motivation came from both internal, body related and external factors. External factors include the community of patients, rehabilitation staff, family and friends who encourage them when they are in the gymnasium. All patients commented that when they improved, they felt more motivated to continue completing their exercises. However, patients also commented that internal factors such as being in pain from exercising the day before or from pre-existing conditions, such as arthritis, affected their motivation as it made it physically more difficult to complete exercises. Some older patients also commented that it had been many years since they had done exercise of that intensity.

Existing literature that looks at patient motivation from the physiotherapists' perspective identifies that providing information about improvements in patient's rehabilitation, as well as setting relevant and realistic goals with patients, can help with motivation [3, 8].

This understanding of patient motivation is of particular importance for patients when they have returned to a home environment and no longer have the help and support of the rehabilitation staff. It is during this time that many patients discontinue their rehabilitation exercises. As a result it is important to be able to design for these changes in motivation so that we can persuade patients to continue with their rehabilitation when they have varying levels of motivation.

6 Design Guidelines

The following design four guidelines (DG) are for the use of researchers and designers wanting to create interactive equipment for stroke rehabilitation.

DG1 – Allow the user to set goals relevant to themselves

The interviews showed that that main goal of all patients is to live unassisted at home. However, patients also discussed the positive affect that improvements and progress have on their motivation. It is therefore important to allow the patients to set and revise their own goals. They should be able to increase or decrease the difficulty of the exercise as well as the number of repetitions. Therefore patients have a goal that is relevant and achievable to them.

DG2 – Give patients feedback on their short-term and long-term improvements

During the interviews, patients discussed how important being able to see feedback of improvements is for their motivation. Showing patients the short-term improvements in their limb movement alongside the larger long-term improvements they have made can help to motivate patients.

DG3 – Create a community

Both the interviews and observations showed the importance of the camaraderie and support that the patients offer each other. Being able to support this sense of community both in the ward and when patients have returned home could allow patients to continue to encourage each other to complete their exercises.

Technology can also be used to facilitate the collaboration between patients and their family members and friends. It was observed that when patient's family members completed their exercises with the patient, they were more motivated and in many cases completed more repetitions of the exercises.

DG4 – Inform patients about the purpose of different exercises

During the interviews, some patients commented that they could not see the point in certain exercises. As an example, patients questioned the value of the peg exercise where the patient is asked to move up to fifteen pegs from the lip of one bucket to the lip of another. However, it was observed that when patients understand the point of an exercise and how it is helping them with their rehabilitation, they are more likely to complete the exercise.

7   Conclusion and Next Steps

This research aims to understand the motivation of stroke patients who are undergoing rehabilitation. By observing and interviewing patients, we gained an understanding of the patient perception of their motivation and how it had changed during their time in the hospital. Our findings show that there are a range of different factors which affect motivation. Some of these factors can be designed for, for example aiding with a sense of community, and some, such as reduction of pain, cannot.

Whilst this paper has touched on the motivation of patients who have left the hospital and are completing their rehabilitation in a home environment, it is important to conduct a similar study interviewing patients participating in rehabilitation at home. There may be differences in what motivates patients when they have returned to a home environment, as they no longer have the support of the rehabilitation team.

This research is part of a larger piece which focuses on motivation, feedback and technology used in the rehabilitation ward from the perspective of the patient and physiotherapist. A model that focuses on feedback and motivation is being developed, for use by designers.

Following this research phase, interactive equipment to help patients with motivation will be designed and prototyped. To validate this equipment, we will use methods such as a motivation questionnaire or an experience sampling method that allows us to collect data at each time point. This technique was not used for this piece of research as we wanted to explore a number of topics around motivation and the use of technology that could not be explored with a questionnaire.

By observing and interviewing patients, we have also been able to understand the context of stroke patient rehabilitation. Using this information we can better design persuasive systems which suit the needs of patients. We can leverage the tools of persuasive technology [23] to aid and encourage patients as they face the highs and lows of motivation during their rehabilitation. The outcome of this study is a set of design guidelines for researchers and designers who are designing interactive equipment for stroke patients undergoing rehabilitation.

Acknowledgements.   We would like to thank all the patients and physiotherapists who contributed to this study. The study is completed under ethics approval (HREC/12/CRGH/185) and (SSA/13/LPOOL/80). This research was supported by STW VIDI grant number 016.128.303 of The Netherlands Organization for Scientific Research (NWO), awarded to Elise van den Hoven.

References

1. Balaam, M., Rennick Egglestone, S., Fitzpatrick, G., Rodden, T., Hughes, A., Wilkinson, A., Nind, T., Axelrod, L., Harris, E., Ricketts, I., Mawson, S., Burridge, J.: Motivating mobility: designing for lived motivation in stroke rehabilitation. In: Proceedings of the SIGCHI Conference on Human Factors in Computing Systems (CHI 2011), pp. 3073–3082. ACM, New York (2011)
2. Holmqvist, L.W., Koch, L.: Environmental factors in stroke rehabilitation: being in hospital itself demotivates patients. Br. Med. J. **322**, 1501 (2001)
3. Maclean, N., Pound, P., Wolfe, C., Rudd, A.: The concept of patient motivation: a qualitative analysis of stroke professionals' attitudes. Stroke **33**, 444–448 (2002)
4. Rosewilliam, S., Roskell, C., Pandyan, A.D.: A systematic review and synthesis of the quantitative and qualitative evidence behind patient-centered goal setting in stroke rehabilitation. Clin. Rehabil. **25**, 501–514 (2011)
5. Hellstom, K., Lindmark, B., Wahlberg, B., Fugl-Meyer, A.R.: Self-efficacy in relation to impairments and activities of daily living disability in elderly patients with stroke: a prospective investigation. J. Rehabil. Med. **35**, 202–207 (2003)
6. Wunsch, M., Stibe, A., Millonig, A., Seer, S., Dai, C., Schechtner, K., Chin, R.C.C.: What makes you bike? Exploring persuasive strategies to encourage low-energy mobility. In: MacTavish, T., Basapur, S. (eds.) PERSUASIVE 2015. LNCS, vol. 9072, pp. 53–64. Springer, Heidelberg (2015)
7. Toscos, T., Faber, A., An, S., Gandhi, M.P.: Chick clique: persuasive technology to motivate teenage girls to exercise. In: CHI 2006 Extended Abstracts on Human Factors in Computing Systems (CHI EA 2006), pp. 1873–1878. ACM, New York (2006)
8. Pickrell, M., Bongers, B., van den Hoven, E.: Understanding persuasion and motivation in interactive stroke rehabilitation. In: MacTavish, T., Basapur, S. (eds.) PERSUASIVE 2015. LNCS, vol. 9072, pp. 15–26. Springer, Heidelberg (2015)
9. Consolvo, S., Klasnja, P., McDonald, D.W., Landay, J.A.: Goal-setting considerations for persuasive technologies that encourage physical activity. In: Proceedings of the 4th International Conference on Persuasive Technology, pp. 1–8, ACM, New York (2009)
10. Fogg, B.J.: Creating persuasive technologies: an eight-step design process. In: Proceedings of the 4th International Conference on Persuasive Technology, pp. 1–6. ACM, California (2009)
11. van den Berg, M., Sherrington, C., Hassett, L., Killington, M., Smith, S.T., Bongers, A.J., Hassett, L., Crotty, M.: Video and computer-based interactive exercises in geriatric and neurological rehabilitation wards. J. Physiotherapy (2016, accepted for publication)
12. Fogg, B.J.: Persuasive Technology: Using Computers to Change What We Think and Do. Morgan Kaufmann, San Francisco (2003)
13. IJsselsteijn, W.A., de Kort, Y.A.W., Midden, C., Eggen, B., van den Hoven, E.: Persuasive technology for human well-being: setting the scene. In: IJsselsteijn, W.A., de Kort, Y.A.W., Midden, C., Eggen, B., van den Hoven, E. (eds.) PERSUASIVE 2006. LNCS, vol. 3962, pp. 1–5. Springer, Heidelberg (2006)

14. Smith, S.T., Schoene, D.: The use of exercise-based videogames for training and rehabilitation of physical function in older adults: current practice and guidelines for future research. Aging Health. **8**, 243–252 (2013)
15. Caplan, L.: Stroke. Demost Medical Publishing, New York (2006)
16. Lincoln, N.B., Kneebone, I.I., Macniven, C.M.: Psychological Management of Stroke, pp. 3–28. Wiley, Malden (2012)
17. Fasoli, S., Krebs, H., Hogan, N.: Robotic technology and stroke rehabilitation: translating research into practice. Top. Stroke Rehabil. **11**, 11–19 (2004)
18. Maclean, N., Pound, P., Wolfe, C., Rudd, A.: Qualitative analysis of stroke patients' in rehabilitation. Br. Med. J. **321**, 1051–1054 (2000)
19. Shaughnessy, M., Resnick, B.M., Macko, R.F.: Testing a model of post-stroke exercise behavior. J. Rehabil. Nurs. **31**, 2048–7940 (2006)
20. Bongers, A.J., Smith, S.T.: Interactivating Rehabilitation through Active Multimodal Feedback and Guidance. In: Rocker, C., Ziefle, M. (eds.) Smart Healthcare Applications and Services: Developments and Practices, pp. 236–260. IGI-Global, Pennsylvania (2010)
21. Hilland, T., Murphy, R., Stratton, G.: The Feasibility and Appropriateness of Utilising the Nintendo Wii during Stroke Rehabilitation to Promote Physical Activity, A report by the Liverpool John Moores University (2011)
22. Orji, R., Vassileva, J., Mandryk, R.: LunchTime: a slow-casual game for long-term dietary behaviour change. Pers. Ubiquit. Comput. **17**, 1211–1221 (2013)
23. Froehlich, J., Findlater, L., Landay, J.: The design of eco-feedback technology. In: Proceedings of the SIGCHI Conference on Human Factors in Computing Systems (CHI 2010), pp. 1999–2008. ACM, New York (2010)
24. Bongers, A.J., Smith, S.T., Donker, V., Pickrell, M., Hall, R.: Interactive infrastructures – physical rehabilitation modules for pervasive healthcare technology. In: Holzinger, A., Ziefle, M., Röcker, C. (eds.) Pervasive Health – State of the Art and Beyond, pp. 229–254. Springer, London (2014)
25. Cockrell, J., Folstein, M.F.: Mini-mental state examination. In: Copeland, J.R.M., Abou-Saleh, M.T., Blazer, B.G. (eds.) Principles and Practice of Geriatric Psychiatry, 2nd edn, pp. 140–141. Wiley, Chichester (2002)
26. House, A.: Mood disorders after stroke a review of the evidence. Int. J. Geriatr. Psychiatry **2**, 211–221 (1987)

Developing a Virtual Coach for Chronic Patients: A User Study on the Impact of Similarity, Familiarity and Realism

Arlette van Wissen[(⊠)], Charlotte Vinkers, and Aart van Halteren

Philips Research, High Tech Campus 34, 5656 AE Eindhoven, The Netherlands
{Arlette.van.Wissen, Charlotte.Vinkers,
Aart.van.Halteren}@philips.com

Abstract. Healthcare costs are increasing dramatically due to disproportional consumption of healthcare resources by chronic patients. Automated forms of health coaching can contribute to improved patient self-management while reducing costs due to increased scalability and availability of the use of human health coaches. Embodied Conversational Agents (ECAs) seem to be good candidates to function as automated coaches, as they introduce a social component to human-computer interactions which makes them particularly suitable to influence a user's attitude or behavior. To date, there is limited knowledge on the impact of appearance-related characteristics of an ECA as a virtual coach among a chronically ill elderly population. The primary aim of this study is to investigate the impact of three appearance cues on user acceptance: (i) similarity; (ii) familiarity; and (iii) realism. Findings demonstrate that patients (a) preferred the realistic-looking ECA over the more stylized one; (b) showed no preference for the familiar over the unfamiliar ECAs (but did evaluate the unfamiliar ECAs as more positive than the familiar one); and (c) evaluated an ECA as virtual coach for self-management support as useful.

Keywords: Persuasive technology · Socially influencing systems · Human-computer interaction · Virtual coaching · Embodied conversational agent

1 Introduction

The prevalence of chronic illnesses, such as diabetes and heart failure, has strikingly increased in the past decades [35]. One viable way to keep healthcare costs within bounds is to help patients better manage their health and illness through health coaching (in the context of chronic disease called *self-management support* [17]), which refers to coaching towards a change in lifestyle-related behaviors for improved health and quality of life, or towards establishing and maintaining health promoting goals [7]. In current clinical practice, health coaching is often human effort that is labor-intensive, costly, and therefore less scalable and cost-effective compared to automated forms of health coaching. Moreover, human health coaches (HCs) have limited availability and reach and therefore limited impact (as impact can be considered reach * efficacy). The reach of a virtual agent in the role of a health coach is much broader as it is accessible to patients whenever they require support. As such there is a

© Springer International Publishing Switzerland 2016
A. Meschtscherjakov et al. (Eds.): PERSUASIVE 2016, LNCS 9638, pp. 263–275, 2016.
DOI: 10.1007/978-3-319-31510-2_23

need to develop innovative and interactive virtual HC services that are able to address those limitations associated with human HC support [3, 18].

Embodied Conversational Agents (ECAs) are a promising technique to help balance the desire for human HC involvement with the need to increase automated interventions in healthcare context. In the present work, we describe an ECA that will function as a virtual (health) coach (VC). The discussed prototype is designed to be the core of a more extensive automated coach that can be used to provide advice and guidance in health promotion and aims to persuade users to change their self-management behaviors to engender beneficial health-related outcomes.

For such a VC to be effective, it has to maximize the influence it has on the user. In persuasive communication there are three components (the source, the receiver, and the messages) that can affect the effectiveness of persuasion [20]. In this paper we examine the influence of the source, in particular, of different appearance characteristics of the source, on its persuasiveness and acceptance among elderly chronic patients. The main aim of our work is (1) to develop an ECA that functions as a virtual coach for chronic patients, i.e. that is able to support and stimulate behavior change, and (2) to identify visual characteristics of the agent that yield the highest user acceptance among our target population.

2 Background

ECAs can provide a particularly acceptable form of human-computer interaction for chronic patients, which are primarily older adults (e.g. [19]). ECAs are suitable for older adults and can address challenges such as their declining sensory and physical abilities [34] and their limited comfort with using technology based on text rather than voice [32]. Moreover, interactive automated HC systems have been developed that have shown to be as effective as human healthcare providers and yield advantageous health-related outcomes such as treatment adherence [6, 24].

Despite its potential benefits in terms of ease of use and health outcomes, there is limited evidence about the extent to which chronic patients accept the use of an ECA as health coach, and if they do, what the ECA should look like to engender user acceptance. User acceptance and perceived persuasiveness of an ECA is a crucial determinant of an ECA's effectiveness, as source characteristics can unconsciously affect the human decision making process [22, 23, 29]. Examples of these characteristics are trustworthiness, perceived expertise, likeability, and similarity to the user.

We have designed a user study that will yield the required insights as to which ECA characteristics should be implemented to obtain maximum user acceptance and consequently potential persuasive influence and user adherence.

3 User Acceptance and Engagement

In the study, we will systematically vary (a) familiarity and similarity; and (b) the visual rendering (realistic vs stylized) of the ECA to examine its impact on user acceptance. With user acceptance, we refer to the acceptance of the ECA in the role of a health coach, which means that the ECA should be trustworthy, likeable, and be perceived as having the expertise to be an effective substitute for a human HC. These factors are also known to influence persuasiveness [11, 23, 29]. The effect of these three characteristics have yielded inconclusive and contradictory results in earlier research, which has been primarily conducted with younger highly educated populations and with observational study designs. We therefore use an experimental design to study whether these characteristics influence user acceptance among older patients (i.e. the target group for the virtual health coach).

Similarity. With regard to the ECA's similarity to the user, it is often assumed that the agent should look similar to the user in order to obtain user acceptance and trust (cf. [11, 30, 31]). This is also reflected in consistent findings in research on human-human relationships that similarity breeds attraction, as advocated by the *Similarity Attraction Theory* (see [31, 36]). In this study we will focus on age as proxy for perceived similarity, as age also has consequences for another dimension that determines how people evaluate others: power or perceived competence [13, 28]. In our study the ECA will have the role of an expert, and as such it is important that it is perceived to be competent and trustworthy [4]. As such, users may prefer an older-looking ECA due to perceptions of competence and experience. On the other hand, although our users may identify themselves more with an older-looking ECA, they may prefer to receive health advice from younger-looking ECAs, as younger people are often seen as more attractive, which may yield more liking, user acceptance and persuasiveness [16, 25].

Familiarity. Another question that is not unambiguously answered in the literature is to which extent an ECA should be a representation of a familiar person that exists in real-life. A vast amount of research shows that the more familiar someone is, the more a person will like and trust him or her (e.g. [9, 10]). Literature on the importance of familiarity in ECAs is scarce, but psychologists and counselors have begun to use virtual representations of themselves ('doppelgangers') to deliver therapy to clients, which suggest that familiarity may be an important feature to implement in an ECA as HC for chronic patients. The effect of familiarity on user acceptance is therefore another characteristic we will examine in the present study.

Realism. There are diverging claims in the literature about the impact of realistic versus more stylized appearances in visual rendering [15], but few empirical studies to back up claims on either side. On the one hand, an ECA's strength is that it emulates a human communicator, with all its social and emotional affordances that such a relationship brings (e.g., support) [2, 8]. On the other hand, the 'uncanny valley' demonstrates a thin line between very realistic ECAs and those that look uncomfortably creepy, leading to negative user responses and discontinued system use [21]. Moreover, people expect virtual characters to display behavior that fits their appearance: the more human-like an ECA looks, the less forgiving they are when the ECA does not meet expectations (e.g., [27]).

4   Virtual Coaching: Design and Use

4.1   Technical and Functional Requirements

For a virtual coach to be effective as a health coach of chronic patients, it needs to have functionalities that reach beyond many current approaches of assistance for chronic patients that focus mostly on diagnosis, reminders, and direct feedback of behavior. It should be able to deploy different behavior change techniques and using those, persuade the user to change attitudes and behaviors. Keeping our target functionality and domain in mind, we identified several high-level Virtual Coach Requirements that have to be met in order to achieve this:

1. the agent should support both **user-initiated and system-initiated interactions**. System-initiated interactions enable pro-active pushes of personalized information to the user. User-initiated interactions allow for a degree of control for the user.
2. the agent should be able to **collect personal data** from the patient to assess the current state of the user and to provide the health care professional with up to date information.
3. the ECA should be able to **learn real-time** from user input. That is, it should be able to dynamically update the knowledge base about the user and generate responses on-the-fly based on new information
4. **assessing and reacting to the user state** should be core of the ECA's functionality.
5. the virtual coach should be capable of providing **long-term support**. It should support and guide users through longer periods of change and should aim to form a social bond with the user.

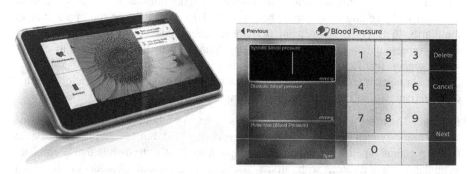

Fig. 1. Tablet with eCareCompanion interface   **Fig. 2.** Measurement entry within eCP

4.2   Integration and Use in a Telehealth Program

The virtual coach is intended to be a fully developed ECA that can be used to provide advice and guidance in health promotion and disease management. As a first step towards realization of such a system, a prototype was developed that is able to talk to the user and respond to touch-based user interactions. The core functionality of this prototype was to provide the user with information about the importance of physical activity, to give encouragement and to support them in setting reminders for medication intake and appointments with health care professionals. This VC is intended to be used in a digital environment called eCareCompanion (eCP), which is realized as a tablet-based interface (see Fig. 1). This interface enables patients to manually enter measurements and respond to survey questions (see Fig. 2). Patients also receive feedback on how their measurements (e.g., blood pressure, weight) change over time. Additionally, patients can use the app to see what consults have been scheduled and to connect to members of their telehealth team through video-chat.

The VC is designed to complement health coaching in a telehealth program. Although for some types of support human coaching and interventions are necessary or preferred, in other cases a virtual coach can take on (parts of) the work of care team members, such as health nurses, health coaches, psychologists, social workers or clinicians. By performing tasks such as scheduling appointments, reminder patients to upload their physiological measurements, providing surveys, or providing some form of social support, the VC will be able to reduce the work load of the care team members, allowing them to focus their efforts where a human touch is most needed and providing them with relevant and regular feedback on the patient status.

5 Method

5.1 Study Aim and Design

The primary aim of the study was to investigate the independent differential impact of the following static ECA characteristics on user acceptance: (a) a younger vs. older appearing ECA (both unfamiliar) vs. an ECA that resembles a familiar person in real-life, and (b) a more realistic vs a more stylized visual rendering of the ECA. These factors were tested in a 3X2 mixed between- and within-subjects design with 3 between-subject conditions: older (unfamiliar) vs. younger (unfamiliar) vs. familiar, and 2 within-subject conditions: stylized vs. photo-realistic. The stylized version of the ECA was created using a software that creates a cartoonized filter on top of the original photographs. We choose this approach because we wanted the stylized version to resemble the realistic one as closely as possible (in order to rule out other effects of appearance). Additionally, we decided on a female representation for the ECA, because prior studies show that people prefer ECAs who conform to stereotypical expectations (e.g., [12]). Given that most (health) coaches in the US are female, these findings suggest that the ECA as HC should be female to induce the most positive responses. Each participant was semi-randomly allocated (in order to guarantee an equal number of participants in the different conditions) to one of the six conditions. The conditions were operationalized as follows (see Fig. 3):

- Younger: a representation of a woman of the age 30–35
- Older: a representation of a woman of the age 55–60
- Familiar: a representation of an actual female health coach/nurse
- "stylized" versions of each picture were created using rotoscoping

5.2 Procedure

Prior to the experiment, a health coach was recruited whose representation we used to create the 'familiar' ECA. Upon arrival at the research facility, participants were asked to sit at a table and were provided a tablet. At this point the experiment leader (i.e. the researcher in the older/younger condition or the health coach in the familiar condition) explained the purpose of the study, after which informed consent was signed.

The Virtual Coach Application was then launched on the tablet, after which participants were presented with the first ECA (photorealistic or stylized), with which they were able to interact via multiple choice responses on the touch screen. The order of presentation of the stylized vs. photo-realistic version of the ECA was counterbalanced between participants. During the interaction with the VC, the VC briefly introduces herself, creates a reminder for medication, and asks the participant a question about physical activity.

After the interaction, participants filled out an evaluation survey on the tablet, and subsequently were presented with the second ECA (photorealistic or stylized) and some final surveys. All versions of the ECA (older, younger, familiar) had the same voice, pushed the same content, and were otherwise matched on appearance features to the extent possible (e.g., hair color, skin color). Finally, the experiment leader returned to the room for a discussion and debriefing.

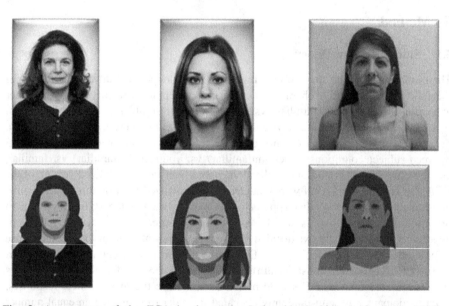

Fig. 3. Appearances of the ECA in the study. Left: older-looking (unfamiliar), middle: younger-looking (unfamiliar), right: familiar. Upper: realistic, under: stylized

5.3 Materials

Tablet. An Android tablet was used to collect data and enable interaction with the VC. The survey data were collected via a secure link; data that participants filled out during the interactions with the VC was not recorded.

Virtual Coach application. The Virtual Coach app presented the torso of a fully animated talking head of an Embodied Conversational Agent. The avatar was generated with a software package called CrazyTalk[1] and deployed on Android using the Unity platform to create the interactive user experience.

Background Survey. Socio-demographic variables such as gender, age, household composition and education level were assessed, as well as relevant psychological constructs, such as social support and ability for self-care.

Manipulation Check. As a manipulation check (younger vs. older vs. familiar; realistic vs. stylized), participants were asked three questions after each presentation of the ECA. Sample item: "How humanlike do you find the virtual health coach?"; all response options ranging from 1 (*not at all*) to 5 (*very*).

Coach Evaluation Survey. To measure user evaluations of the ECA, we used the questions from extensive earlier research on user acceptance of ECAs by Bickmore [5] which are based widely acknowledged models on technology acceptance (Unified Theory of Acceptance and Use of Technology, [33]; Technology Acceptance Model, [1]). Sample item: "How much do you like the virtual health coach?"; all response options ranging from 1 (*not at all*) to 5 (*very*).

Attitudes Towards Use. As the use of a VC for the purpose of support with health-related tasks in a chronically ill population has received limited attention to date, we developed an 8-item survey based on prior research (cf. [16]) about the perceived use and usefulness of the VC. Sample item: "I would find the virtual health coach useful to support me with the management of my health"; all response options ranging from 1 (*not at all*) to 5 (*very*).

6   Study Results

6.1   Participants

In total, 64 participants, of whom 34 female, participated. The majority of participants was between 65–70 years old (62.5 %; > 70 years: 31.3 %; < 65 years: 6.3 %), highly educated (=> associate degree: 59.4 %), living with their spouse (54.7 %), and Caucasian (95.3 %). All participants had one or multiple chronic illnesses for which they had to take medications (e.g. diabetes, cardiovascular disease). Overall, the sample reported to be comfortable with technology ($M = 4.02$, $SD = .88$), to have a high level of social support ($M = 4.13$, $SD = .79$), and indicated a good ability to engage in self-management, such as self-monitoring symptoms and eating a healthy diet (M range 2.83–3.56; SD range .38–.70).

---

[1] https://www.reallusion.com/crazytalk/.

6.2   Manipulation Check

Repeated measures ANOVAs with visual rendering (realistic vs. stylized) as within factor, and Appearance (older vs. younger vs. familiar) and Order (realistic first vs. stylized first) as between factors showed that, as expected, the realistic version was perceived as more human-like, similar, and familiar than the stylized version of the VC, all $p < .01$. No significant differences were found on these three variables between the older, younger, and health coach conditions.

6.3   Coach Evaluation Survey

Separate Repeated Measures ANOVAs were performed for each of the items relating to the users' evaluations of the VCs, with visual rendering (Realistic vs. Stylized) as within factor, and Appearance (Older vs. Younger vs. Familiar) and Order (Realistic first vs. Stylized first) as between factors.

Table 1. Means of evaluations of the coach evaluations of the older, younger and familiar virtual coach

Coach evaluations		Realistic	Stylized
		M (SD)	M (SD)
Friendly	Familiar	3.22 (2.02)	2.92 (2.01)
	Older	4.15 (2.07)	3.44 (2.07)
	Younger	3.68 (1.97)	3.23 (1.96)
Competent	Familiar	3.61 (1.91)	2.92 (1.81)
	Older	3.60 (1.97)	3.28 (1.87)
	Younger	3.50 (1.87)	3.32 (1.77)
Attractive	Familiar	3.32 (1.94)	1.93 (1.85)
	Older	3.41 (1.99)	1.80 (1.90)
	Younger	3.50 (1.89)	2.32 (1.80)
Like	Familiar	3.29 (1.97)	2.51 (1.75)
	Older	3.51 (2.02)	2.84 (1.80)
	Younger	3.59 (1.92)	3.05 (1.71)
Trust	Familiar	3.34 (1.67)	2.84 (1.98)
	Older	3.43 (1.72)	3.00 (2.03)
	Younger	3.68 (1.64)	3.32 (1.93)
Follow advice	Familiar	3.58 (1.57)	3.04 (2.01)
	Older	3.54 (1.62)	3.17 (2.07)
	Younger	3.77 (1.53)	3.64 (1.96)
Continue interaction	Familiar	3.35 (2.16)	2.47 (2.17)
	Older	3.40 (2.22)	2.77 (2.24)
	Younger	3.82 (2.11)	3.27 (2.13)
Satisfied	Familiar	3.31 (2.06)	2.36 (2.18)
	Older	3.39 (2.11)	2.87 (2.25)
	Younger	3.68 (2.01)	3.23 (2.13)

For all outcome variables, a significant difference between evaluations of the stylized compared to the realistic appearances were found. Specifically, the participants evaluated the realistic version more positively with respect to characteristics such as likeability, competency, trustworthiness (all p's < .01; see Table 1).

For one outcome variable, 'friendly', a marginally significant main effect of Appearance (older vs. younger vs. familiar) appeared, $F(2, 57) = 2.64$, $p = .08$, $p\eta^2 = .08$. Post hoc analysis (Least Square Difference Test) revealed that participants in the older condition ($M = 3.80$, $SD = 1.80$) found the VC significantly friendlier than participants in the familiar HC condition ($M = 3.07$, $SD = 1.75$, $p = .03$). There were no differences between the younger condition ($M = 3.46$, $SD = 1.71$) and the other two conditions (p's > .21). For all other outcome variables, no differences between the older, younger, and familiar VC were demonstrated (all p's > .14).

6.4   Attitudes Towards Use of a Virtual Coach

Again, separate Repeated Measures ANOVAs were performed for each of the items relating to the users' evaluations of the VCs, with visual rendering (realistic vs. stylized) as within factor, and Appearance (older vs. younger vs. familiar) and Order (realistic first vs. stylized first) as between factors. No main effects of visual rendering were demonstrated. However, for four of seven outcome variables, a main effect of Appearance (older vs. younger vs. familiar) appeared, all p's <= .05.

We found differences between participants in the extent to which they evaluated the (intended) functionality of the VC as useful, easy to use, enabling better health goal achievement, supporting their health management, and whether they liked working with it (see Table 2). Post-hoc analyses revealed that for 'easy to use', 'like working with', and 'enable health goal achievement', the younger VC was evaluated as significantly more favorable than the familiar VC (p's < = .03), whereas no differences were found between the younger and older, and older and familiar VC. For 'easier to manage health' and 'useful', a significant difference was also found between the older and familiar VC, with the older VC evaluated as more favorable than the familiar VC.

Table 2. Means of evaluations of the usefulness of the older, younger and familiar virtual health coach

Survey item	Familiar	Older	Younger	$p\eta^2$
	M (SD)	M (SD)	M (SD)	
Easy to use	4.05 (.97)	4.43 (.68)	4.55 (.51)	
Like working with	3.29 (.96)[a]	3.71 (.64)[a,b]	4.05 (.84)[b]	.13
Useful to support health management	3.48 (.93)	3.76 (.89)	4.05 (.84)	
Enable health goal achievement	3.38 (.92)[a]	3.71 (.78)[a,b]	4.00 (.69)[b]	.10
Easier to manage health	3.24 (.77)[a]	3.52 (.98)[a]	4.09 (.61)[b]	.17
Useful	3.24 (.83)[a]	3.52 (.93)[a]	4.05 (.72)[b]	.15
Make life more interesting	3.00 (.84)	3.00 (.89)	3.50 (1.01)	
Help when necessary	3.76 (.70)	3.95 (.87)	4.27 (.63)	

Note. Values with different superscripts differ at $p < .05$

7 Discussion and Future Work

Our results show that using a familiar face for a virtual coach may pose challenges. Compared to the other appearances, the familiar virtual coach received lower evaluations. One hypothesis for these results is that people are disappointed by a virtual representation of someone they know, as it emphasizes technological limitations (such as imperfect lip synchronization, lack of shared knowledge between virtual and actual coach) and the mismatch with reality (different voice, different movements). An alternative explanation for our findings could be that they can be contributed to the particular images that were used. Future work could explore this further. Furthermore, our results indicate that people have slight preference for a younger appearance over an older one. It could be that they found her more attractive and as such they might have a cognitive bias in favor of her (see [16, 25]).

Overall, people were positive about their interaction with the Virtual Health Coach and they have a positive attitude towards the deployment of an ECA to support with health related tasks. This indicates that such a virtual coach can indeed be deployed as an aid to an elderly chronic patient population with respect to behavior change and self-management support. This is in line with results found in [14, 26], in which the use of ECAs as a medium for persuasive dialogue was examined. Future research will have to show whether the ECA will be preferred over merely text- or voice-based interactions, given that the acceptance of voice-based assistants has improved dramatically over the last years (e.g. Siri by Apple, Google Now, and Cortana by Microsoft).

With respect to our study design, some limitations have to be noted. With respect to the analyses, we are aware of the discussion as to whether 5-point Likert scales should be considered ordinal or interval data, and analyzed as such. In this case we argue that the items can be considered symmetric and equidistant and as such will behave like an interval-level measurement which measures continuous concepts. Furthermore, in the study we chose to create an environment in which patient and health coach could become familiar with each other, rather than working with someone who was actually known to the patients. This was decided because of (a) scalability of the study (so as not to have to create 64 different ECAs from photos of different health coaches), and (b) participants' opinions about their health coach, which may bias their evaluations of the ECA resembling this person. We do however acknowledge that the degree of familiarity is somewhat limited and as such we would in the future like to explore setups with truly familiar subjects and ECAs.

8 Conclusion

This paper discusses part of the development process of a virtual coach for elderly chronic patients. The virtual coach will be a tablet-based application integrated in a telehealth program where it will function to monitor the patient and support with taking measurements, as well as to use more complex intervention strategies to provide (pro) active and persuasive coaching and social support. In order to achieve maximum user acceptance and persuasive potential, a study was conducted in which the effects of changes in familiarity, similarity and visual rendering of the ECA were examined. Findings demonstrated that participants preferred the realistic-looking ECA over the more stylized one; as well as had a slight preference for the unfamiliar ECAs over the familiar ones. These findings suggest that when designing ECAs as virtual coaches, their appearance should be realistic in order to mimic human coaching relationships, and that using representations of loved/familiar ones is not (yet) recommended due to the heightened expectations that current state-of-the-art technology has difficulty to address. Additionally, the participants considered a virtual coach for self-management beneficial to their health. As user acceptance of technology among the target population is a requirement for (long-term) system use, we consider this user study a crucial step in the development of virtual health coaches for chronic patients.

References

1. Bagozzi, R.P., Davis, F.D., Warshaw, P.R.: Development and test of a theory of technological learning and usage. Hum. Relat. **45**(7), 659–686 (1992)
2. Bailenson, J., Swinth, K., Hoyt, C., Persky, S., Dimov, A., Blascovich, J.: The independent and interactive effects of embodied conversational agent appearance and behavior on self-report, cognitive, and behavioral markers of copresence in virtual immersive environments. Presence **14**, 379–393 (2005)
3. Barlow, J., Wright, C., Sheasby, J., Turner, A., Hainsworth, J.: Self-management approaches for people with chronic conditions: a review. Patient Educ. Couns. **48**, 177–187 (2002)
4. Beishuizen, J., Hof, E., Putten, C., Bouwmeester, S., Asscher, J.: Students' and teachers' cognitions about good teachers. Br. J. Educ. Psychol. **71**, 185–201 (2001)
5. Bickmore, T., Caruso, L., Clough-Gorr, K., Heeren, T.: It's just like you talk to a friend: relational agents for older adults. Interact. Comput. HCI Older Popul. **17**, 711–735 (2005)
6. Bickmore, T., Giorgino, T.: Health dialog systems for patients and consumers. J. Biomed. Inform. **39**, 556–571 (2006)
7. Butterworth, S., Linden, A., McClay, W., Leo, M.: Effect of motivational interviewing-based health coaching on employees' physical and mental status. J. Occup. Health Psychol. **11**, 358–365 (2006)
8. Campbell, R.H., Grimshaw, M.N., Green, G.M.: Relational agents: a critical review. Open Virtual Reality J. **1**, 1–7 (2009)
9. Chu, S., Fedorovskaya, E., Quek, F., Snyder, J.: The effect of familiarity on perceived interestingness of images. In: Human Vision and Electronic Engineering, vol. 8651 (2013)
10. Cialdini, R.B., Goldstein, N.J.: Social influence: compliance and conformity. Ann. Rev. Psychol. **55**, 591–621 (2004)
11. Fogg, B.J.: Persuasive Technology: Using Computers to Change What We Think and Do. Morgan Kaufmann Publishers, San Francisco (2003)
12. Forlizzi, J., Zimmerman, J., Mancuso, V., Kwak, S.: How interface agents affect interaction between humans and computers. In: Proceedings of the 2007 Conference on Designing Pleasurable Products and Interfaces, pp. 209–221. ACM (2007)
13. Georgesen, J., Harris, M.: The balance of power: interpersonal consequences of differential power and expectancies. Pers. Soc. Psychol. Bull. **26**, 1239–1257 (2000)

14. Grolleman, J., van Dijk, B., Nijholt, A., van Emst, A.: Break the habit! designing an e-therapy intervention using a virtual coach in aid of smoking cessation. In: IJsselsteijn, W.A., de Kort, Y.A., Midden, C., Eggen, B., van den Hoven, E. (eds.) PERSUASIVE 2006. LNCS, vol. 3962, pp. 133–141. Springer, Heidelberg (2006)

15. Haake, M., Gulz, A.: Visual realism and virtual pedagogical agents. In: The 3rd International Design and Engagability Conference@ NordiCHI 2006 (2006)

16. Khan, R., De Angeli, A.: The attractiveness stereotype in the evaluation of embodied conversational agents. In: Gross, T., Gulliksen, J., Kotzé, P., Oestreicher, L., Palanque, P., Prates, R.O., Winckler, M. (eds.) INTERACT 2009. LNCS, vol. 5726, pp. 85–97. Springer, Heidelberg (2009)

17. Lorig, K., Holman, H.: Self-management education: history, definition, outcomes, and mechanisms. Ann. Behav. Med. **26**, 1–7 (2003)

18. Lorig, K., Ritter, P., Stewart, A.L., Holman, R.: Chronic disease management program: 2-year health status and healthcare utilization costs. Med. Care **39**, 1217–1223 (2001)

19. Mendis, S., Puska, P., Norrving, B.: Global Atlas on Cardiovascular Disease Prevention and Control, pp. 2–14. World Health Organization, Geneva (2011)

20. Miller, G.R.: On being persuaded: some basic distinctions. In: Roloff, M.E., Miller, G.R. (eds.) Persuasion: New Directions in Theory and Research, pp. 11–28. Sage, Beverly Hills (1980)

21. Mori, M.: The uncanny valley (K.F. MacDorman and N. Kageki, Trans.). IEEE Robot. Autom. Mag. **19**(2), 98–100 (1970/2012)

22. Nguyen, H., Masthoff, J.: Is it me or is it what i say? source image and persuasion. In: de Kort, Y.A., IJsselsteijn, W.A., Midden, C., Eggen, B., Fogg, B.J. (eds.) PERSUASIVE 2007. LNCS, vol. 4744, pp. 231–242. Springer, Heidelberg (2007)

23. O'Keefe, J.D.: Persuasion: Theory and Research. Sage, Newbury Park (1990)

24. Revere, D., Dunbar, P.: Review of computer-generated outpatient health behavior interventions: clinical encounters in absentia. J. Am. Med. Inform. Assoc. **8**, 62–79 (2001)

25. Ring, L., Utami, D., Bickmore, T.: The right agent for the job? In: Bickmore, T., Marsella, S., Sidner, C. (eds.) IVA 2014. LNCS, vol. 8637, pp. 374–384. Springer, Heidelberg (2014)

26. Schulman, D., Bickmore, T.W., Sidner, C.L.: An intelligent conversational agent for promoting long-term health behavior change using motivational interviewing. In: AAAI Spring Symposium: AI and Health Communication, March 2011

27. Slater, M., Steed, A., Chrysanthou, Y.: Computer Graphics and Virtual Environments: From Realism to Real-Time. Pearson Education, Boston (2002)

28. Svennevig, J.: Getting Acquainted in Conversation: A Study of Initial Interactions, vol. 64. John Benjamins Publishing, Amsterdam (2000)

29. Stiff, J.B., Mongeau, P.A.: Persuasive Communication. Guilford Press, New York (2003)

30. Van Vugt, H., Bailenson, J., Hoorn, J.F., Konijn, F.: Effects of facial similarity on user responses to embodied agents. ACM Trans. Comput. Hum. Interact. **17**, 7 (2010)

31. Van Vugt, H.C., Konijn, E.A., Hoorn, J.F., Keur, I., Eliéns, A.: Realism is not all! User engagement with task-related interface characters. Interact. Comput. **19**(2), 267–280 (2007)

32. Vardoulakis, L.P., Ring, L., Barry, B., Sidner, C., Bickmore, T.: Designing relational agents as long term social companions for older adults. Intell. Virtual Agents **7502**, 289–302 (2011)

33. Venkatesh, V., Zhang, X.: Unified theory of acceptance and use of technology: US vs. China. J. Glob. Inf. Technol. Manage. **13**(1), 5–27 (2010)

34. Wallace, J., Mulvenna, M., Martin, S., Stephens, S., Burns, W.: ICT interface design for ageing people and people with dementia. In: Mulvenna, M.D., Nugent, C.D. (eds.) Supporting People with Dementia Using Pervasive Health Technologies. Advanced Information and Knowledge Processing, pp. 165–188. Springer, Heidelberg (2010)

35. Ward, B., Schiller, J., Goodman, R.: Multiple chronic conditions among U.S. adults: A 2012 update. Prev. Chronic Dis. **11**, E62 (2014)
36. Zhou, S., Bickmore, T., Paasche-Orlow, M., Jack, B.: Agent-user concordance and satisfaction with a virtual hospital discharge nurse. In: Bickmore, T., Marsella, S., Sidner, C. (eds.) IVA 2014. LNCS, vol. 8637, pp. 528–541. Springer, Heidelberg (2014)

Improving Adherence in Automated e-Coaching

A Case from Insomnia Therapy

Robbert Jan Beun[1(✉)], Willem-Paul Brinkman[2], Siska Fitrianie[1],
Fiemke Griffioen-Both[1], Corine Horsch[2], Jaap Lancee[3], and Sandor Spruit[1]

[1] Utrecht University, Utrecht, The Netherlands
{r.j.beun,s.fitrianie,f.griffioen-both,a.g.l.spruit}@uu.nl
[2] Delft University of Technology, Delft, The Netherlands
w.p.brinkman@tudelft.nl,corinehorsch@gmail.com
[3] University of Amsterdam, Amsterdam, The Netherlands
j.lancee@uva.nl

Abstract. Non-adherence is considered a problem that seriously undermines the outcome of behavior change therapies, in particular of self-help therapies delivered without human interference. This paper presents the design rationale behind a computer system in the domain of adherence enhancing strategies in automated e-coaching. A variety of persuasive strategies is introduced and implemented in a mobile e-coaching system in the domain of insomnia therapy. The system integrates two types of interface elements, i.e. dedicated tools and natural language conversation, to simplify therapy related activities and to include social strategies to improve motivation. We focus on the crucial role of communication and adaptation.

Keywords: e-Coaching · Adherence · Persuasive strategies · Insomnia therapy · Conversation · Tools · Behavior change systems

1 Introduction

One of the first software programs that automatically mimicked the behavior of a therapist is the digital Rogerian psychoanalyst 'Eliza' [26]. Eliza simulates a simple question-answer conversation in natural language by rephrasing many of the patient's statements into questions. The program showed that a digital therapist could be implemented in a computer system that has strong positive emotional effects with relatively simple means.

Since the appearance of Eliza the world changed radically. In the digital world, powerful mobile systems support the majority of the population with a wide range of activities; in health care, awareness increased that our health can be positively influenced by our behavior and activities. In the field of consumer health care, these developments resulted in a variety of products, ranging from various types of monitoring systems to self-help apps that aim to change an individual's behavior and cognition. Today over 100,000 health apps exist in the Apple and Google stores that support all types of health related activities, but a major problem is that a proliferation of consumer health care

© Springer International Publishing Switzerland 2016
A. Meschtscherjakov et al. (Eds.): PERSUASIVE 2016, LNCS 9638, pp. 276–287, 2016.
DOI: 10.1007/978-3-319-31510-2_24

applications arises regardless of real user needs [21]. Potentially, we now have the knowledge and the technology to build interventions and coaching principles in smartphones that are far beyond the capabilities of Weizenbaum's Eliza, but the design of these systems should be preceded by careful analysis of the coaching process.

In this paper, we present the design rationale behind a fully automated coaching system that supports an intervention for behavior change in the domain of insomnia therapy – we refer to this system as the 'SleepCare-system'. The system behaves as a digital agent, the so-called e-coach, and integrates various types of interaction, in particular natural language conversation and graphical interaction with various tools. We focus in particular on the requirements and the generic elements in the design that were included to improve exercise adherence.

We first elaborate on the coaching process and some existing e-coaching implementations. We then turn to the domain of the application, insomnia therapy, and the problem of exercise adherence within the domain. Next, we discuss various adherence enhancing strategies to improve behavior change. We then turn to the design elements of the system that support these strategies and consider some aspects of testing. We finish this paper with a discussion about the relevant design elements.

2 Coaching and e-Coaching

Central to most definitions of coaching is that coaching is a goal-oriented activity to help people enhance aspects of both their personal and professional lives by fostering self-directed learning through collaborative goal setting, action planning and feedback [14]. Assumptions in the coaching process are the absence of serious mental health problems [6] and the notion that the client – or coachee – is resourceful and motivated to engage in finding solutions [1, 17]. In the coaching process, two learning dimensions are essential: (1) learning through individual subjective experiences and (2) learning as a social and collaborative practice. The first dimension refers to the experiential and action oriented process of the coachee; the second refers to the idea of a collaborative dialogue that unfolds between the coaching parties and where the coachee learns in interaction with the coach.

Since current society and daily lives of people are highly contextual and characterized by a growing degree of uncertainty, a coach will be cautious in offering solutions. What counts as a solution for one person, not necessarily counts as a solution for another. Therefore, coaching involves a collaborative approach and respect of the coachee's autonomy. Personalization, contextualization and frequent adaptation are necessary prerequisites of the coaching process. In that respect, the role of a coach seems an excellent candidate for a digital agent that supports automated self-help therapies; we will refer to these systems as *e-coaches*.

Examples of e-coaches that apply methods from behavior medicine cover a wide range of therapy domains, ranging from obesity to depression and insomnia treatment. In [5], for example, an e-coach was developed to support overweight people improving their lifestyle. The e-coach is able to help motivated participants adhere to the program and lose weight. In [7], an e-coach is described that offers a fully automated treatment for depression, based on behavioral activation, a form of psychotherapy. In [9] an e-coach is described that offers an insomnia treatment in six weekly sessions. The authors successfully tested the intervention against a placebo and treatment as usual in a randomized controlled trial.

Previous studies mainly focus on one specific domain. An important exception to domain specificity is the work described in [4] who describe a theory-driven computational model to deliver health behavior change counseling. The authors present an ontology containing concepts from behavioral medicine and communication. Various models are introduced that enable the representation of knowledge about, for instance, the user and the underlying theory of the intervention. We also aim at developing a reusable mobile framework based on generic coaching principles, but in contrast to [4] who focuses on modeling counseling knowledge from which dialogue actions can be inferred, our perspective starts from communication and cybernetics theory, and is based on concepts such as alignment, negotiation, evaluation, feedback and adaptation. This enables us to include persuasive strategies such as tunneling, adaptation, reduction and increase of motivation. The insomnia domain will be used as a proof of concept.

3   Insomnia and Insomnia Therapy

Insomnia is a sleep disorder with a high prevalence (about 10 % of the population) and can have severe individual and societal consequences (e.g., concentration problems, increased risks of accidents, depression); people with insomnia have difficulty initiating and/or maintaining sleep. Today, it is widely accepted that behavior change treatments such as Cognitive Behavior Therapy (CBT) produce sustainable positive changes in the condition of insomnia [22].

CBT for insomnia (CBT-I) offers a variety of exercise types that differ in aim and properties [23]: sleep restriction, stimulus control, relaxation, cognitive therapy and sleep hygiene. Sleep restriction involves curtailing the time spent in bed to stabilize the sleep pattern and lengthening sleep time as sleep efficiency improves. Stimulus control aims at restoring the coachee's positive association of the bed and the bedroom with sleep. Relaxation training involves methods aimed at reducing somatic tension. Cognitive therapy aims at changing dysfunctional beliefs and attitudes. Sleep hygiene education aims to make the person aware of practices and environmental factors that may either be detrimental or beneficial for sleep. Treatment protocols usually take between 6 and 10 weekly consultation sessions. The actual intervention is preceded by a one- or two-week baseline sleep diary monitoring period.

4   Exercise Adherence

Central in self-management approaches to behavior change for health – and CBT-I is no exception to this – is the idea that the individual invests a reasonable amount of effort and time in the activities. However, people have many reasons not to perform the assignments: lack of energy, motivation and willpower, mistrust, procrastination, simply forgetting, etcetera. As a result, low *adherence* rates are an ever present and complex problem, and seriously undermine the outcome of CBT [25]. In [15], it has been shown that the average treatment adherence for technology mediated insomnia treatments is approximately 52 %, meaning that almost half of the people did not finish the treatment.

It may even be expected that in reality these rates are considerably lower. First, since these results were based on self-reports and user logs, the reports by the participants may be overrated and based on a positive answer bias. Second, adherence is a complex notion and has no clear-cut boundaries (e.g., total time in bed, number of relaxation exercises per day, completion of the assignments). Low adherence rates can be expected in particular with exercise types that require strong willpower.

Preventing the process of a downward motivation spiral and adequately responding to it is a mandatory element in any behavior change intervention. For that, we should realize that the exercises in insomnia treatment include a large variation of activities in terms of actual content, duration, timing, frequency, presentation and intensity (cf. [12]). Some of these activities take time and should be performed on a daily or weekly basis such as relaxation exercises or consults. Sleep restriction and stimulus control require a great deal of willpower and can even be dangerous, but may have high treatment effects if well adhered to. The sleep hygiene exercise may require changing habits such as refrain from drinking coffee or alcohol before bedtime; in other cases, the exercise requires a one-time behavior such as cleaning the bedroom or changing the bedroom temperature. Improving adherence to this variation of therapy elements requires a well-dosed combination of various adherence enhancing strategies.

5   Adherence Enhancing Strategies

5.1   Tunneling, Feedback and Adaptation

Basically, every CBT-coach offers evidence based behavior change techniques that should be experienced by the coachee for a particular period of time. The behavior in the CBT-I domain consists of introducing or changing activities in the coachee's daily life such as filling in a sleep diary, having a conversation for consultation or changing bedtime; in other cases, activities and habits are discouraged such as drinking coffee or alcohol just before bedtime. In other words, a coach tunnels therapy related activities: it determines the exercise types, the properties of these exercises and communicates this information to the coachee. We call this process *tunneling* (cf. [11]).

In contrast to self-help books, a human coach adds an important quality to the tunneling process: a *feedback loop*. To cope with the many uncertainties, a frequent feedback loop is included to reshape the offered techniques and the communication about these techniques. Hence, the information flow between coach and coachee not only pertains to tunneling (e.g., 'Go to bed at 12', 'Fill in your sleep diary before 8'), but also to the adaptation process. A human coach observes, asks questions, negotiates, agrees, aligns and tailors the exercises to the multifarious coachee characteristics such as age, habits, preferences, intermediary results and experiences [3]. Adaptation is a crucial element in the tunneling process. A person who, for whatever reason, is unable to go to bed at twelve and repeatedly hears from her coach that she should go to bed at twelve, most likely decides that the therapy is not applicable and may even consider the coach as ignorant or unreliable. This is one of the reasons that the results of many self-help books are rather disappointing [24]: they are targeted at large user groups and do not offer information or exercises tailored to the individual.

5.2 Persuasive Strategies

Coaches also apply a range of behaviors to support the behavior change: they motivate, encourage, challenge, and explain; they show progress and confront with discrepancies in real and committed behaviors. In that sense, coaching is a constant process of tunneling, tailoring and support. We refer to a collection of coherent activities that support the process of behavior change as a *persuasive strategy*. In line with [13, 20], we assume that persuasive strategies aim at increasing the ability and/or motivation of the coachee with respect to the intended behavior change. Loosely speaking, improving ability implies that the coachee may decrease the amount of effort that should be put into the therapy; improving motivation implies that the coachee is willing to put more effort into the therapy. The distinction between the two concepts is not always that clear, however.

We assume that the coachee is located in a complex multidimensional space, the current state, and aims to achieve another complex space, the desired state. In insomnia therapy, both states can be expressed in concrete values for sleep variables such as total sleeping time and quality of sleep. In the desired state, the coachee has 'improved' on at least some of these values. To stress the importance of the difference between the use of tools and language (cf. [11]), persuasive strategies are now classified in two categories (cf. [16]): (1) polishing strategies and (2) meta-level strategies.

ad 1. The road to the desired world is full of obstacles. An important function of the coach is to take away these obstacles and polish the way to success. Metaphorically speaking, the coach offers a slide to improve the flow of activities that have to be performed to achieve the desired world. It may simplify behavior and help to avoid boredom and stress; it may include beauty or a positive user experience to attract attention and willingness to participate. In practice, this may imply that the coach offers tools, e.g., an electronic sleep diary, an agenda, relaxing music or a game. This is also related to what is often called 'reduction' and 'nudging'. In insomnia therapy, for instance, a tool may be implemented that automatically lowers the intensity or changes the color of the light to induce homeostatic processes in the body for bedtime preparation.

ad 2. The meta-level adds a symbolic level to the previous category. It is what we often call 'social influence' and may, for instance, be represented in the interface as an embodied character that uses natural language dialogue and nonverbal signs. The coach is now able, for instance, to communicate that 'if the coachee performs an activity, then the coachee will be rewarded'. The use of symbols enables the coach to approve or disapprove the coachee's behavior, to communicate about the road to the desired state and to explain matters in terms of cause and consequence. The meta-level also enables to negotiate the intensity of the intervention, or to show some type of authority (e.g., 'This is an evidence based intervention'). Including the meta-level enables us to incorporate social elements that have a high impact on a person's behavior: collaboration, transparency, competition, trust, commitment, reciprocity (see e.g., [8]) and accompanying speech acts such as promise, praise, welcome, bid, finish the conversation, etcetera. The meta-level substantially increases the expressivity of the coaching system; in practice, the levels are constantly intertwined.

In CBT-I two types of activities can be distinguished: a. *main* activities that have to be experienced by the coachee such as sleep restriction and b. *supporting* activities such as activity scheduling. To restructure the coachee's sleep architecture, it is important to experience sleep pressure, but it is unimportant to experience calculating sleep efficiency. Consequently, all activities that are part of CBT-I and that do not have to be experienced by the coachee can be simplified. In CBT-I, for instance, sleep data can be registered by means of an electronic diary instead of paper and pencil notation; calculations of sleep efficiency can be automated and integrated in a proposal for wake up and bedtimes. In the ideal case, supporting activities are fully automated. Because main activities, such as decreasing total bedtime, should be experienced, it is important to increase motivation for these types of activities.

To conclude, an e-coach that is intended to offer an intervention for behavior change should include a variety of adherence enhancing strategies that aim at:

- tunneling the intended activities,
- adaptation of exercises and interaction,
- reduction by simplification of supporting activities,
- increasing motivation to perform main activities (cf. [19]).

We now turn to the design of the SleepCare-system and explain how these requirements were applied in the system.

6 The SleepCare System

6.1 The Functionality of the e-Coach

The SleepCare-system offers a therapy on an Android smartphone that includes a variety of CBT-I exercises: relaxation, sleep restriction and sleep hygiene. Sleep restriction has been chosen, because it is an effective element of CBT-I; relaxation and sleep hygiene were chosen because these exercises were relatively easily to implement and vary substantially from sleep restriction. Exercises consist of *assignments* that have to be carried out during the therapy. There are five types of assignments: going to bed, getting out of bed, filling in the sleep diary, doing a relaxation exercise and taking part in a consult. A consult is a conversational activity about various therapy related topics such as the introduction and evaluation of a particular exercise type.

In the therapy, three interaction stages are distinguished: opening, intervention and closure [3]. The goal of the opening phase is twofold: improving transparency through a process of alignment and establishing commitment to the therapy. In the intervention phase the actual therapy is conducted and the coachee is supposed to carry out the assignments. The closure phase starts when all assignments have been performed or when the coachee indicates the desire to withdraw. In this phase, the e-coach and coachee evaluate the offered therapy and may say goodbye.

6.2   Tunneling the Coachee's Activities

A fundamental element in the process of tunneling is the activity schedule that is introduced by the e-coach in one of the early introduction sessions. The primary task of the
activity schedule is to keep track of the various assignments that have been or should
be carried out during the therapy. All scheduled assignments result from an agreed
contract between coach and coachee. The end time of the activities is usually unknown,
but in practice the time interval of assignments is relatively short (e.g., between 1 and
16 min). Scheduled assignments may trigger the generation of reminders and other
communication acts. Activities by the e-coach may also be triggered by non-scheduled
events, in particular when the system detects violations of pre-defined 'constraints' such
as obvious non-adherence of the coachee [3].

   To observe the properties of the scheduled assignments, such as starting-time and
performance status, there exists a corresponding interaction tool. The most important
function of the tool is to display the coachee's previous commitments and adherence to
the assignments. For that, the interaction tool not only displays the scheduled starting
time and date in the past, present or future, but also the performance status of an assign-
ment by a colored line in front: red means missed, orange means near missed, green
means completed and grey means planned or actual. The left picture in Fig. 1 shows a
part of the interaction tool presented in the system's home screen. As a consequence,
the tool not only enables a coachee to have a prompt overview of the future commitments, but also of the (non-)adhered assignments in the past. In that way, the schedule-
tool not only tunnels the coachee's activities, but also refers to meta-level properties
such as agreed commitments.

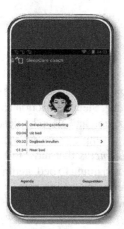 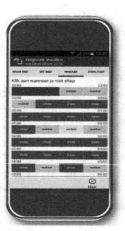 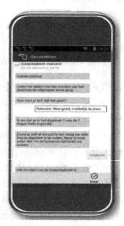

Fig. 1. The left picture depicts the home screen of the SleepCare-system and a part of the schedule
tool; colored vertical lines indicate the performance status of the exercises. The middle and right
picture show examples of the sleep diary tool and an evaluation dialogue about the use of the sleep
diary. On top of the interface notification icons appear in the notification area (the small black
beam).

6.3 Feedback and Adaptation

Starting from the opening phase, there is a constant activity of feedback and adaptation. From the e-coach's point of view, the goal of the opening phase is to construct a user model to adapt the therapy to the characteristics of the coachee. The adaptation process pertains to information at both the therapy and the communication level (e.g., sleep characteristics, age and name). Based on a set of exclusion criteria, the coach may also advise the coachee to withdraw from the therapy; the coachee, however, makes the final decision about continuation.

During the intervention phase, exercises always follow the same four steps [3]: 1. introduction, 2. planning and commitment, 3. task execution and 4. evaluation. In the introduction step, the exercise type is explained. In the planning and commitment step, e-coach and coachee aim at agreement about the exercise properties. During task execution the coachee performs the assignments. In the evaluation step, results are discussed and the exercise properties may, in deliberation with the e-coach, be adapted to the coachee's desires. In case of exercise adaptation, the process is repeated, starting from the planning and commitment phase. If no constraints are violated, the planning-evaluation cycle takes about one week. All exercise steps are included in the activity schedule, but in the course of the therapy, assignments may be added, rescheduled or even be removed in deliberation with the e-coach.

6.4 The User Interface

In the system, four categories of interface elements are distinguished: conversations, tools, notifications and the menu. Conversations enable the e-coach to perform meta-level natural language interaction activities such as introductions and weekly consults. Tools are relatively independent modules that are less language oriented and contain graphical elements such as buttons, wheels and tables; we included the schedule-tool, an electronic sleep diary and a relaxation tool. Notifications function as attention grabbers to start a particular activity and are displayed outside the system's normal user interface (see Fig. 1 middle and right pictures). The menu offers access to the various tools, performed conversations, sleep exercises, advice and information, and general issues such as notification settings, privacy and safety.

Although simplistic compared to human F2F-conversations, the use of natural language interaction enables us to include a plethora of conversational structures that resemble well-known collaboration and persuasion strategies at the meta-level. As such, conversations are the central interaction concept in the system. They not only explain the assignments (what, how and why) and what can be expected (e.g., difficulties, results), but also function as an instrument for adaptation, shared commitment and explicit motivational support such as praise and encouragement.

To elucidate a conversational interaction, we briefly focus on one of the meta-level strategies used in the SleepCare-system: the establishment of a shared commitment by negotiation. An adapted version of a conversation about the sleep restriction exercise is shown in the dialogue fragment below (translated from Dutch; E: e-coach, C: coachee). In this fragment, the coachee options are given between brackets (selected options in bold); values of variables based on the e-coach's knowledge base are represented in italics. In this case, we have chosen a persuasive strategy of shared decision making, because sleep restriction is an intensive exercise and can even be dangerous in certain circumstances (e.g., [18]). The negotiation space depends on the user model, in particular total bedtime and sleep efficiency, and a number of rules, for instance, total bedtime should never be shorter than 5 h.

E   *Good morning John.* This week we will start the sleep restriction exercise. You have to keep regular bed times and should shorten the total time in bed. Because you have less time to sleep, you will be more tired and that helps for a better sleep. Would you like to know more before we start?
C   [**Let's start**] [What do I have to do?] [What can I expect?]
E   We will now determine your bedtimes. On the basis of your sleep diary I suggest that the total bedtime will be *5* h. Do you agree?
C   [Yes] [**I prefer longer**][I don't want to do bedtime restriction]
E   How long do you want to stay in bed?
C   [*5.30*][*6.00*][*6.30*]
E   You suggested *6.30* h. The exercise works better when you stay in bed as long as your mean sleeping time last week. I therefore suggest that the total time in bed will be *5.30*. Do you agree?
C   [Yes][**I prefer longer**]
E   ...

To cover the main interaction needs in CBT-I, 18 different conversational types were included (e.g., intro, planning and commitment, evaluation). These conversations can be considered as tree like structures where selections of the coachee or the value of particular sleep and behavior data causes a branch. Half of them are scheduled based, and the others are constraint-based conversations. Conversations are generated using XML-based predefined templates for describing the discourse moves of the e-coach [10]. All conversations (including the branches) were evaluated by an expert in Dutch communication and a sleep therapist.

6.5   Testing

The complex nature of the system and the application domain, the multimodal nature of the interaction, the large amounts of collected user knowledge and the many uncertainties in the use of mobile applications make the testing procedure a challenge. In particular, the variety in the circumstances of use is one of the main difficulties in the development of a smartphone application. Different versions of Android and smartphone manufacturers and changes thereof during use, network availability, unexpected user behavior and changes in the environment may cause a great deal of uncertainty in the outcome of the offered therapy. This not only requires that the system functions flawlessly, but also that the e-coach offers a therapy that is safe and in line with the advice of human therapists even under extreme circumstances.

For testing purposes, scenarios were written together with a sleep psychologist, making sure that the scenarios and user data covered the most common sleeping patterns and extremes on both ends as well. The scenarios were simulated and recorded in videos. A group of four sleep experts watched and commented on the behavior of the e-coach in the videos, providing us with information on the validity of the offered therapy. They focused in particular on the critical scenarios in which people sleep less than five hours per night.

Next, a pilot experiment was organized to test the SleepCare-system with intended users. 24 people asynchronously started using the app in their daily life and focused in particular on usability issues, the interaction with the e-coach and the circumstances of a possible system break down. Main success criteria for continuation were: a. no decrease in sleep efficiency and sleep quality, and b. no technical failure. The results gave us enough confidence in the system and the training program to execute a randomized controlled trial (RCT) as a next step in the research process.

7   Discussion

In this paper, strategies were discussed for enhancing adherence in behavior changing therapies delivered by digital systems. As a proof of concept, some of the strategies were implemented in an automated e-coaching system that supports insomnia therapy – the so-called SleepCare-system. An interface was realized that distinguishes between graphical tools and natural language conversations. Conversations enable us to include meta-level persuasive strategies based on social influence, such as commitment and shared decision making. We have stressed the importance of a design rationale and a careful analysis of the coaching process.

We briefly recapitulate the strategies discussed in this paper and their implementation in the SleepCare-system:

Tunneling: the e-coach should communicate the intended activities at the right moment in the right form. In SleepCare a sophisticated activity schedule, notifications and reminders were included.

Adaptation: exercises and interaction should be personalized and adapted to the circumstances. In SleepCare an explicit alignment phase and frequent feedback loops were included.

Reduction: therapy related activities that do not have to be experienced can be supported by tools or automated. In SleepCare tools were included for handling sleep data (e.g., registration, overviews), scheduling and relaxation.

Increasing motivation: therapy related activities that must be experienced can be supported by increasing the coachee's motivation. Examples in SleepCare are: showing (non-)adherence, performance and progress, shared decision making, explicit user commitment, explanation of therapy and exercise rationale, and expectation management.

Our first activity for the future is experimental verification of the SleepCare-system by means of the RCT. Next we will extend the adherence enhancing strategies to other domains and user groups, for example shift workers, and include automated sleep registration by non-obtrusive sensor information.

Finally, we may ask what we have learned since the appearance of Weizenbaum's digital therapist Eliza. We believe that in the future, consumers in e-health will not only be confronted with a variety of tools for monitoring health related characteristics and telecommunication with human caretakers, but also with automated e-coaches or e-doctors that direct a user's behavior. Computer systems aiming at behavior change will be equipped with adherence enhancing techniques to 'seduce' their users to do the therapy activities. This not only raises interesting philosophical questions, but also questions with respect to ethical design. Clearly, extensive testing is a mandatory element, but we also believe that explicit strategies should be included that protect the user's autonomy. We have the tools and the language, we now need the knowledge.

Acknowledgements. This research is supported by Philips and Technology Foundation STW, Nationaal Initiatief Hersenen en Cognitie NIHC under the Partnership programme Healthy Lifestyle Solutions.

References

1. Berg, I.K., Szabo, P.: Brief Coaching for Lasting Solutions. W.W. Norton, NY (2005)
2. Beun, R.J.: Persuasive strategies in mobile insomnia therapy: alignment, adaptation, and motivational support. Pers. Ubiquit. Comput. **17**(6), 1187–1195 (2013)
3. Beun, R.J., Griffioen-Both, F., Ahn, R., Fitrianie, S., Lancee, J.: Modeling interaction in automated e-coaching: a case from insomnia therapy. In: 6th International Conference on Advanced Cognitive Technologies and Applications (2014)
4. Bickmore, T.W., Schulman, D., Sidner, C.L.: A reusable framework for health counseling dialogue systems based on behavioral medicine ontology. J. Biomed. Inform. **44**, 183–197 (2011)
5. Blanson Henkemans, O.A., van der Boog, P.J.M., Lindenberg, J., van der Mast, C.A.P.G., Neerincx, M.A., Zwetsloot-Schonk, B.J.H.M.: An online lifestyle diary with a persuasive computer assistant providing feedback on self-management. Technol. Health Care **17**(3), 253–257 (2009)
6. Bluckert, P.: The similarities and differences between coaching and therapy. Ind. Commercial Training **37**(2), 91–96 (2005)
7. Both, F., Cuijpers, P., Hoogendoorn, M., Klein, M.: Towards fully automated psychotherapy for adults: BAS - behavioral activation scheduling via web and mobile phone. In: 3rd International Conference on Health Informatics 2010, pp. 375–380 (2010)
8. Cialdini, R.B.: Influence: Science and Practice. Pearson, New York (1993)
9. Espie, C.A., Kyle, S.D., Williams, C., Ong, J.J., Douglas, N.J., Hames, P., Brown, J.S.L.: A randomized, placebo-controlled trial of online cognitive behavioral therapy for chronic insomnia disorder delivered via an automated media-rich web application. Sleep **35**(6), 769–781 (2012)
10. Fitrianie, S., Griffioen-Both, F., Spruit, S., Lancee, J., Beun, R.J.: Automated dialogue generation for behavior intervention on mobile devices. Procedia Comput. Sci. **63**, 236–243 (2015)
11. Fogg, B.J.: Persuasive Technology: Using Computers to Change What We Think and Do. Morgan Kaufmann, San Francisco (2002)
12. Fogg, B.J.: The behavior grid: 35 ways behavior can change. In: Persuasive 2009. Claremont, California (2009a)

13. Fogg, B.J.: A behavioral model for persuasive design. In: Persuasive 2009. Claremont, California (2009b)
14. Greene, J., Grant, A.M.: Solution-Focused Coaching: Managing People in a Complex World. Momentum Press, London (2003)
15. Horsch, C.H.G., Lancee, J., Beun, R.J., Neerincx, M.A., Brinkman, W.P.: Adherence to technology-mediated insomnia treatment: a meta-analysis, interviews with users, and focus groups with users and experts. J. Med. Internet Res. **17**(9), e214 (2015)
16. Horsch, C.H.G., Brinkman, W.P., van Eijk, R.M., Neerincx, M.A.: Towards the usage of persuasive strategies in a virtual sleep coach. In: UKHCI 2012 Workshop on People, Computers and Psychotherapy (2012)
17. Hudson, F.M.: The Handbook of Coaching. Jossey-Bass, San Francisco (1999)
18. Kyle, S.D., Miller, C.B., Rogers, Z., Sirwardena, A.: Sleep restriction therapy for insomnia is associated with reduced objective total sleep time, increased daytime somnolence, and objectively-impaired vigilance: implications for the clinical management of insomnia disorder. Sleep **37**(2), 229–237 (2014)
19. Lancee, J., van den Bout, J., Sorbi, M.J., van Straten, A.: Motivational support provided via email improves the effectiveness of internet-delivered self-help treatment for insomnia: a randomized trial. Behav. Res. Ther. **51**, 797–805 (2013)
20. Michie, S., van Stralen, M.M., West, R.: The behavior change wheel: a new method for characterizing and designing behavior change interventions. Implementation Sci. 6(42) (2011)
21. Middelweerd, A., Mollee, J.S., van der Wal, N., Brug, J., te Velde, S.J.: Apps to promote physical activity among adults: a review and content analysis. Int. J. Behav. Nutr. Phys. Act. **11**(1), 97 (2014)
22. Morin, C.M., Bootzin, R.R., Buysse, D.J., Edinger, J.D., Espie, C.A., Lichstein, K.L.: Psychological and behavioral treatment of insomnia: update of the recent evidence (1998–2004). Sleep **29**, 1398–1414 (2006)
23. Morin, C.M., Espie, C.A.: Insomnia: A Clinical Guide to Assessment and Treatment. Springer, New York (2003)
24. Van Straten, A., Cuijpers, P., Smit, F., Spermon, M., Verbeek, I.: Self-help treatment for insomnia through television and book: a randomized trial. Patient Educ. Couns. **74**(1), 29–34 (2009)
25. Vermeire, E., Hearnshaw, H., Van Royen, P., Denekens, J.: Patient adherence to treatment: three decades of research a comprehensive review. J. Clin. Pharm. Ther. **26**, 331–342 (2001)
26. Weizenbaum, J.: ELIZA – a computer program for the study of natural language communication between man and machine. Commun. ACM **9**(1), 36–45 (1966)

Online Peer Groups as a Persuasive Tool to Combat Digital Addiction

Amen Alrobai[✉], John McAlaney, Keith Phalp, and Raian Ali

Faculty of Science and Technology, Bournemouth University, Bournemouth, UK
{aalrobai,jmcalaney,kphalp,rali}@bournemouth.ac.uk

Abstract. Digital Addiction (DA) denotes a problematic usage of digital devices characterised by properties such as being compulsive, impulsive, excessive and hasty. DA is associated with negative behaviours such as anxiety and depression. "Digital Detox" programs have started to appear and are mainly based on a relatively expensive and heavyweight in-patient care utilising traditional solutions such as motivational interviews and cognitive behavioural therapies. For moderate addiction, persuasive technology could have potential, as a brief intervention, to assist users to regulate their usage. This paper explores the design of online peer groups as a persuasive technique that puts together people who share a common interest in combating their DA or in helping others to do so. We conducted empirical research to explore design aspects of this mechanism. The results raise a range of questions and challenges to address when developing such a technique for the behaviour change needed against DA.

Keywords: Digital addiction · Digital health persuasion · Online peer groups

1 Introduction

Despite obvious benefits, the emergence of digital technologies and social networking services has also led to negative consequences on modern societies. A recent meta-analysis study covered 80 empirical reports from 1996 to 2012 and concluded that Internet Addiction, which is a form of digital addiction, affects 6 % of people worldwide [1]. In 2013, 3.2 % of British students were considered to be addicted [2]. In South Korea, over 140 Internet Addiction treatment recovery centres opened by 2011 [3]. According to the recent statistics from the China Youth Association for Network Development, the number of Chinese teenage addicts increased to 24 million (14.1 %) by 2009 [4]. This is over double the number in 2005, which was around 10 million (13.2 %). It is worth noting that these studies followed different criteria on assessing addictive usage.

These trends have led to growing interest in research to combat DA using self-regulation systems. These systems are seen as supportive means and emphasize that addicts have an active role in changing their own behaviour. These systems could include for example interactive warning labels containing persuasive techniques like timers and avatars to combat DA, as proposed in [5]. In another study [6], a new approach to ICT-facilitated self-regulation was proposed based on social cognitive theory to limit smartphone usage. The approach facilitates creating groups of users to share their usage

© Springer International Publishing Switzerland 2016
A. Meschtscherjakov et al. (Eds.): PERSUASIVE 2016, LNCS 9638, pp. 288–300, 2016.
DOI: 10.1007/978-3-319-31510-2_25

information. Generally, these systems are based on the assumption that people have the individual ability to adjust and optimise their own behaviour to maximise their gains according to their particular circumstances.

Despite such efforts, the introduction of these software systems to health-related behaviour, including addictive behaviours such as DA, has led to many controversial arguments. Most notable is the lack of strong scientific proof for their potential effectiveness. In a recent study [7], researchers found that many app-based psychological interventions including those hosted by governmental bodies, such as the National Health Service in the UK, fail to demonstrate clinical evidence of a long term change. A longitudinal research study found that delivering interventions within peer group settings could be harmful due to different factors relevant to group structure, which led to reinforcing the negative behaviour [8] such as loafing and compensation [9], and conformity effect [10]. Some negative attributes of persuasive technologies were also reported in [11], such as frustration, anxiety, peer pressure and feeling of guilt for the participants. This suggests a need for further research on the design of such software-based solutions in order to exploit their power whilst attempting to avoid or reduce negative side effects.

In this paper, we introduce online peer groups as a persuasive mechanism based on self-regulation systems, to support an effective and long-term behavioural change to combat DA. This paper conducts an exploratory research on the different aspects that need to be considered when designing online peer groups and reflects on the applicability and potential as well as risks of such a mechanism.

2   Background and Research Motivation

A motivational peer group is where people "voluntarily come together to help each other address common problems or shared concerns" [12]. Linking addicts to peer support groups prior to the professional treatment may reduce the duration needed in the initial episodes of treatment and increase recovery rates [13]. Also, extending the participation in peer support groups reduced the need for subsequent treatment episodes [13]. The peer groups approach can also be utilised in the post-treatment to reduce relapse rates [14]. The strength of this approach lies in its distinct persuasive and motivational mechanisms to sustain behavioural change; mainly commitment and consistency, reciprocity, and social proof [15] as well as surveillance which reinforce all these mechanisms. Peer groups technique could utilize the helper-therapy principle [16] which suggests that it can be personally beneficial for addicts to assist others deal with own addictions.

Behavioural change theories such as the theory of planned behaviour [17] and goal-setting theory [18] are used to bridge the gap between attitudes and behaviours. These theories aim at reducing discrepancies between these two conceptual constructs such as, for example, the gap between the intention to change a behaviour and the act of actually doing so [19]. This is achieved by encouraging individuals to create a plan to achieve the targeted behaviour. In self-regulation systems, monitoring is a fundamental design element. It provides a useful basis for effective intervention design by enabling users to track their performance and support them in achieving their goals, whilst also maintaining their regulated behaviours [20]. Self-monitoring is a "process of having individuals record data regarding their own behaviour for the purpose of changing its rate" [21]. When doing so, correctly in social settings, such as peer groups, it can further support the positive change.

Goal setting is a key element to guide monitoring processes and make it more meaningful. In DA, it is still a research question as to which type of goals, i.e. proximal and distal, would be more effective to develop self-efficacy and be easier for users to setup. Proximal goals are essential sub-goals to achieve the distal goals. For example, increasing offline social connection is a proximal goal to regulate digital usage and combat DA, the associated distal goal. In DA, we still have no models on the decision rights of goal settings for a particular group and whether it should be set up by the individuals or an authorized moderator or perhaps collectively. Likewise, the decision on setting up the goals is still a research issue, e.g., whether it should be self-set, provider-set, participatory-set, or set up by recommender systems [22].

Self-regulation systems can either monitor behaviour, e.g., the user shared 40 posts this week on their social network, or monitor change in the behaviour, e.g., the user shared fewer posts than last week [23]. It is fundamental to investigate which type of monitoring would motivate users. Some studies, such as [24], concluded that intervention systems for addictive behaviours may fail due to poor application of goal-setting theory, e.g., difficulty in setting standards as well as poor consideration of *conflicting goals*, such as regulating mobile usage and enjoying the moment, and also *distorted goals*, such as surfing the Internet to improve mood. These risks pose challenges for group's governance. While there are some successful intervention cases, they are often short term, as such interventions are expensive and hard to maintain [25]. This suggests the need for complementary strategies to support long-term interventions and to reduce relapse rate. This could be achieved through in-patient care, which is expensive and heavy weight for the early stages of DA.

Hence, we suggest investigating a persuasive technique that combines technology with human support to achieve sustainable behaviour change in a flexible and efficient style, hence the suggestion of online peer groups. Peer groups approach can be an appropriate program for users in the transition to addiction stage due to their need for less action-oriented strategies in which immediate change is not expected [26]. It can also benefit those who are also unaware of their level of addiction as it can make them more informed of the consequences occurred to their peers. This paper will explore the potential of online peer groups as a persuasive technique in that regard and focus on different design aspects.

3   Method and Research Settings

This paper reports upon work to explore users' perceptions of online peer groups, with respect to their possible use to help digital addicts. We adopted several qualitative methods in two studies to triangulate the findings and to generate more comprehensive understanding.

For the first study, we had a relatively broad remit, to investigate how users would perceive self-monitoring and peer monitoring to combat DA. We first conducted a diary study with 14 participants, 5 male and 9 female, aged between 18 and 50. A convenience-sampling technique was used. A pre-selection questionnaire test was used to ensure that participants had at least one aspect of problematic usage of their smart phones. The pre-selection test was an adapted version of the CAGE questionnaire customized to fit the properties and remit of DA [27].

The participants were asked to install one of three commercial digital diet smart-phones applications and use it for 14 days, and to record their observations and feelings about the application and their usage style. These diaries were used to guide the follow-up interviews with the same participants. To be selected, the application needed to have a rating of at least three stars out of five, a high number of downloads (no less then 500); at least 5 persuasive techniques, e.g. goal-settings, monitoring reminders, and rewarding, coercion and surveillance. This was to allow users to engage with a wide range of persuasive features in order to assess their influence and suitability for DA. After 14 days of usage and writing reflections and feedback, we conducted semi-structured inter-views with the same participants to elaborate on their diaries. One of the interviews questions was about the social features of the applications, which represent various aspects of online peer groups.

The second study focused on understanding different perspectives on online peer groups and their interactive design. We conducted a two sessions focus group study. The first one included 6 participants, 3 males and 3 females. The participants had pre-existing social relationships with each other so they aligned with the concept of a peer group, which requires some degree of shared interest and trust. Ages ranged between 20 and 26. The CAGE-like questionnaire was again used as a pre-selection test. Partic-ipants were given an engaging task in which they had to comment on and construct different online peer group designs and interaction styles including the use of persuasive techniques to regulate addiction.

We used all obtained data in the first session to come up with a new peer group design and made it the subject of discussion in the next session in which the same participants would engage as potential users of such online peer group aiming to regulate their addiction. However, one of the participants, who could not participate, was replaced with another one who met the selection criteria and had good experience in 3D anima-tion, which was advantageous to give some ideas on a creative design.

Finally, we performed a survey study to get further confirmation and insights through comments from a wider sample on our findings. A total of 73 completed responses were returned from the sample of 42 male and 31 female, aged between 18 and 65, recruited through an open call via several academic mailing lists.

In order to scope our analysis and as an initial template, we used the Cialdini's six principles of influence [15] to investigate the potential influential aspects in social settings from users' perspective as well as Fogg's behavioural model [28] to focus on the technology-facilitated features that can maximise the persuasion of online peer groups.

4   Results

Different aspects and areas of concerns about peer groups have been explored such as the study in [8]. This includes the personal characteristics that can heavily influence the effectiveness of ex-addicts and non-professional participation in counselling activities [29]. In online peer groups, such concerns need to be revisited by exploring what digital addicts prefer in terms designing online peer groups. Figure 1 presents the main aspects of online peer groups for DA. This conceptual map reflects the areas of concerns that are considered important from users' perspective. Governance, Structuring and Moderation will be discussed in separate subsections while Risks will be discussed as a cross-cutting aspect through all subsections.

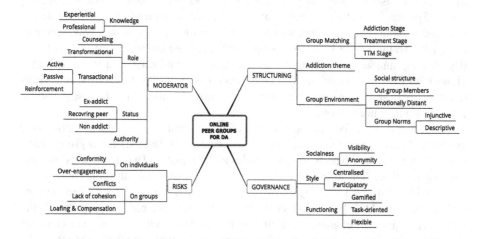

Fig. 1. Online peer groups for digital addiction

In the next subsections, we present general findings including the usefulness of peer groups to regulate DA, users' motivations to join them and how group structuring is seen and preferred by the users. We will also discuss various concerns and design issues related to the role of groups' moderators and the application of behaviour change theories and persuasive techniques within social settings including social norms.

4.1   Attitudes to the Overall Concept of on-Line Peer Groups

In our study, we assessed the perception of digital addicts of the usefulness of peer groups to regulate their usage. The overall impression was positive, and 71 % felt that a peer group would be useful (26 % certainly, 45 % somehow). Participants liked the idea of technology-limiting technology and found *"online system to cure online addiction is an interesting concept"*. However, it had not escaped the authors, nor had it escaped some of the participants, that there is a paradox in supporting online addiction by inviting people to partake of online support, as part of another community. Perhaps one of the comments that highlight this best was one person who likened the approach *"inviting alcoholics down the pub to chat about their alcoholism*". Of course, there are key differences here. Firstly, the medium, the online, is for many, something that they cannot choose to avoid. As such, being connected is a fundamental part of their life, or indeed, for many, their professional life. Secondly, digital addiction is a software-mediated behaviour. Hence, with the aid of software means, it is possible to actively monitor and intervene when necessary.

To identify the primary appealing characteristics of online peer groups, participants were asked about their motivation to join peer groups. Interestingly, most of the comments were clearly stating that providing moral support to others would be the main motivation. This motivation can be triggered by *reciprocity* norm [15] which suggests that the equality of power and exchanging help are the essential ingredients to build effective groups. This is well understood in the "helper therapy" principle [16]. That is, participants find it more motivating to be also useful for others, not only addicts who are seeking for help. This is perhaps the key element of peer groups.

Some other techniques used in persuasive systems seem not to be an important aspect for online peer groups used to assist the behavioural change for combating DA. For example, the Cialdini's Liking principle suggests that people are easily influenced by those who they admire, such as celebrities. That is to say popular persuasive techniques may not be seen efficient and even accepted when applied for behavioural change in addictive behaviours, such as DA, and they need to be revisited for that context of use.

4.2   The Moderation Role in Online Peer Groups

Participants highlighted the important role of having the human element such in software systems advocating techniques like peer groups to build a sense of trust and commitment to support long-term change. For example, one participant commented that in young age groups, having parental involvement would benefit more as they have a *sense of authority* to regulate the usage. For all of the individuals within the group, the role of the moderator was clearly understood as of paramount importance.

For example, there was a legitimate concern that there is a high risk factor of peers developing deviant behaviours due to normative influence [30]. This is one of the main reasons to introduce the *moderation* as an essential process in online peer groups. Moderator can also play other typical governance roles such as those related to member-ships and rewards allocation as well as addressing the influence of the non-matched members such as grouping members who belong to different levels of change.

Characteristics of Moderators. Participants were asked to consider a range of poten-tial characteristics for the crucial role of moderator. Of these, only one question gained greater than 50 % agreement, 58 % believing the moderator must be *"accredited/profes-sional/should be professional for [advanced digital] addiction"*. The comment above appears to endorse the need for a 'professional' moderator, though an exception was highlighted when groups or moderators have *"successful support history"* regardless of their *professional knowledge*. Thus, the *experiential knowledge* was perceived as an appealing attribute of the moderation role. In addition, two further clear themes are clear from the comments.

The first observation is that the participants made a distinction between 'light' and 'advanced stage' digital addiction. That is, they suggest that for early stage addiction, friends or less qualified people might be helpful in a peer group, and this further suggests that such a peer group approach as an early, low cost, intervention is something that they consider to be useful even among genuine peers. Two comments exemplify this commonly stated view: (1) *"for groups with advanced addiction, moderator should be a therapist or a digital addict or an ex digital addict but with therapist expertise so they know what to say and how to say it"*, and (2) *"For light addiction anyone really, does not matter, I would say the same for early addiction that means to prevent it first or to recover from it. I see difference"*.

The second observation is that the attitude or approach of the moderator is seen as paramount, friendliness and liberal styles being mentioned, one argued that *"friendliness in the group is a main requirement"*. However, again these comments being qualified by those cases where 'professional treatment', requires a therapist.

Finally, the question of whether moderators should themselves be ex-addicts drew far more mixed response. While some, 20 % of the survey, considered that ex-addicts would have more empathy, a greater number suggested that the moderator should not be an ex-addict, *"addicts might dictate their opinion and be biased to their own experience"*.

The Role of Moderators. Participants wanted to have collaborative moderators, who have the ability to guide the behavioural change by providing inspirational motivation. For example, a participant commented that a moderator should be *"someone who is respectable and can take charge; but also sympathises"*. The most positive responses for activities of the moderator, were: create and suggest rules (of engagement) 58 %, support motivation (55 %), provide advice to members (54 %), and create real life events (54 %) – but of course this final suggestion contrasts with anonymity, and reward members for complaint behaviour/usage (though note this is taken on trust) 50 %.

Hence, the moderator's role was seen, as in other forms of addiction, as primarily about setting out and controlling how people interacted, suggesting rules, motivating members, and giving advice. A perhaps surprising finding is that many wanted moderators to create real life events, contrasting with other questions for anonymity. Finally, while the moderator giving some kind of rewards was favoured by 50 % of the survey respondents, penalties was, a much lower score, with only 30 % believing that the moderator should give penalties. An interesting comment from the survey, which again tallied with our other studies was: *"No penalty but probably confrontation with their status"*, since one of the perceived benefits is concrete evidence and heightened awareness of actual usage. These characteristics of the role of moderation align well with the *transformational* leadership paradigm [31].

The use of "rational or economic means" to strengthen the probability of members' compliance with group's goals, suggests a moderation role that follows *transactional* leadership paradigm [31]. In this type of moderation, two approaches can be taken. The first is about active moderation and requires monitoring groups' interaction to ensure continued enhancement of the performance through applying corrective actions. Second is a passive moderation in which a moderator intervenes and applies operant conditioning when group's goals and standards are violated [31]. Other users preferred to have the moderator as a councillor, so members request their interventions when needed. As such, no monitoring and direct intervening are required.

Using persuasive techniques for behavioural change might lead some design issues related to the moderator role in peer groups. Participants argued that in some groups a moderator should be enabled to guide the change through positive reinforcements and light penalties as persuasive techniques. For example, one participant commented: "*people may leave a peer group if too much penalty is enforced*". Another one highlighted that if penalties must be implemented should take more influential approach such as "*confrontation members with their status*".

The careful implementation of persuasion techniques and moderation role will have profound a impact on groups' self-esteem. One of main components in Fogg's model for persuasive design [28] is the ability to perform the targeted behaviour or to reduce negative behaviour. When reducing the negative behaviour is very challenging goal such as in severe addiction, we would expect the design of online peer groups to increase the motivational influence and to apply the right triggers. This is to increase the probability of behavioural change to occur. For example, providing means to express the confidence in member's ability to change or applying the right social norm would increase the perceived self-efficiency which will act as a powerful motivational tool [32]. Peer group design should provide moderators with means to enact such policies and enable an effective persuasion to change behaviour.

4.3 Structuring of Online Peer Groups

Professional involvement in severe addiction cases suggests that the stage of addiction, i.e. early, intermediate and advanced, has an influence on how to customise online peer groups. Thus, we would expect the design on online peer groups to sense users' addiction status and adapt different facets of this mechanism accordingly to provide more persuasive effects.

Ultimately, each stage of addiction represents different level of self-control and distinct attitudes and behaviours. Regardless of the extent to which the object of addiction dominates decision-making processes, individuals with less severe addictive behaviour can be guided through the stage of change [26]. The stage of change, correspond to the stages of the Transtheoretical model (TTM) to behavioural change [26].

A critical assumption is that persuasive software-mediated interactions are more suitable for those who are open to the change, honest and do not have denial of reality. On the other hand, users who exhibit severe addiction symptoms require different course of action and more comprehensive treatment regardless of the stage of change they are at [26]. However, peer groups can still play a role in different phases of that comprehensive treatment, e.g. pre-treatment phase to support problem recognition "*non-addicts have no idea but they may give a perspective and may learn how it feels*" and post-treatment phase to support relapse avoidance as highlighted in [13]. Structuring peer groups should also consider the theme of addiction. For example addiction to online pornography would require certain degree of anonymity. This aspect will be discussed in the next section.

The social structure within online peer groups seems a very important aspect to be considered in the design. For example, a participant commented *"friends are not always the good thing here but unknown people with no direct contact or a friend of friend might be better and more relaxed"* and he continued, *"family members would be distracting in the group as I may need to behave differently"*. Only, 9 % of the responses were in favour of having family members. However, another one commented: *"family members are fine to have in the online peer groups but not as moderators"*. This suggests that the design needs to consider the impact of including family and friends versus unknown individuals in the group. This could be linked to the severity and domain of DA. Thus, the design of online peer groups must also consider the domain of addictions, such as gambling and pornography, which would require higher level of anonymity.

The social norms approach has become a major focus of research in recent years and is widely adopted in different developmental sectors such as educational settings in the United States [33]. The approach has been successfully used for behavioural change in the domain of addiction as well as a number of health and socially relevant behaviours [33].

As has been demonstrated extensively throughout social psychological research, individuals are strongly motivated to alter their own thoughts and behaviours to match the norms of the group [34]. This can include *descriptive norms*, which refers to how often or extensively we perceive our peers to engage in a behaviour or *injunctive norms*, which refers to the attitudes we believe our peers to hold. In a case of reciprocal causality individuals will also seek out social groups whose behaviours and attitudes they perceive to reflect their own [35]. Explicit attempts to manipulate groups, particularly by *out-group members*, can lead what known as a reactance response in which individuals engage even more strongly in the original behaviour [36]. However people also tend to underestimate how easily influenced they are by the groups they belong to [37]. As such by challenging the perceived norms within a group or encouraging the group to aspire towards a healthier norm behaviour change may be achieved.

Research into the use of peer networks to bring about behaviour change would suggest that they can indeed create new and more positive social norms [38]. There is overall though a lack of research on how social norms may operate within online peer groups.

The degree to which social norms may operate differently in online groups could be expected to reflect the complexity of the social relationships between the members of the peer groups. In the case of peer groups where members feel *emotionally distant* from one another they are less likely to conform to the norm [39]. However conformity to the social norm is more likely to occur in groups where there is a shared sense of a common goal and a belief that each member plays an important role in the achievement of this goal [10]. If peer groups are therefore to be used to address DA it is important that this is done in a way that engages the group, creates an agreed norm to aspire too and involve all the members of this group into the process. A participant commented, *"if a group of people I knew were all trying to cut down their phone usage then I think it would [motivate me to cut down my usage"*.

4.4   Governance and Social Aspects in Online Peer Groups

Enabling computer-mediated interactions among peers raises several social-related concerns. Participants highlighted the level of *anonymity as* key motivation to join peer groups. Several participants commented that such platforms should be a *"safe space"* in which users can maintain certain level of anonymity not necessarily complete, as self-disclosure is a key aspect in such social software platforms. For example, anonymity might need to be maintained at the level of members' interactions only, i.e. a member cannot be identified by other members but still identifiable by the system to monitor his progress over time. As such, online peer groups should accommodate various degrees of anonymity [40]. We expect the design of online peer groups to consider the *addiction theme as* an important aspect in deciding the suitable levels of privacy. More work is still needed to look into how addicts perceive anonymity and the influential privacy aspects that plays a role in persuading them to join and sustain their participation.

The *experiential knowledge* attribute mentioned in Sect. 4.2 suggests *visibility* concept in groups functioning as an important persuasive feature to enhance the intra-group's trust. Participants used the visibility term to denote the notion of having accessible service history and overall performance of groups and moderators. In this sense, anonymity and visibility are not conflicting requirements as the latter revolves around participation visibility rather than participant's visibility.

Other participants showed interest in sharing the role of moderator to maximise group's outcomes. The observation from the lack of having a particular trend in electing moderators is perhaps due to people in peer groups wanting a *participatory style* and to hear from peers rather than *authority* figures, such as parents, which take more *centralised style.*

As with the whole concept of using online to regulate DA drew some mixed views, and many noted the apparent paradox of having gamification and online approaches due to the risk from over-engagement. However, on the whole participants were positive about bringing some 'fun' to the peer group, and transfer of activities is often something useful within traditional addictions. On the whole, competition inside the group was seen as potentially problematic whereas they wanted to support rather than to compete other members. However, from all stages of the research there was a mention of the possibility of the group having an overall usage, from all members, and that they might wish to see this as a collective goal, or even compete with other groups. Clearly, this is an often used gamification tactic, call centre teams compete with each other, and often weight loss has been tackled with such an approach. Having the element of competition suggests that the group functioning can take *task-oriented approach* to either meet individuals' or collective goals. Other users wanted more flexible and supportive medium that is free from competition to *"support rather than beat each other".*

In terms of specific tactics, 53 % wanted points for compliance with 'healthy' activity, whereas only 40 % were happy with the idea of something like a leader board. Of course one person noted the monitoring issue, stating *"points are good but how will you monitor off-line behaviour?"*

Finally, and perhaps to be expected for peer support, the most desirable feature, (64 %), was online chat, further reinforcing the impact of people in support.

5   Conclusions and Future Work

In this paper we explored different aspects of online peer groups, as a motivational mechanism, from users perspectives. We demonstrated its prominent persuasive considerations. Although peer groups technique aims at supporting individuals in all addiction levels, we argue the need for careful re-evaluation of the online version of it from the perspectives of behavioural change theories. We also argue that tailoring such social software platform to support those with advanced stage addiction would be a very challenging task. Users who exhibit severe addiction are more vulnerable to relatively unconscious distorted, conflicting, changing requirements and could be accompanied with denial of reality. Our understanding of how social norms operate within peer groups is based primarily on offline interactions. Online environments may have unique characteristics that need to be better understood if change is to be achieved.

The current state of classical methods in software development, e.g. requirements engineering, is not efficient enough to deal with users in that stage. Thus, to design persuasive systems for DA, future studies are required to re-visit software engineering methods to customise existing elicitation models to the domain of behavioural addiction. Ultimately, adapting online peer groups to different users' needs and expectations should eventually produce more persuasive effects. Using simple metrics such as time and frequency to measure the level of addiction would perhaps provide misleading assertions. As such, we argue that measurement models should consider the psychological research on the addiction severity based on clinical criteria, such as salience, conflict and relapse [41]. Thus, users feedback should feed into future measurement models to provide meaningful and suitable configurations for online peer groups. The design of such user feedback acquisition and its peculiarities in this domain, e.g. to detect and react against denial of reality, is a challenge to address.

Acknowledgment.   The research was supported by Bournemouth University through the PGR Development fund. We would like also to thank Asad Khan and Yasmeen Abdalla for their valuable contributions in conducting the focus group and diary studies in the early stages of this research.

References

1. Cheng, C., Li, A.Y.-L.: Internet addiction prevalence and quality of (real) life: a meta-analysis of 31 nations across seven world regions. Cyberpsychology Behav. Soc. Netw. **17**, 755–760 (2014)
2. Kuss, D.J., Griffiths, M.D., Binder, J.F.: Internet addiction in students: prevalence and risk factors. Comput. Hum. Behav. **29**, 959–966 (2013)
3. Young, K.S., de Abreu, C.N. (eds.): Internet Addiction: a Handbook and Guide to Evaluation and Treatment. John Wiley & Sons (2010)
4. China Youth Association for Network Development. 2009 statistical Report on Internet? Addictions of Chinese Adolescents. Beijing (In press, 2010)

5. Ali, R., Jiang, N., Phalp, K., Muir, S., McAlaney, J.: The emerging requirement for digital addiction labels. In: Fricker, S.A., Schneider, K. (eds.) REFSQ 2015. LNCS, vol. 9013, pp. 198–213. Springer, Heidelberg (2015)

6. Ko, M., Yang, S., Lee, J., Heizmann, C., Jeong, J., Lee, U., Shin, D., Yatani, K., Song, J., Chung, K.-M.: NUGU: a group-based intervention app for improving self-regulation of limiting smartphone use. Presented at the February (2015)

7. Leigh, S., Flatt, S.: App-based psychological interventions: friend or foe? Evid. Based Mental Health 18, 97–99 (2015)

8. Dishion, T.J., McCord, J., Poulin, F.: When interventions harm: peer groups and problem behavior. Am. Psychol. 54, 755–764 (1999)

9. Karau, S.J., Williams, K.D.: Social loafing: a meta-analytic review and theoretical integration. J. Pers. Soc. Psychol. 65, 681–706 (1993)

10. Allen, V.: Situational factors in conformity. Adv. Exp. Soc. Psychol. 2, 133–170 (1965)

11. Hamari, J., Koivisto, J., Pakkanen, T.: Do persuasive technologies persuade? - a review of empirical studies. In: Spagnolli, A., Chittaro, L., Gamberini, L. (eds.) PERSUASIVE 2014. LNCS, vol. 8462, pp. 118–136. Springer, Heidelberg (2014)

12. Davidson, L., Chinman, M., Kloos, B., Weingarten, R., Stayner, D., Tebes, J.K.: Peer Support among individuals with severe mental illness: a review of the evidence. Clin. Psychol.: Sci. Pract. 6, 165–187 (2006)

13. Moos, R.H., Moos, B.S.: Help-seeking careers. J. Subst. Abuse Treat. 26, 167–173 (2004)

14. Moos, R.H., Moos, B.S.: Paths of entry into alcoholics anonymous: consequences for participation and remission. Alcohol. Clin. Exp. Res. 29, 1858–1868 (2005)

15. Cialdini, R.B.: Influence. HarperCollins, New York (2009)

16. Riessman, F.: The "helper" therapy principle. Soc. Work 10, 27–32 (1965)

17. Ajzen, I.: The theory of planned behavior. Organ. Behav. Hum. Decis. Process. 50, 179–211 (1991)

18. Locke, E.A., Latham, G.P.: A Theory of Goal Setting and Task Performance. Prentice-Hall, Englewood Cliffs (1990)

19. Webb, T.L., Sniehotta, F.F., Michie, S.: Using theories of behaviour change to inform interventions for addictive behaviours. Addiction 105, 1879–1892 (2010)

20. Torning, K., Oinas-Kukkonen, H.: Persuasive system design: state of the art and future directions. In: PERSUASIVE, p. 30 (2009)

21. Coleman, M.C., Webber, J.: Emotional and Behavioral Disorders: Theory and Practice. Allyn & Bacon, Boston (2002)

22. Strecher, V.J., Seijts, G.H., Kok, G.J., Latham, G.P., Glasgow, R., DeVellis, B., Meertens, R.M., Bulger, D.W.: Goal setting as a strategy for health behavior change. Health Educ. Behav. 22, 190–200 (1995)

23. Maitland, J., Chalmers, M.: Self-monitoring, self-awareness, and self-determination in cardiac rehabilitation. In: CHI, pp. 1213–1222 (2010)

24. Vohs, K.D., Baumeister, R.F.: Handbook of Self-Regulation, 2nd edn. Guilford Press, New York (2013)

25. Green-Demers, I., Pelletier, L.G., Ménard, S.: The impact of behavioural difficulty on the saliency of the association between self-determined motivation and environmental behaviours. Can. J. Behav. Sci./Revue Canadienne des sciences du comportement. 29, 157–166 (1997)

26. Prochaska, D.J.O.: Transtheoretical model of behavior change. In: Gellman, M.D., Turner, J.R. (eds.) Encyclopedia of Behavioral Medicine, pp. 1997–2000. Springer, New York (2013)

27. Ewing, J.A.: Detecting alcoholism: the CAGE questionnaire. JAMA 252, 1905–1907 (1984)

28. Fogg, B.J.: A behavior model for persuasive design. In: PERSUASIVE, p. 40 (2009)

29. Snowden, L., Cotler, S.: The effectiveness of paraprofessional ex-addict counselors in a methadone treatment program. Psychotherapy: Theor. Res. Pract. **11**, 331–338 (1974)
30. Allen, J.P., Chango, J., Szwedo, D., Schad, M., Marston, E.: Predictors of susceptibility to peer influence regarding substance use in adolescence. Child Dev. **83**, 337–350 (2011)
31. Bono, J.E., Judge, T.A.: Personality and transformational and transactional leadership: a meta-analysis. J. Appl. Psychol. **89**, 901–910 (2004)
32. Shamir, B., House, R.J., Arthur, M.B.: The motivational effects of charismatic leadership: a self-concept based theory. Organ. Sci. **4**, 577–594 (1993)
33. McAlaney, J., Bewick, B., Hughes, C.: The international development of the "social norms" approach to drug education and prevention. Drugs. Educ. **18**, 81–89 (2011)
34. Kelman, H.C.: Interests, relationships, identities: three central issues for individuals and groups in negotiating their social environment. Annu. Rev. Psychol. **57**, 1–26 (2006)
35. Ennett, S.T., Bauman, K.E.: The contribution of influence and selection to adolescent peer group homogeneity: the case of adolescent cigarette smoking. J. Pers. Soc. Psychol. **67**, 653–663 (1994)
36. Fuegen, K., Brehm, J.W.: The intensity of affect and resistance to social influence. In: Resistance and Persuasion, pp. 39–64 (2004)
37. Darley, J.M.: Social organization for the production of evil. Psychol. Inq. **3**, 199–218 (1992)
38. Wright, K.B., Bell, S.B., Wright, K.B., Bell, S.B.: Health-related support groups on the internet: linking empirical findings to social support and computer-mediated communication theory. J. Health Psychol. **8**, 39–54 (2003)
39. Greene, J.D., Sommerville, R.B., Nystrom, L.E., Darley, J.M.: An fMRI investigation of emotional engagement in moral judgment. Science **293**, 2105–2108 (2001)
40. Kobsa, A., Schreck, J.: Privacy through pseudonymity in user-adaptive systems. TOIT **3**, 149–183 (2003)
41. Griffiths, M.: A "components" model of addiction within a biopsychosocial framework. J. Subst. Use **10**, 191–197 (2005)

Design Strategies and Techniques

Red Radiators Versus Red Tulips: The Influence of Context on the Interpretation and Effectiveness of Color-Based Ambient Persuasive Technology

Shengnan Lu$^{(\boxtimes)}$, Jaap Ham, and Cees Midden

Human Technology Interaction, Eindhoven University of Technology,
P.O.Box 513, 5600 MB Eindhoven, The Netherlands
{s.lu,j.r.c.ham,c.j.h.midden}@tue.nl

Abstract. Colors are widely used as feedback in ambient persuasive technology. In current research, we argue that the information that color-based feedback carries is highly context dependent. Two studies investigated effects of context (in which color-based feedback was presented) on user's interpretation of feedback messages, and more importantly, on the effectiveness of this feedback (for influencing energy conservation behavior). Results of both studies showed that participants perceived the color red in an energy-related context to be warmer and as related to a higher energy consumption level than red in an energy-unrelated context. Also, participants receiving color-based feedback in an energy-related context consumed the lowest amount of energy. These findings extend our insight into the psychological mechanisms of ambient persuasive technology by making clear that ambient stimuli (e.g., color) are part of a broader context (e.g., projected on a radiator) that influences user's interpretation and the effectiveness of these stimuli.

Keywords: Ambient persuasive technology · Context · Color · Sustainability

1 Introduction

In day-to-day life, people constantly interact with and reflect on their surroundings [1]. Indeed, the physical environment has a strong influence on how people experience the world, and also on how people function in many ways [2]. In other words, people's subjective experiences are dependent on their bodily sensations and their perceptions of their physical environments [3].

The other way around, psychological factors including subjective experiences can also influence people's assessment of their physical environments [4,5]. For example, earlier research showed that social exclusion experiences can make people literally feel colder [6]. Likewise, other research showed that people's beliefs regarding the current temperature settings and their own abilities

© Springer International Publishing Switzerland 2016
A. Meschtscherjakov et al. (Eds.): PERSUASIVE 2016, LNCS 9638, pp. 303–314, 2016.
DOI: 10.1007/978-3-319-31510-2_26

to adjust to warm or cold conditions can influence their thermal experiences [7,8]. Also, research showed that a reported (relatively) high temperature can increase perceived comfort even when the actual room temperature remained the same [9]. Moreover, recent research showed that a sustainable mindset (e.g., people being aware of acting environmentally friendly) can induce people to perceive the room temperature to be physically higher [10].

In this interaction between physical and psychological factors, colors presented in the physical environment play an important role [11,12]. Various earlier theories and research studying the influence of color on people presented evidence for a link between colors and temperature-related experiences. For example, Bennett and Rey [13] argued that colors with 'cold' hues (e.g., blue, green and violet), lead to the perception of temperatures being lower, while colors with 'warm' hues (e.g., red, yellow and orange), lead to the perception of temperatures being higher (known as "Hue-Heat" hypothesis). Confirmed by Franger and colleagues [14], a red room led to the perception of higher temperature, whereas a blue room created the perception of a colder temperature (even though room temperature was objectively the same). Also, earlier research showed that yellow can induce a higher perceived room temperature than blue [15].

However, in some other studies that also used colors to test the "Hue-Heat" hypothesis, different results have been reported refuting or not confirming this hypothesis [16]. For instance, Ho and colleagues [17] found effects apparently in contrast with the red-hot/blue-cold association, which indicated that a blue object is more likely to be judged as warm than a red object of the same physical temperature. Also, several studies were unable to demonstrate that colors had any effect on the perception of temperature [16,18]. Separate from the "Hue-Heat" hypothesis literature, other research also showed results that conflict. That is, some studies presented evidence in line with this hypothesis by indicating that warm colors can evoke more arousal than cool colors [19]. Still other research presented evidence opposing this hypothesis, that is, brain research showed that blue light (in comparison to red light) leads to more arousal [20]. In addition, several researchers pointed out that red enhances cognitive performance [21,22] while, in contrast, others found that red reduces cognitive performance [21,23], or no relation between color and performances [12,24,25]. Finally, some earlier research showed that colors can influence human emotional state [26], while others studies did not find such evidence [27].

These conflicting results might be due to various causes. In the current research, we explore as a reason Elliot and Moller's Color-in-Context Theory [28]. This theory proposed that the effects of colors are highly context dependent. That is, it argues that color is an integrated part of the environment and cannot be separated from its form, texture and other surroundings. Therefore, influences of colors can only be observed in its context. For instance, the color red can carry a negative meaning (failure, danger, threat) for individuals in achievement contexts [28]. That is, research [21] showed that in a context in which people have to avoid making mistakes, priming them with the color red made participants more afraid to make mistakes. In other contexts, the color red can carry a positive meaning and have affiliation-related implications, for example in contexts involving heterosexual interaction [28].

2 Current Research

The current research was designed with the aim to investigate the influence of a color's context (i.e., the context in which colors were presented as energy feedback) on the interpretation of the information that color-based persuasive technology carries, and furthermore on the effectiveness of this color-based persuasive technology to influence users' energy consumption behavior.

In the research area of persuasive technology [29], colors have been widely used as media to support behavioral changes (e.g., [30,31]). Midden and colleagues [31] indicated that persuasive technologies, that utilize forms of sensory information like changing colors, can inform users at an intuitive level, demanding little cognitive effort. The colors, such as red and green, have been employed to present energy feedback to promote energy conservation behavior [32–34]. For example, earlier research provided individual comparison feedback by changing the shirt color of onscreen avatars that represented participants. The avatar with a red shirt represented the person who used the largest amount of energy, while the avatar with the green shirt represented the person who used the smallest amount of energy. Results suggested that using these colors as feedback in this context was very effective for motivating participants to save energy [35]. Likewise, Jentsch and colleagues [33] used colored ambient display to convey information about energy consumption in office environments. That is, green was used to convey that an office environment did not have energy-saving potential, and red meant that an office environment did have energy-saving potential. More recent research showed comparable results, now using colored lighting to provide feedback [36,37]. More specifically, Lu and colleagues [37] used red and green lighting to provide ambient lighting feedback about energy consumption. Their results indicated that colors that have pre-existing associations with energy consumption (e.g., red/green that is associated with high/low energy consumption) can enhance the persuasive power of ambient feedback.

Importantly, in the current research we argue that the meanings that colors carry may vary dependent on the context in which a color is perceived. So, although in certain context colors such as red are interpreted to indicate high energy consumption and thereby help users to understand the feedback messages, in different context the color red can be interpreted as indicating good and alive, as for example, in a nature context (e.g., when detecting ripe fruit) [28].

Based on a pretest, we specified two contexts: one is an energy-related context in which colors were projected on the form of a heating radiator, and the other is an energy-unrelated context in which colors were projected on the form of a tulip. We based these context choice on a pretest, in which participants had indicated that an heating radiator is an object is strongly associated with energy consumption, whereas a tulip is an object that is weakly associated with energy consumption.

Specifically, in the first study, we argue that presenting colors (e.g., red) in an energy-related context (e.g., projecting red on an object – the form of a radiator – to indicate high energy consumption) will make feedback messages (e.g., high energy consumption level) more clear and can enhance the correct interpretation of the color (e.g., warm), compared to presenting colors in an energy-unrelated context (e.g., projecting red on an object – the form of a tulip – to indicate high energy consumption). In the second study, we aim to replicate the effects of a color's context on the interpretation of the information that colors carries (as in the first study), and more importantly, we argue that presenting colors in energy-related contexts can increase the effectiveness of the color-based ambient persuasive technology, leading to stronger energy conservation behavioral changes

3   Study 1

In Study 1, we focused on the influence of context (in which colors were perceived) on the messages and users' interpretations of the color when using it as a feedback mechanism in colored-based ambient persuasive technology. Two specific colors (i.e., red and blue) were presented in either an energy-related context or an energy-unrelated context respectively. We expected (H1.1) that participants would interpret the color red in an energy-related context as indicating the highest energy consumption level, compared to the color red in an energy-unrelated context and the color blue in an energy-related or energy-unrelated context. Also, we expected (H1.2) that participants would perceive the color red in an energy-related context to be the warmest, compared to the participants in other conditions.

3.1   Method

Participants and Design. Fifty-one students (average age 21.6 years old, $SD = 2.15$) of Eindhoven University of Technology (23 male and 28 female) were recruited by using a local participant database. We invited only participants who were not color blind. All participants were native Dutch speaker and were randomly assigned to one of the four experimental conditions: 2 (context: energy-related vs. energy-unrelated)×2 (color: red vs. blue). The experiment lasted approximately 15 min, and participants received 3 euros for their participation.

Experimental Procedure. Before participants entering the lab, each participant was asked to read and sign an informed consent form stating the general purpose of the research and their willingness to participant in this research. Meanwhile, the room was changed to fit one of the four experimental conditions, that is, we changed only the picture presented on the TV screen present in the room to show the related lighting stimulus (i.e., a red radiator, a red tulip, a blue radiator or a blue tulip; see Fig. 1).

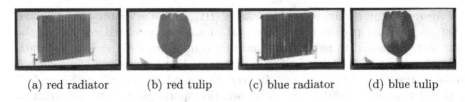

(a) red radiator   (b) red tulip   (c) blue radiator   (d) blue tulip

Fig. 1. Four experimental conditions: (a) the color red in an energy-related context, (b) the color red in an energy-unrelated context, (c) the color blue in an energy-related context and (d) the color blue in an energy-related context (Color figure online).

First of all, participants were asked to look around the room and then remember (for later recall) as many objects in this room as possible (with the purpose of making them spend attention to the ambient environment). Then, participants were asked to fill out a questionnaire. This questionnaire contained a variety of questions (in a random order) about the ambient environment and the object on the TV screen, amongst them the two questions of focus. That is, this questionnaire asked participants for their interpretations of the color (i.e., either red or blue) on either the radiator or tulip (using the question "How do you judge the meaning that this object conveys? I think this object means...", to which participants could answer by choosing an option on a 7-point bipolar scale ranging from 1 = very low energy consumption to 7 = very high energy consumption). Also, the questionnaire asked participants for the warmth perception of the color on either radiator or tulip (using the question "How warm do you feel the object projected on the screen is? I feel the object is something...", to which ranging from 1 = very cold to 7 = very warm). Finally participants were debriefed and thanked for their participation.

3.2 Results and Discussion

To analyze the effects of the context in which colors were presented on participant's interpretation of the color meaning and warmth of the object, we used an analysis of variance (ANOVA), in which 2 (context: energy-related vs. energy-unrelated)×2 (color: red vs. blue) experimental conditions were manipulated between participants.

Confirming our first hypothesis (H1.1), planned contrasts revealed that participants interpreted the color red in an energy-related context as indicating the highest energy consumption level, compared to participants in other conditions, $t(47) = 4.2, p < .001$. Furthermore, an additional analysis using a two-way ANOVA confirmed that participants reported the color red as related to a higher energy consumption level ($M = 4.98, SE = .30$) than the color blue ($M = 3.59, SE = .31$), $F = 10.5, p = .002, \eta^2 = .18$. Also, participants interpreted the color in an energy-related context (i.e., radiator) as indicating a higher energy consumption ($M = 4.78, SE = .29$) than in an energy-unrelated context (i.e., tulip) ($M = 3.79, SE = .31$), $F = 5.31, p = .026, \eta^2 = .10$.

Also, confirming our second hypothesis (H1.2), planned contrasts supported that participants perceived the color red in an energy-related context as the warmest, compared to participants in other conditions, $t(47) = 7.10, p < .001$. Likewise, two-way ANOVA confimed that participants perceived the color red to be warmer ($M = 5.64, SE = .24$) than the color blue ($M = 3.00, SE = .24$), $F(1, 47) = 59.5, p < .001, \eta^2 = .56$. In addition, participants rated the color in an energy-related context (i.e., radiator) as warmer ($M = 4.72, SE = .24$) than in an energy-unrelated context (i.e., tulip) ($M = 3.92, SE = .25$), $F(1, 47) = 5.46, p = .024, \eta^2 = .10$.

In sum, results of Study 1 showed that presenting colors (e.g., red) in an energy-related context indeed made the feedback message (e.g., high energy consumption) more clear, and moreover, enhanced the correct interpretation (e.g., warmer) represented by the color.

Still, although Study 1 showed that participants can easily understand the information that color-based persuasive technology conveys in a fitting context, the important question remains of whether this fitting context (in which the color-based persuasive technology was presented) can influence users' energy conservation behavior. Therefore, the second study was designed with the following two purposes: (1) to replicate the effect of context on users' interpretation of the feedback messages that color-based persuasive technology carries, and (2) to further investigate the influence of the context on the effectiveness of color-based ambient feedback for promoting users' energy conservation behavior.

4   Study 2

In the second study, first of all, to replicate effects of the context on users' interpretation of feedback messages found in Study 1, we argue that a fitting context would strengthen the associations of color with high energy consumption and the concept of warmth, which makes the feedback messages directly understandable. Therefore, we expected (H2.1) that participants would interpret the color red in an energy-related context to indicate a higher energy consumption level than the color red in an energy-unrelated context. Also, we expected (H2.2) that participants would perceive the color red in an energy-related context as being warmer than the color red in an energy-unrelated context.

Secondly, and more importantly, to investigate the context effect on behavioral change, we argued that a fitting context can increase the effectiveness of this color-based energy feedback to facilitate energy conservation behavior. Therefore, we developed an interactive energy feedback system, in which the object (i.e., either a radiator or tulip) could show colors varying from very weak red to very intense red depending on people's energy use. And we expected (H2.3) that participants would save the most energy when they receive the color-based ambient feedback in an energy-related context.

4.1   Method

Participant and Design. Fifty students (average age 23.1 years old, $SD =$ 3.14) of Eindhoven University of Technology (32 male and 18 female) were recruited by using a local participant database. We invited only participants who were not color blind. They participated in the current experiment in either an energy-related context (i.e., projecting red as energy feedback on the radiator) or an energy-unrelated related context (i.e., projecting red on the tulip). All participants were native Dutch speakers. The experiment lasted approximately 30 min, and participants received 5 euros for their participation.

Experimental Procedure. Participants were welcomed at the entrance of the lab. Each participant was asked to read and sign an informed consent form stating the general purpose of the research and their willingness to participate in this research.

After entering the lab, participant was seated in front of a laptop on a desk. All the instructions and tasks we used in this experiment were fully computerized and were all in Dutch. First of all, participants were asked to read a magazine for a period of five minutes, while either a red radiator (in the energy-related context condition) or a red tulip (in the energy-unrelated context condition) was presented on the TV (see Fig. 2). After five minutes, the computer indicated that the reading period was over and participants were asked to fill out a questionnaire (similar one as used in Study 1) about the object on the TV screen and the ambient environment.

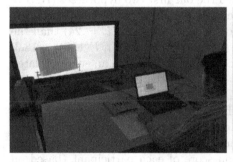
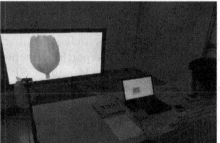
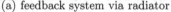

(a) feedback system via radiator   (b) feedback system via tulip

Fig. 2. The interactive ambient energy feedback system by presenting colors in (a) an energy-related context and in (b) an energy-unrelated context.

After answering these questions, we assessed energy consumption behavior by asking participants to perform a virtual thermostat task on the laptop while immediately receiving the interactive color-based energy feedback (see Fig. 3). That is, participants received instructions on how to program a virtual room thermostat interface, and were asked to program this thermostat for two practice scenarios. After two practice scenarios, participants completed programming tasks on the thermostat for ten experimental scenarios. For each scenario, the scenario itself was first described to the participants (e.g., It is night and you are going to bed. It is −10°C outside), and then participants were asked to program the thermostat by setting the temperature for the each room, while receiving feedback (see Fig. 3) after each change of the temperature settings, until they pressed the 'Ready' button. Finally, participants were asked to answer several demographic questions, thanked for participation, and debriefed.

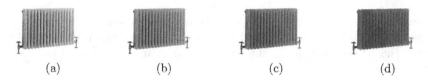

(a)   (b)   (c)   (d)

Fig. 3. The interactive color-based energy feedback system showed colors varying between very weak and intense red depending on people's energy use from (a) indicating very low energy consumption to (d) very high energy consumption (Color figure online).

4.2   Result and Discussion

Replicating the effects of context on user's interpretation of the feedback messages (found in Study 1), results confirmed the our first two hypotheses (H2.1 & H2.2). That is, participants interpret the color red in an energy-related context as indicating a higher energy consumption level ($M = 6.12, SE = .24$) than the color red in an energy-unrelated context ($M = 4.68, SE = .24$), $F(1, 48) = 18.3$, $p < .001, \eta^2 = .28$. Also participants perceived the color red in an energy-related context to be warmer ($M = 6.44, SE = .17$) than the color red in an energy-unrelated context ($M = 5.64, SE = .17$), $F(1, 48) = 10.7, p = .002, \eta^2 = .18$.

Most importantly, to analyze the influence of the context (in which color-based ambient feedback was presented) on the effectiveness of this color-based ambient persuasive technology (for influencing user's energy conservation behavior), we collected the energy consumption score of each participant (based on his or her performance during the thermostat task) as dependent variable. These dynamic energy consumption scores were based on their actions during the thermostat task and were submitted to a linear mixed effects analysis to assess the relationship between the manipulation factor *context* (radiator vs. tulip) and a participant's scores of energy consumption. So, as fixed effects, we entered *context* into the model. As random effects, we entered scenario items. Confirming our third hypothesis (H2.3), results showed that participants who received color-based energy feedback in an energy-related context (i.e., radiator) decreased their energy consumption more ($M = −13.6, SE = 2.25$) than participants who received color-based energy feedback in an energy-unrelated context (i.e., tulip) ($M = −10.1, SE = 2.3$), $F(1, 1715.9) = 4.84, p = .028$.

So, results of Study 2 showed that participants could clearly interpret the information of color-based energy feedback carries (e.g., red indicated high energy consumption and was more associated with warm) in an energy-related context. Furthermore, color-based energy feedback in an energy-related context led to the most energy conservation behavior. Thereby, these findings revealed that color context can help users to correctly interpret the information that color-based feedback carries, and moreover, can increase the effectiveness of this ambient persuasive technology to facilitate energy consumption behavior.

5   General Discussion

Colors have been widely used as media to promote behavioral changes. In the current research, we argue that the information that color-based ambient persuasive technology carries is highly context dependent. Two studies were designed to investigate the effects of a color's context (i.e., the context in which colors were presented as energy feedback) on users' interpretation of the information that colors carried. Also, we investigated the effect of color context on the effectiveness of this color-based ambient persuasive technology to influence users' energy consumption behavior. Results of both studies showed that participants to whom we presented colors in an energy-related context (e.g., projecting red on an object in the form of a radiator in indicate high energy consumption) could most optimally interpret the information of a color carried (e.g., red indicated high energy consumption and was more associated with warm). More importantly, results showed that participants to whom we presented colors in an energy-related context saved the most energy when they were receiving color-based energy feedback as compared to participants in an energy-unrelated context.

In line with earlier research and the Color-In-Context theory [28,38], our findings confirmed that the context can shape the associations of color. In addition, using colors as ambient feedback to promote energy conservation behavior, we found that a fitting context (in which this color-based ambient persuasive technology is presented) can strengthen the associations of the color red with high energy consumption (or concept of warm), and subsequently can enhance the energy-saving performance. Importantly, the current research implies that by taking into consideration the context of ambient persuasive technology, the effectiveness of ambient persuasive technology (e.g., colored lighting ambient feedback used in [37]) could be increased.

The current research opens up a new field of research. That is, based on the first findings of the current studies, future research might investigate the influence colors, in context, on user comfort perceptions and thereby on user's (energy consumption) behavior. Indeed, comfort experience was stated as one of the dominant influences on people's (energy conservation) behavior [39,40]. Besides using colors (in different context) as feedback to indicate energy information, future research can also investigate whether user's comfort experiences will be influenced by using color-based persuasive technology, via a comfort-experience-based persuasive strategy [41].

Another important consideration related to studying conform experience is that in our second study, participants performed the temperature-setting task on a simulated thermostat without the physical room temperature being adapted. However, in a day-to-day environment, changes on the settings of a heating thermostat directly lead to changes in room temperature. Future research could investigate the relationship between ambient persuasive technology, comfort experiences and energy consumption behavior, in an environment in which these variables are connected to one another. For example, room temperature changes after people change settings of a thermostat. In such research, a simulated thermostat could be connected to the heating system in the lab. In addition, by applying this thermostat system and color-based energy feedback in real setting, future research can also compare the effect size between lab studies and field studies.

Additionally, future research may extend the current findings by not only presenting color-based ambient energy feedback on a TV screen. That is, future research might replicate and also extend these findings by investigating the influencing of colors and the role of their context when colors are presented in a more ecological context, for example when presenting an actual red glow on an actual physical radiator.

In sum, our studies showed that a fitting context in which ambient persuasive technology is presented can shape the associations of color with high energy consumption and the concept of warm, which makes the feedback messages directly understandable. And more importantly, this fitting context can increase the persuasive power of ambient persuasive technology to promote energy conservation behavior. These findings extend our insight into the psychological mechanisms of ambient persuasive technology by making clear that contextual stimuli (e.g., colored lighting used as ambient feedback) are part of a broader context (e.g., projected on a radiator vs. a tulip) that influences user's interpretation and the effectiveness of these stimuli. This could also have implications for the design of future ambient persuasive technology as the current findings show that such design should take into consideration the context in which ambient persuasive technology is used.

References

1. Ford, F.L.: Political Murder: From Tyrannicide to Terrorism. Harvard University Press, Cambridge (1987)
2. Schneider, W.: Sinn und Un-Sinn: Umwelt Sinnlich Erlebbar Gestalten in Architektur und Design. Bau-Verlag, Berlin (1957)
3. Barsalou, L.W.: Perceptual symbol systems. Behav. Brain Sci. **22**(04), 577–660 (1999)
4. Helson, H., Blake, R.R., Mouton, J.S., Olmstead, J.A.: Attitudes as adjustments to stimulus, background, and residual factors. J. Abnorm. Soc. Psychol. **52**(3), 314 (1956)
5. Sherif, M.: An Outline of Psychology. Sage Publications, New York (1948)
6. Zhong, C.B., Leonardelli, G.J.: Cold and lonely does social exclusion literally feel cold? Psychol. Sci. **19**(9), 838–842 (2008)

7. Howell, W.C., Kennedy, P.A.: Field validation of the fanger thermal comfort model. Hum. Factors: J. Hum. Factors Ergon. Soc. **21**(2), 229–239 (1979)

8. Howell, W.C., Stramler, C.S.: Contribution of psychological variables to the prediction of thermal comfort judgments in real world settings. ASHRAE Trans. **87**(5), 609–619 (1981). (United States)

9. Stramler, C.S., Kleiss, J.A., Howell, W.C.: Thermal sensation shifts induced by physical and psychological means. J. Appl. Psychol. **68**(1), 187 (1983)

10. Strack, F., Deutsch, R.: Acting green elicits a literal warm glow. Nat. Clim. Change **5**, 37–40 (2014)

11. Tofle, R.B., Schwarz, B., Yoon, S.Y., Max-Royale, A., Des, M., Thanks, S.: Color in healthcare environments-a research report (2004)

12. Elliot, A.J., Maier, M.A., Moller, A.C., Friedman, R., Meinhardt, J.: Color and psychological functioning: The effect of red on performance attainment. J. Exp. Psychol.: Gen. **136**(1), 154–168 (2007)

13. Bennett, C.A., Rey, P.: What's so hot about red? Hum. Factors: J. Hum. Factors Ergon. Soc. **14**(2), 149–154 (1972)

14. Fanger, P., Breum, N., Jerking, E.: Can colour and noise influence man's thermal comfort? Ergon. **20**(1), 11–18 (1977)

15. Winzen, J., Albers, F., Marggraf-Micheel, C.: The influence of coloured light in the aircraft cabin on passenger thermal comfort. Lighting Research and Technology 1477153513484028 (2013)

16. Candas, V., Dufour, A.: Thermal comfort: multisensory interactions? J. Physiol. Anthropol. Appl. Hum. Sci. **24**(1), 33–36 (2005)

17. Ho, H.N., Iwai, D., Yoshikawa, Y., Watanabe, J., Nishida, S.: Combining colour and temperature: A blue object is more likely to be judged as warm than a red object. Sci. Rep., vol. 4 (2014)

18. Berry, P.C.: Effect of colored illumination upon perceived temperature. J. Appl. Psychol. **45**(4), 248 (1961)

19. Jacobs, K.W., Suess, J.F.: Effects of four psychological primary colors on anxiety state. Percept. Motor Skills **41**(1), 207–210 (1975)

20. Yoto, A., Katsuura, T., Iwanaga, K., Shimomura, Y.: Effects of object color stimuli on human brain activities in perception and attention referred to eeg alpha band response. J. Physiol. Anthropol. **26**(3), 373–379 (2007)

21. Mehta, R., Zhu, R.: Blue or Red? Exploring the effect of color on cognitive task performances. Sci. **323**, 1226–1229 (2008)

22. Kwallek, N., Lewis, C.M., Robbins, A.S.: Effects of office interior color on workers' mood and productivity. Percept. Motor Skills **66**(1), 123–128 (1988)

23. Soldat, A.S., Sinclair, R.C., Mark, M.M.: Color as an environmental processing cue: External affective cues can directly affect processing strategy without affecting mood. Soc. Cogn. **15**(1), 55–71 (1997)

24. Etnier, J.L., Hardy, C.J.: The effects of environmental color. J. Sport Behav. **20**(3), 299 (1997)

25. Ainsworth, R.A., Simpson, L., Cassell, D.: Effects of three colors in an office interior on mood and performance. Percept. Motor Skills **76**(1), 235–241 (1993)

26. Kaya, N., Epps, H.: Relationship between color and emotion: A study of college students. Coll. Student J. **38**(3), 396 (2004)

27. O'Connor, Z.: Colour psychology and colour therapy: caveat emptor. Color Res. Appl. **36**(3), 229–234 (2011)

28. Elliot, A.J., Maier, M.A.: Color-in-context theory. Adv. Exp. Soc. Psychol. **45**, 61–125 (2012)

29. Fogg, B.: Persuasive Technology: Using Computers to Change What We Think and Do. Morgan Kaufmann, San Francisco (2003)

30. Arroyo, E., Bonanni, L., Selker, T.: Waterbot : Exploring Feedback and Persuasive Techniques at the Sink. In: Proceedings of the SIGCHI Conference on Human Factors in Computing Systems, pp. 631–639 (2005)

31. Midden, C., Kaiser, F.G., Mccalley, L.T.: Technology's four roles in understanding individuals' conservation of natural resources. J. Soc. Issues **63**(1), 155–174 (2007)

32. Maan, S., Merkus, B., Ham, J., Midden, C.: Making it not too obvious: The effect of ambient light feedback on space heating energy consumption. Energy Effi. **4**(2), 175–183 (2011)

33. Jentsch, M., Jahn, M., Pramudianto, F., Simon, J., Al-Akkad, A.: An energy-saving support system for office environments. In: Salah, A.A., Lepri, B. (eds.) HBU 2011. LNCS, vol. 7065, pp. 83–92. Springer, Heidelberg (2011)

34. Merkus, B., Ham, J., Midden, C.: A Shower Meter to Save Water and Energy : the Influence of Two Feedback Sources, Goals, and the Role of Comfort on Conservation Behavior in a Lab and Field Experiment in partial fulfilment of the requirements for the degree of Master of Science in Human. Ph.D. thesis (2012)

35. Midden, C., Kimura, H., Ham, J., Nakajima, T., Kleppe, M.: Persuasive power in groups: the influence of group feedback and individual comparison feedback on energy consumption behavior. In: Proceedings of the 6th International Conference on Persuasive Technology: Persuasive Technology and Design: Enhancing Sustainability and Health, p. 1. ACM (2011)

36. Ham, J., Midden, C.: A persuasive robotic agent to save energy: the influence of social feedback, feedback valence and task similarity on energy conservation behavior. In: Ge, S.S., Li, H., Cabibihan, J.-J., Tan, Y.K. (eds.) ICSR 2010. LNCS, vol. 6414, pp. 335–344. Springer, Heidelberg (2010)

37. Lu, S., Ham, J., Midden, C.J.H.: Using ambient lighting in persuasive communication: the role of pre-existing color associations. In: Spagnolli, A., Chittaro, L., Gamberini, L. (eds.) PERSUASIVE 2014. LNCS, vol. 8462, pp. 167–178. Springer, Heidelberg (2014)

38. Busch, M., Schrammel, J., Flu, M.A., Kruijff, E., Tscheligi, M.: Persuasive strategies report. CURE-Center for Usability Research & Engineering (2012)

39. Becker, L.J., Seligman, C., Fazio, R.H., Darley, J.M.: Relating attitudes to residential energy use. Environ. Behav. **13**(5), 590–609 (1981)

40. Heijs, W., Stringer, P.: Research on residential thermal comfort: Some contributions from environmental psychology. J. Environ. Psychol. **8**, 235–247 (1988)

41. Lu, S., Ham, J., Midden, C.: Persuasive technology based on bodily comfort experiences: the effect of color temperature of room lighting on user motivation to change room temperature. In: MacTavish, T., Basapur, S. (eds.) PERSUASIVE 2015. LNCS, vol. 9072, pp. 83–94. Springer, Heidelberg (2015)

Investigating Politeness Strategies and Their Persuasiveness for a Robotic Elderly Assistant

Stephan Hammer[1]([✉]), Birgit Lugrin[2], Sergey Bogomolov[1], Kathrin Janowski[1], and Elisabeth André[1]

[1] Human Centered Multimedia, Augsburg University, Augsburg, Germany
{hammer,janowski,andre}@hcm-lab.de
[2] Human Computer Interaction, University of Wuerzburg, Wuerzburg, Germany
birgit.lugrin@uni-wuerzburg.de

Abstract. This work is targeted towards the development of a Robotic Elderly Assistant (REA) system that provides assistance in the form of recommendations to support single-living elderly people in their domestic environment. To avoid potential face threats the REA should be as polite as possible whilst keeping a certain persuasiveness to promote its recommendations. This paper investigates different verbalizations of the REA's recommendations regarding their perceived politeness as well as their persuasiveness. We present the results of a laboratory study with younger adults and a user study with the inhabitants of a retirement home. Results suggest that the different politeness strategies reflected different levels of politeness in both studies, while their perceived persuasiveness needs further investigation in the domain of elderly care.

Keywords: Elderly people · Social robots · Recommendations · Politeness strategies · Persuasiveness

1 Motivation

The demographic change, especially in industrialized countries, results in important societal challenges to be dealt with. Since elderly people often suffer from physical and mental restrictions, they lose living independence. Especially single-living elderly often lack societal interactions and thus get isolated. Both problems get amplified if the elderly are inactive and lack self-initiative.

Studies have shown that regular physical and cognitive activities can help mitigate many age-related diseases [1,2]. For example, pain due to arthrosis could be alleviated by moving the affected joints on a regular basis, and activities, such as gardening or painting, can positively influence elderly people's well-being [3]. However, some seniors tend to not engage in these activities. Therefore, Seiderer et al. [4], for example, tried to promote a healthier lifestyle and to increase seniors' overall well-being by providing concrete recommendations. However, developing such systems for seniors should be done with care, as people of their generation may be less familiar with newer electronic devices and thus have a rather high barrier of use or, even worse, are afraid of using them [5,6].

© Springer International Publishing Switzerland 2016
A. Meschtscherjakov et al. (Eds.): PERSUASIVE 2016, LNCS 9638, pp. 315–326, 2016.
DOI: 10.1007/978-3-319-31510-2_27

Through their embodiment, among other features, social robots are very well suited to support socio-emotional factors. There is evidence that humans perceive them as social actors and are likely to respond to them in a similar way that people respond to each other [7]. Furthermore, through their ability to adapt to a large variety of users and remain attractive to users on a long-term basis, social agents are typically useful for intuitive and persuasive interaction [8]. Therefore, it seems to be promising to develop a Robotic Elderly Assistant (REA) that could contribute to the establishment of a positive emotional and social relationship between user and system.

A number of studies have been conducted that explore social robots, such as the iCat or Nao, in terms of their acceptance by older adults, e.g. [9,10]. In general, seniors seem to evaluate social robots mainly in terms of appearance, intellectuality, and friendliness [11]. Robots should appear less threatening, but kind-hearted [12,13] and more realistic faces are perceived as more trustworthy and sociable [11]. Elderly people prefer discrete and small robots with human or pet-like traits over large humanoid robots [12,14]. Furthermore, robots are more likely to be accepted if they move slowly, act less autonomously, have a female voice and a monochrome and serious appearance [12]. There is also evidence that elderly people respond positively to robotic companions if they emulate social behavior that matches the seriousness of a current task or situation [15]. However, if robots look too human-like, but do not match the high expectations in terms of behavior, people tend to get disappointed and distrustful of them [16].

Special attention should be paid to the fact that many elderly find themselves in a situation where they can no longer take full care of themselves and need the help of others to accomplish daily tasks. Consequently, the feeling of embarrassment or loss of control over their lives become important issues. Therefore, providing recommendations often comes along with a certain threat of the users' face. For example, the statement "Drink some water." could invoke the feeling of being patronized. In contrast, the question "How about drinking some water?" would keep the users in control whilst reminding them to drink enough water. Therefore, we think that verbal politeness strategies, as an aspect of social and respectful behavior, can further enhance the acceptance of a REA and can foster a good working relationship between the elderly user and the REA.

In the following we will introduce related work that investigated the role of politeness in verbal social interactions. Afterwards, our approach to a REA will be presented. The main part of the paper will explain details on two studies that were performed to investigate the perception of different politeness strategies and their persuasiveness. The second study was conducted in a local retirement home with our REA system and also investigated the elderly participants' reaction to the robot. The paper concludes with a discussion and some lessons learned from the observations made during our studies.

2   Politeness as a Social Factor

Sidner and Lee [17] designated politeness as an important factor when robots initiate engagement with people, and Nomura et al. [18] showed that even small differences in a robot's non-verbal behavior, such as motions, could influence people's perception of it as well as their behavior towards it. In the domain of elderly care, politeness seems to be of special importance, as the perceived politeness of a system varies with the user's experience with technical systems [19].

We think that the way recommendations are verbalized by the robotic companion can help mitigating facial threats, e.g. by using suggestions, hints or proposals instead of commands. Brown and Levinson [20] describe politeness as a means to preserve the reputation of conversation partners even in critical situations. Their politeness theory builds on the fact that every interlocutor has two basic wants concerning their face or public self-image: (1) to be approved of by the conversation partner (positive face) and (2) to be unrestricted by the conversation partner (negative face). In order to avoid threads to their (positive or negative) face during a conversation, interlocutors tend to apply different types of politeness strategies: (1) to emphasize approval (positive politeness), (2) to emphasize the interlocutor's freedom of choice (negative politeness) and (3) indirect statements in case an action is necessary (off-record statements).

Johnson et al. [21] incorporated these politeness strategies in different verbalizations of an artificial tutor that used politeness for motivating a learner to accomplish different tasks. Eight categories of verbalizations were presented that relate to Brown and Levinson's notation of positive and negative face. These categories are: (A) direct commands, (B) indirect suggestions, (C) requests, (D) actions expressed as the tutor's goals, (E) actions as shared goals, (F) questions, (G) suggestions of student goals, and (H) Socratic hints.

Results of Johnson's experiment showed that participants rated positive and negative politeness with a high degree of consistency and that their ratings were consistent with Brown and Levinson's assessment of the strategies' politeness.

In the context of an elderly care assistant, it should be noted that depending on the importance of the given advice, more or less polite wordings might be required. Thus, the present contribution investigates all eight categories and rates them with regard to their perceived politeness as well as their perceived persuasiveness.

3   The REA System

Our overall goal is to develop a sensitive and personalized system to support elderly people who would generally be able to live independently, but lack a certain autonomy due to forgetting appointments, daily tasks or not showing the initiative for activities. Assistance is given in the form of situationally appropriate recommendations to encourage physical, mental, and social activities, all aimed at increasing the users' well-being. To ensure an interaction that is as natural and intuitive as possible, and to reduce barriers to entry, the system is impersonated by an expressive robot that acts like a social companion. The robot chosen for the REA system was a *Robopec Reeti*[1], see Fig. 1. It meets the

---

[1] http://www.reeti.fr.

most important criteria that were mentioned in Sect. 1. It is comparatively small (44 cm), plain white and, apart from the head, it does not have any movement capabilities that could be perceived as threatening. Its basic appearance is that of a cartoon-like extraterrestrial or fantasy creature. The facial expressions are human-like, which allows the user to relate to the robot more easily, yet stylized enough to reduce expectations about realistic behavior. For German speech synthesis, Reeti uses the Loquendo text-to-speech software by Nuance[2].

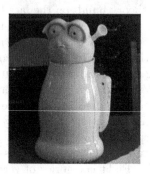

Fig. 1. Reeti, a social robot with an expressive head created by Robopec. It supports gaze behavior with three movement axes in the neck and two in each eye, as well as eight degrees of freedom for animating the mouth, eyelids and ears.

Based on Brown and Levinson's politeness strategies and Johnson et al.'s taxonomy of verbalizations (see Sect. 2), we prepared three recommendations

Table 1. Different wordings of the recommendation 'Drink some water'

Politeness strategy	Verbalization	Translation
Direct command	Trinken Sie etwas Wasser	Drink some water
Indirect suggestion	Ihr Ernährungsplan sieht vor, dass Sie etwas Wasser trinken	Your dietary plan suggests that you drink some water
Request	Ich hätte gern, dass Sie etwas Wasser trinken	I would like you to drink some water
Actions expressed as the system's goals	Ich würde etwas Wasser trinken	I would drink some water
Actions expressed as shared goals	Wir sollten etwas Wasser trinken	We should drink some water
Questions	Wie wäre es, wenn Sie etwas Wasser trinken würden?	How about drinking some water?
Suggestions of user goals	Sie möchten bestimmt etwas Wasser trinken	You would probably like to drink some water
Socratic hints	Haben Sie daran gedacht etwas Wasser zu trinken?	Did you think about drinking some water?

---

[2] http://www.nuance.com.

that would naturally fit in a scenario of a REA: 1) drink some water, 2) open the window, and 3) go for a walk. Examples of the different wordings can be seen in Table 1. The German version as used in our system is included, since an equally perceived degree of politeness of the translations cannot be guaranteed.

For presenting the recommendations, the *VisualSceneMaker* tool [22,23] was used to implement a semi-automatic dialog application. Via keyboard inputs the experimenter was able to move to the next phrase, to repeat the current phrase, or to stop the whole process.

4 Laboratory Study

To ensure that our experiment is not too subtle or too abstract to grasp for the inhabitants of an elderly home, we conducted a text-based study at our lab first to verify that the different verbalizations are perceived as expressing different levels of politeness and persuasiveness.

4.1 Participants and Procedure

The study was conducted with 5 female and 15 male native German speakers aged from 25 to 45, in a lab environment. After a short introduction, participants answered a few demographic questions. Then they were shown eight textual verbalizations for each of the implemented recommendations (1: drink some water, 2: open the window, and 3: go for a walk) in an incomplete counterbalanced order. For each verbalization, participants had to rate their perceived politeness as well as persuasiveness on a 7-point Likert-scale from 1 = "not polite/persuasive at all" to 7 = "very polite/persuasive".

4.2 Results

An analysis of the mean ratings, see Fig. 2, showed that *questions* were rated as most polite. Actions that were expressed as *shared goals* or *the system's goals*, and *requests* were perceived as polite, too. In contrast, *direct commands* were assessed as impolite. Interestingly, *direct commands* were perceived to have a similar degree of persuasion as *questions*. *Socratic hints* and *suggestions of user goals* were rated as least convincing. Strategies that were perceived as polite as well as persuasive were *actions expressed as shared goals* and *requests*.

A repeated-measures ANOVA analysis of the provided ratings for all recommendations showed significant differences for the perceived politeness ($F(7,308) = 37.82, p < .001$) as well as the perceived persuasiveness ($F(5.25, 231.05) = 8.14, p < .001$). A subsequent Bonferroni post-hoc test, see Table 2, confirmed the impressions of the descriptive analysis. Amongst others, *questions* were perceived as significantly more polite than any other strategy, and *direct commands* scored significantly worse on politeness than the other strategies.

All Recommendations

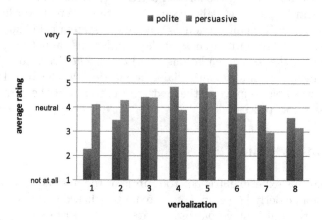

Fig. 2. Results of the laboratory study (Mean ratings for all recommendations). 1: direct command, 2: indirect suggestions, 3: requests, 4: actions as system goals, 5: actions as shared goals, 6: questions, 7: suggestions of user goals, 8: Socratic hints

Thus, the study showed that the investigated politeness strategies were perceived as significantly differently polite as well as persuasive. However, strategies that were perceived as polite were not necessarily perceived as persuasive or unpersuasive. Therefore, a good strategy for a REA might be to (1) choose verbalizations that are both, polite and persuasive, (2) neglect verbalizations that are neither polite nor persuasive, and (3) adapt verbalizations to the current situation to keep a certain variability in behavior, e.g., by choosing the verbalization depending on the importance of the given recommendation. For example, in cases where it is necessary to follow the advice of the robotic companion (such as remembering to take the prescribed medicine), a more convincing strategy

Table 2. Results of the laboratory study: M = Mean; SD = Standard Deviation; Sig = significantly better than

	Politeness			Persuasiveness		
	M	SD	Sig	M	SD	Sig
1. Direct command	2.27	1.03		4.11	1.76	
2. Indirect suggestion	3.47	1.41	1**	4.29	1.63	7**; 8*
3. Request	4.42	1.60	1***	4.40	1.48	7***;8**
4. Actions expressed as system goals	4.84	1.11	1,2,8***	3.89	1.45	7*
5. Actions expressed as shared goals	4.98	1.22	1,2,8***	4.64	1.45	7***; 8**
6. Questions	5.78	1.11	5*; 1,2,3,4,7,8***	3.76	1.32	7*
7. Suggestions of user goals	4.09	1.41	1***	2.96	1.38	
8. Socratic hint	3.58	1.20	1***	3.16	1.51	

*significant with p <.05; **significant with p <.01; ***significant with p <.001

could be chosen over a more polite but less persuasive version. In other cases, such as a suggestion to drink water regularly, the recommendation should focus more on politeness than on persuasiveness.

5   Study with Target User Group

After the politeness strategies were evaluated by younger adults in text form in a laboratory environment, a second study was conducted with the target user group, elderly inhabitants of a local retirement home who are needing assistance in certain daily situations, but do not suffer from serious mental diseases such as dementia. This time, the recommendations were presented by the REA described in Sect. 3. The aim was to investigate whether the elderly would distinguish between the perceived politeness and persuasiveness of the different verbalizations. Furthermore, we wanted to observe the seniors' acceptance of the presented REA system.

5.1   Participants and Procedure

In cooperation with the retirement home's head, we recruited 11 female and three male native German speakers aged between 50 and 100 that required care, but were still capable of accomplishing many of their daily tasks themselves. To facilitate the questionnaires' completion for the elderly, they were adapted to their requirements. Questions were formulated shortly and clearly, and whenever possible the Likert-Scales were reduced to five options. Each item of the questionnaire was printed on a separate page. Thus, at any time, participants only had to deal with the information that was necessary for rating the current verbalization.

Figure 3 shows the experimental setup. After a short introduction to the REA system, the robot introduced itself and allowed the participant to choose a comfortable volume and speed of its voice, to ensure that the recommendations were easy to understand. Then the robot explained the course of the study. In the next phase, the robot presented the eight different wordings for each of the three recommendations. To reduce the risk of order effects, the verbalizations were presented in an incomplete counterbalanced order. After each item the dialog paused while the participant answered the related questions. During the explanation and the waiting phases, the robot's head and face were subtly animated with idle movements such as blinking or moving its head to make it appear more alive and therefore more accessible. To avoid an influence on the ratings, the robot stopped moving and returned to a neutral position when presenting a recommendation. At the end, the robot thanked the participants for their help and said goodbye. This last phase could be triggered earlier in case a participant did not want to complete the entire study.

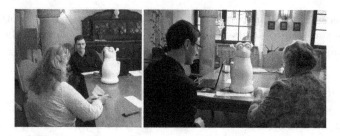

Fig. 3. Experimental setup: The study took place in a dining room at the retirement home. The REA was placed on a table in front of the participant. The application controlling the REA was running on a laptop which was positioned behind the robot and turned away to hide the screen and keyboard from the participant's view.

5.2 Results

Ten of the elderly people finished the study which took 45 to 60 min to complete. Unfortunately, four participants wanted to terminate their participation early because the procedure was too tiring for them.

In general, the participants provided relatively high ratings for the perceived politeness as well as the perceived persuasiveness for all verbalizations. The mean ratings of both criteria are graphically represented in Fig. 4. Similarly to the first study, *questions* were perceived as most polite. *Actions expressed as the system's goal* also received high ratings regarding the perceived politeness. However, *Socratic hints* were perceived as much more polite than in the first study. *Direct commands* also received much higher ratings, but were still perceived as least polite. Regarding the perceived persuasiveness, most of the verbalizations scored around 5.00. Only *suggestions of user goals* achieved a slightly lower mean rating of 4.73. Strategies that achieved high ratings concerning both criteria include indirect *suggestions*, *requests* and *Socratic hints*.

A repeated-measures ANOVA analysis showed significant differences between the different wordings for the perceived politeness ($F(7, 203) = 4.69, p < .0001$), but not for the perceived persuasiveness ($F(4.39, 127.38) = .53, p > .05$). A subsequent Bonferroni post-hoc test showed that *questions* and *actions expressed as the system's goals* were rated significantly more polite than *direct commands*, see Table 3. Nevertheless, the three strategies were rated as equally persuasive.

Observations of the seniors interacting with the REA indicated that none of them was afraid of the robot or rejected it, although most of them had never seen a system like REA before. After a few minutes of skepticism and doubts ("That's a machine. I can't talk to it.") almost all seniors did like the REA and talked to it as if it would understand them. They stated that the robot is "very friendly", "very nice", or even "really polite". Several participants complimented it directly and told stories about their families, their own childhood, adolescence, or current life. One woman even wanted to hug it. Furthermore, some of the elderly people tried to interpret the REA's random non-verbal behavior when it incidentally moved its head after they had talked to it.

All Recommendations

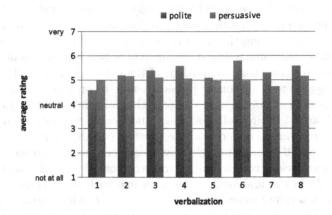

Fig. 4. Results of the field study (Mean ratings for all recommendations). 1: direct command, 2: indirect suggestions, 3: requests, 4: actions expressed as system goals, 5: actions as shared goals, 6: questions, 7: suggestions of user goals, 8: Socratic hints

Table 3. Results of the user study: M = Mean; SD = Standard Deviation; Sig = significantly better than

	Politeness			Persuasiveness		
	M	SD	Sig	M	SD	Sig
1. Direct command	4.58	1.37		4.98	1.39	
2. Indirect suggestion	5.19	1.04		5.16	1.13	
3. Request	5.40	1.28		5.10	1.21	
4. Actions expressed as system goals	5.58	.96	1**	5.06	1.18	
5. Actions expressed as shared goals	5.10	1.38		4.97	1.58	
6. Questions	5.80	.96	1**	4.97	1.38	
7. Suggestions of user goals	5.30	1.47		4.73	1.66	
8. Socratic hint	5.58	1.28		5.16	1.25	

*significant with $p < .05$; **significant with $p < .01$; ***significant with $p < .001$

5.3   Discussion

The studies' results showed that people do distinguish between the perceived politeness and persuasiveness of different politeness strategies. However, compared to the study with younger adults, with inhabitants of an retirement home we found smaller and fewer significant differences concerning the perceived politeness and no significant differences concerning the perceived persuasiveness.

One reason could be that the interrelation between politeness and persuasiveness was perceived differently by the seniors. There is evidence that, while several people found wording that they rated more polite also more persuasive, other people rated wording that they found more polite less persuasive.

Furthermore, the comparably small differences between ratings of verbalizations may be caused by some limitations of the elderly. For example, since two of the participants were no longer physically able to open a window, or go for a walk, it was difficult for them to compare the different wordings. In addition, some participants felt tired after a while, and people suffering from impaired hearing had problems to understand the robot at certain points.

Nevertheless, all ratings provided by the elderly were relatively high and all politeness strategies received higher ratings from the elderly than from the younger people in the first study. This is in line with the findings of Nomura et al. [24]. In a series of experiments they found that elderly people have more positive impressions of a robot than younger people. Some interactions such as telling private stories to the REA showed that, despite the short interaction time, the elderly people already established some trust in the robot, which is an important prerequisite to apply recommendations provided by a robotic system.

6   Conclusion

In the present contribution, we investigated linguistic variations to convey different levels of politeness in human-robot interaction. In the long run, a Robotic Elderly Assistant (REA) should provide assistance for elderly people in the form of recommendations to support them in their domestic environment. When robots provide recommendations to the user, they permanently risk threatening the user's face. For example, a recommendation such as "You should be more active." could be perceived as offensive and demotivate users. Politeness strategies may help mitigate face threats that might arise in such situations.

The results of a laboratory study with younger adults and a study with elderly people in a retirement home showed that different politeness strategies were perceived differently. In the laboratory study some wordings were perceived neither polite nor persuasive, e.g. *suggestions of user goals* and *Socratic hints*. Therefore, we think that these verbalizations should be ignored by a REA. In contrast, wordings such as *requests* and especially *actions formulated as shared goals* were perceived as polite and persuasive. They could be utilized as standard strategies whenever a recommendation should be applied. Other wordings that were not rated as very polite or very persuasive could nevertheless be applied by a REA, e.g., to maintain the seniors' interest in the REA by providing a wider variety of behavior that could be adapted on the current situation. For example, wordings that were perceived as being polite but not very persuasive, such as *questions* or *actions expressed as the system's goal*, could be utilized in uncritical situations, where the recommendation does not necessarily have to be applied. In this way, the relationship between the elderly person and the REA could be further established. Vice versa, in critical situations, the system could emphasize the need to apply a specific action by utilizing, for example, *direct commands* or *indirect suggestions* that were assessed rather impolite, but convincing.

While some of the findings from the laboratory study could be confirmed in the study with elderly users regarding the perceived politeness, the perceived persuasiveness of the recommendations needs further investigation. Hence, we will refine our studies to better match the requirements of our target user group. For example, some ratings seemed to be influenced by the fact that certain recommendations were not suitable for some of the participants due to physical impairments, e.g. not being able to go for a walk. In a follow-up study, more recommendations will be included that will be chosen based on the participant's preferences and abilities. Furthermore, it would be of interest to investigate which of the recommendations of the REA will be carried out. It seems likely that there is a gap between the abstract thinking of rating a recommendation as being convincing and the real drive to carry out an action.

Serendipitously, the elderly people's behavior during the user study showed that they were very open minded towards our REA system and acted very positively during the interaction. Therefore, we think that elderly people are generally willing to accept recommendations provided by our REA, and aim on contributing to the field of robotic elderly assistant systems by sharing our insights on the usage of different politeness strategies in this domain.

Acknowledgments. The authors would like to thank the staff and inhabitants of the retirement home "Paritätisches St. Jakobs-Stift Seniorenheim" in Augsburg, Germany, for enabling the main study and providing valuable feedback on the design of the REA. This research was partly funded by the Bavarian State Ministry for Education, Science and the Arts (STMWFK) as part of the ForGenderCare research association.

References

1. Teri, L., Lewinsohn, P.: Modification of the pleasant and unpleasant events schedules for use with the elderly. J. Consult. Clin. Psychol. **50**(3), 444–445 (1982)
2. Mahncke, H.W., Bronstone, A., Merzenich, M.M.: Brain plasticity and functional losses in the aged: scientific bases for a novel intervention. In: Møller, A.R., (ed.): Reprogramming of the Brain, Progress in Brain Research, vol. 157, pp. 81–109. Elsevier (2006)
3. Schmid, T. (ed.): Promoting Health Through Creativity: For Professionals in Health, Arts and Education. Whurr Publishers, London (2005)
4. Seiderer, A., Hammer, S., André, E., Mayr, M., Rist, T.: Exploring digital image frames for lifestyle intervention to improve well-being of older adults. In: Proceedings of the 5th International Conference on Digital Health, DH 2015, pp. 71–78. ACM, New York (2015)
5. Phang, C.W., Sutanto, J., Kankanhalli, A., Li, Y., Tan, B., Teo, H.H.: Senior citizens' acceptance of information systems: A study in the context of e-government services. IEEE Trans. Eng. Manage. **53**(4), 555–569 (2006)
6. Monk, A., Hone, K., Lines, L., Dowdall, A., Baxter, G., Blythe, M., Wright, P.: Towards a practical framework for managing the risks of selecting technology to support independent living. Appl. Ergon. **37**(5), 599–606 (2006)
7. Reeves, B., Nass, C.: The Media Equation: How People Treat Computers, Television, and New Media Like Real People and Places. Cambridge University Press, New York (1998)

8. Fong, T., Nourbakhsh, I., Dautenhahn, K.: A survey of socially interactive robots. Robot. Auton. Syst. **42**(3–4), 143–166 (2003)
9. Heerink, M.: Assessing acceptance of assistive social robots by aging adults. Ph.D. thesis, University of Amsterdam (2010)
10. Looije, R., Neerincx, M.A., Cnossen, F.: Persuasive robotic assistant for health self-management of older adults: Design and evaluation of social behaviors. Int. J. Hum. Comput. Stud. **68**(6), 386–397 (2010)
11. Spiekman, M.E., Haazebroek, P., Neerincx, M.A.: Requirements and platforms for social agents that alarm and support elderly living alone. In: Mutlu, B., Bartneck, C., Ham, J., Evers, V., Kanda, T. (eds.) ICSR 2011. LNCS, vol. 7072, pp. 226–235. Springer, Heidelberg (2011)
12. Broadbent, E., Stafford, R., MacDonald, B.: Acceptance of healthcare robots for the older population: Review and future directions. Int. J. Soc. Robot. **1**(4), 319–330 (2009)
13. Frennert, S., Östlund, B., Eftring, H.: Would granny let an assistive robot into her home? In: Ge, S.S., Khatib, O., Cabibihan, J.-J., Simmons, R., Williams, M.-A. (eds.) ICSR 2012. LNCS, vol. 7621, pp. 128–137. Springer, Heidelberg (2012)
14. Wu, Y.H., Fassert, C., Rigaud, A.S.: Designing robots for the elderly: appearance issue and beyond. Arch. Gerontol. Geriatr. **54**(1), 121–126 (2012)
15. Goetz, J., Kiesler, S., Powers, A.: Matching robot appearance and behavior to tasks to improve human-robot cooperation. In: The 12th IEEE International Workshop on Proceedings of Robot and Human Interactive Communication, ROMAN 2003, pp. 55–60, October 2003
16. Walters, M., Syrdal, D., Dautenhahn, K., te Boekhorst, R., Koay, K.: Avoiding the uncanny valley: robot appearance, personality and consistency of behavior in an attention-seeking home scenario for a robot companion. Auton. Robot. **24**(2), 159–178 (2008)
17. Sidner, C., Lee, C.: The initiation of engagement by a humanoid robot. In: AAAI Spring Symposium on Multidisciplinary Collaboration for Socially Assistive Robotics (2007)
18. Nomura, T., Saeki, K.: Effects of polite behaviors expressed by robots: A psychological experiment in Japan. Int. J. Synth. Emot. **1**(2), 38–52 (2010)
19. Mayer, R., Johnson, W., Shaw, E., Sandhu, S.: Constructing computer-based tutors that are socially sensitive: Politeness in educational software. In: Conference of the American Educational Research Association (2005)
20. Brown, P., Levinson, S.: Politeness: Some Universals in Language Usage. Studies in Interactional Sociolinguistics. Cambridge University Press, Cambridge (1987)
21. Johnson, W.L., Mayer, R.E., André, E., Rehm, M.: Cross-cultural evaluation of politeness in tactics for pedagogical agents. In: Proceedings of the 2005 Conference on Artificial Intelligence in Education: Supporting Learning Through Intelligent and Socially Informed Technology, Amsterdam, Netherlands, IOS Press, pp. 298–305 (2005)
22. Gebhard, P., Mehlmann, G., Kipp, M.: Visual Scenemaker - a tool for authoring interactive virtual characters. Multimodal User Interfaces **6**(1–2), 3–11 (2012)
23. Mehlmann, G., Janowski, K., André, E.: Modeling grounding for interactive social companions. KI - Künstliche Intelligenz **30**, 1–8 (2015)
24. Nomura, T., Takeuchi, S.: The elderly and robots: From experiments based on comparison with younger people (2011)

RightOnTime: The Role of Timing and Unobtrusiveness in Behavior Change Support Systems

Piiastiina Tikka[✉] and Harri Oinas-Kukkonen

Oulu Advanced Research on Service and Information Systems Research Group (OASIS),
University of Oulu, Oulu, Finland
{piiastiina.tikka,harri.oinas-kukkonen}@oulu.fi

Abstract. Influencing people's behavior by means of technology is achievable under many technological guises from websites to mobile devices to activity trackers, making them practically ubiquitous. The timing of persuasive messages has been found to be influential in itself, but the omnipresence of modern computing also raises questions about the effects of randomly timed interruptions and perceived obtrusiveness. The presented research is an explorative experiment regarding the unobtrusiveness of a behavior change support system. The study compares two timing strategies: random timing and user-defined timing for system interaction. While the results of the mixed ANOVA analyses in this pilot study did not yield statistically significant results between the timing strategies, the correlations found do seem to indicate that random interruptions are perceived as more obtrusive than user-timed interaction. Furthermore, a correlation was observed between task success, task satisfaction and perceived unobtrusiveness.

Keywords: Persuasive systems · Behavior change · Timing strategies · Interruptions · Persuasive systems design · User experience · Unobtrusiveness

1 Introduction

Use of information systems to influence behavior has been increasing in popularity in recent years. These systems are available in various forms both on desktops and in mobile devices and range from applications in the realm of the quantified self movement to applications and systems aimed at helping with lifestyle changes such as weight loss or even clinical or therapeutic systems that deal with conditions such as depression [1, 2] or diabetes management [3]. The behavioral problem domains addressed by the many systems are various, but in persuasive technology research the concept of Behavior Change Support System (BCSS) [4, 5] draws together the key elements of the systems themselves as information systems that are designed to form, alter and/or reinforce compliance, attitudes, and/or behaviors, and do so without using coercion or deception [5].

In the present experiment the research focuses on one important element of persuasive systems: the timing of persuasive communications. Such timing of persuasive messages has been suggested to have an effect on behavior [6, 7]. How the timing

© Springer International Publishing Switzerland 2016
A. Meschtscherjakov et al. (Eds.): PERSUASIVE 2016, LNCS 9638, pp. 327–338, 2016.
DOI: 10.1007/978-3-319-31510-2_28

of persuasive messages is managed can also affect an end-user's experience of obtrusiveness, since system-originated messages can produce interruptions and demand attention at moments that an end-user deems irritating [8].

The aim of the present study, therefore, is to shift the focus away slightly from trying to accurately spearfish for those opportune moments, and instead try and trawl for a coarser understanding of how persuasive message timing strategies affect behavior, behavior change and the user experience as regards the system. The key research question in the present pilot study, then, is: How do timing strategies affect behavior change and perceived unobtrusiveness when using BCSSs?

2 Background

There are essentially two perspectives on persuasive message timing that are present in this paper: the perceived interruptions from a system demanding attention, and the search for the opportune moment for demanding that attention. The objective here is not to pinpoint those opportune moments as such, but rather that the need to find them should be taken into account when studying timing issues. The present study aims to support that quest by exploring the broader scope of timing strategies. First, there is the effect of increased cognitive load that results from random interruptions demanding active attention [e.g. 8–10]. The second element is the concept of "an opportune moment" (or 'kairos' from the Greek) in the design of persuasive systems: the problem of when best to communicate a persuasive message to the system user for maximum effect [6, 7].

Cognitive load theory [11, 12] proposes that high working memory effort will have a negative effect on problem solving and other cognitive processes. The implications are notable for, say, learning [11] and decision-making [13]. Research into attention and interruptions has shown that attention is a limited cognitive capacity and that switching attention from one task to another comes at a cost to task performance [14]. Randomly timed interruptions have been found to have a negative effect on the performance of a main task [8, 9, 15] and such interruptions also increase negative affect as regards the system [8, 9]. Even in a broader context than specific tasks, some research suggests that extended and continuous exposure to constant interruptions by messaging and social media can have a detrimental effect on learning [16].

Miyata and Norman [10] argue that notifications from a system would have a lower interruption cost if delivered at a moment of lower mental workload. In other words, they advocate identifying kairos for sending a notification to a system user. Drawing upon this, a host of further research aims at identifying such moments for various systems to make use of [8, 9, 15]. For persuasive systems, the other type of 'opportune moment' has been identified as a factor in increasing the persuasive power of a message [6, 7]. Using the definition by Kinneavy [17], 'kairos' indicates an opportune moment and also the right measure of action. How much, how often and how frequently would all seem reasonable measures when discussing elements affecting perceived unobtrusiveness.

Earlier studies into factors affecting use and intention to use persuasive systems indicate that perceived unobtrusiveness affects at least the intention to use, if not the actual use of a system [18], and that it has an effect also on perceived persuasiveness of a persuasive system [19]. The PSD model [20] proposes that unobtrusiveness should be a key consideration in the design of persuasive systems: these systems should not disturb or interrupt users when they are carrying out their main tasks, and poorly executed timing of persuasive communications can lead to less than ideal results. Irritation resulting from interruptions may lead to levels of negative affect that influence one's intention to use a system or its actual use. The balance between too low involvement, where the necessary effort associated with learning and reflection (both in-action and on-action) [21] does not take place, and too active demand on attention through interruptions is of great interest in efforts to design better persuasive systems. A balance between reflection as a behavior change tool and the level of attention demand is necessary: after all, for self-reflection to take place at all, some attentional resources must be allocated to the process.

Context-aware systems are an absolute necessity in ensuring at least a minimum level of control over interruptions [22]. Irritation or frustration from interruptions is not conducive to successful persuasion, as we have been found to be more open to persuasion when we are in a good mood [6]. Furthermore, having control over when to take a break has been found to produce better problem-solving results than if break times are dictated by someone else [23].

3   Research Setting

3.1   Hypothesis

The research aimed at discovering whether the type of persuasive communication timing strategy had any affect on persuasion outcome and Perceived Unobtrusiveness (PU) of the system. Based on earlier research on the topic, as presented in the Background section, the following hypotheses were formed: (1) Random Timing (RT) is perceived to be more obtrusive than User-defined Timing UT; (2) RT has a stronger positive influence on behavior change both in self-assessed task success than UT; and (3) UT results in a more positive response in terms of Perceived Unobtrusiveness than RT.

Should the presented hypotheses hold true, an interesting conflict emerges in persuasion outcome and perceived unobtrusiveness: a better result in terms of behavioral influence may lead to higher perceived irritation associated with the system in question. The discussion should then focus on how to address this imbalance in persuasive systems design.

3.2   Study Design

The experiment was a mixed design (N = 13) comparing two timing strategies, implemented in a purpose-built iPhone app. The experimentation period was five days, with additional days for pre- and post-test assessments. For the basic analysis of how the different types of interruption affected punctuality performance and perceived satisfaction over a period of time, a mixed ANOVA (analysis of variance) design was selected. The within-subjects factor was self-assessment ratings collected over the experimentation period, with the between-subject factor being the timing strategy. The dependent variables there were self-reported success ratings and perceived satisfaction ratings. Participants were divided into one of two groups as per timing strategy.

Five measures of both dependent variables were used. The participants reported on more than one punctuality task each day, and the average of the ratings for each day was used as the daily score. As the daily tasks were carried out independently by each participant without close supervision by researchers there were individuals who did not always complete three tasks per day and individuals who may have reported more than three tasks on some days. Listwise deletion approach was deemed most suitable for handling missing values.

3.3 Procedure (Data Collection)

Participants (N = 13) in the experiment represent a sample of opportunity. As an incentive to take part, completion of the experiment entered participants in a prize draw. At the time of recruitment participants were not told what the exact topic of the experiment was: the only information offered was a broad outline of the effort expected of them and the explanation that the experiment was to do with behavior change. As participants signed up, they were informed that they could withdraw from the study at any time if they so wished.

The participants were screened for punctuality schematicism. In short, self-schema refers to a person's perception of his or her self in terms of his or her specific environment [24] and it is a construct linked with transition of intention into behavior [24–26]. Research into behavioral intention and self-schemas have established that a positive self-schema towards a specific behavior acts as a moderator in turning intention into behavior [25] and that schema-matched persuasion can result in more effective change [e.g. 27]. The purpose of using such an attitude scale was to ensure that there were participants who would fall within the target group for an app that addressed punctuality problems. Short of finding volunteers who freely admitted to having problems with time keeping, using a punctuality self-schema assessment meant that we were able to identify participants who did not, perhaps, have the need to be on time as a prominent part of their self-identity; we could then assign such participants to both test conditions (RT and UT).

While the sample size in the present experiment is not overly large (N = 13), it was estimated using G*Power analysis tool [28]. Initially, 40 potential participants signed up, but for varying (personal) reasons many of them dropped out and did not complete the experiment. Aiming at effect size of .4 and power of .95 for two groups and five measures, the estimated total sample size required was 14. We were unable to meet this target minimum sample size in the time available for the study. Latin squares were used for balancing punctuality schematics and non-schematics between the conditions (Group A and Group B) at the start of the experiment, but owing to participants' freedom to drop out of the experiment at any time it was not possible to control the final outcome of schematics/non-schematics per condition or to keep the test groups exactly the same size. Overall, 14 participants completed the tasks in a satisfactory manner, but one participant failed to complete the required information regarding schematicism and therefore had to be dropped from the analysis (Table 1).

Table 1. Schematic and non-schematic test participants in the experiment's timing conditions.

Timing/punctuality type	Schematic	Non-schematic	Total
Random	5	3	8
User-defined	3	2	5
Total	8	5	13

After the schematicism screening the participants also filled in a background information questionnaire and were instructed how to download the app and use it with the relevant settings. Finally, after completing the tasks on the app, the participants were sent links to the final questionnaires by e-mail.

The two groups of participants were each instructed as to the specific settings they had to use on the test app in the experiment. Group A were the 'Random Timing' group, where the system would send them tips and hints throughout the day and also query their responses regarding task success and satisfaction some time after the completion of each task. Group B were asked to set one time for daily interactions with the system; in this way all the communications and requests to fill in the self-assessments were sent to the user once a day at a time of the user's own choosing. For both groups the number of tips and hints was limited to three so that frequency would remain the same between the groups.

During the five experiment days all participants set themselves three timed tasks per day and one time-estimation practice task per day. The timed tasks could be anything that the participants determined they needed to be on time for or anything that they decided they wanted to do at some specific time. In the practice task the participants were asked to select some routine such as breakfast, journey to work, etc. and learned to estimate how long the activity actually took. The participants submitted the self-evaluations to the research database using a 'send' button in the test app.

3.4 Materials

Mobile Device Test App. A purpose-made native iOS app called 'RightOnTime' was designed and developed by the research team and was entered into Apple Store as a free download. The particular purpose of the app was to help in rehearsing time management skills that are associated with many cases of chronic tardiness and it also provided features for actively practicing time-awareness and to encourage personal time-management related self-reflection. The app, then, was designed to support users in developing and/or maintaining punctual behavior patterns by making them see when their behavior was not based on realistic perceptions of time (or, indeed, when they were punctual and timely). The problem-domain content used in the app was a collection of existing knowledge and suggestions from the literature [29] and self-help websites[1]. In the experiment the app's two settings configuration possibilities were used in studying the difference in response as regards perceived unobtrusiveness (Fig. 1).

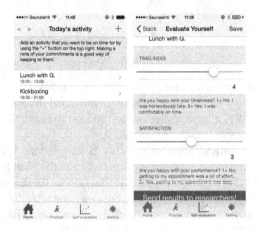

Fig. 1. RightOnTime app: Home screen (left) for setting tasks, and an example of a self-evaluation view (competed after a task is done).

The app had two main parts: user-set punctuality targets/tasks and time-awareness practice. In the first category the user would set a number of timed events for each day. These could be any tasks or activities that the user wanted to be on time for. Each activity would be given an exact starting time and an estimation of duration. The main objective was to increase awareness of important meetings or tasks and to learn in that way to make the effort of getting there on time. Once the task was over, the system would prompt users to evaluate their performance in terms of timeliness. The prompt was set to appear within a 15-min frame after completion of the task so that it was not entirely predictable. Time-awareness assessments were not in the focus of the present pilot study.

A selection of Persuasive Systems Design [20] features was used in the design of the app: reflection (in action as well as on action [21]) is very much in the foreground not only in the form of *Self-monitoring* as such, but by generally offering the user ways of keeping the behavior change target in mind through continuous interactions, practice, etc. Further PSD features [20] used in the app included *reduction*, *reminders*, *suggestion* and *real-world feel* (see Table 2).

The app itself was constructed using iOS components and style as much as possible in order to minimize the effect of design on UX while maintaining an acceptable level of interface familiarity, functionality and usability.

---

[1] How To Be Punctual. http://www.wikihow.com/Be-Punctual. (Date of reference 4.8.2015). Prolific Living. The Importance of Being Punctual. http://www.prolificliving.com/the-importance-of-being-punctual/ (Date of reference 4.8.2015).

Table 2. Persuasive system design features used in the RightOnTime app.

Primary task support	Reduction	An overall goal of "be more punctual" may seem too big to manage, so it is good to split the target into smaller and more manageable individual tasks
	Self-monitoring	Self-assessment data and summaries offer an opportunity to monitor one's development as regards the behavior change targets
Computer-human dialogue support	Reminders	The system reminds the user to complete the self-assessments and to view daily assessment summaries
	Suggestion	The system sends the user tips and hints (information, encouragement and guidance) as push notifications
System credibility support	Read-world feel	An "About" section in the system provides information about the designers, the origins and the purpose of the app

Attitude Questionnaire Development. A self-schema assessment questionnaire was devised based on an established model by, for example, [24]. The questionnaire gauged each participant's self image as regards punctuality by querying representative punctuality statements (measures). The use of an 11-point scale on the two measures ("describes me/does not describe me" and "is important to me/is not important to me") has been used in earlier research on the relationship between self-schemas and behavior by, for example, [24, 30]. As such, the questionnaire style both in the listed studies and in the present experiment is a direct measure, but filler items were used in order to disguise the focus of the questionnaire at the beginning of the experiment. Also, the participants were not told what behavior specifically was going to fall within the scope of the test and the filler items referred to other lifestyle topics such as healthy eating. As mentioned, attitude was queried.

Perceived Unobtrusiveness UX Questionnaire Development. In order to gauge the final experience of unobtrusiveness after using the test app for five days, a questionnaire to that effect was developed. By using established UX questionnaires[2,3] a perceived persuasiveness questionnaire [19, 31] the PSD model [20] and other related material [32, 33], five expert evaluators scored the statements, directing thus which statements were included in the final questionnaire. Again, when administering the questionnaire, filler items were added so as to diffuse the focus of the respondents.

4 Results

4.1 Participants and Sample Characteristics

Initially, a total of 40 people signed up to take part in the experiment initially. Of those, 31 completed the schematicism screener and were assigned to the test groups. Subsequently, more than half dropped out at various stages during the experiment period. 13 participants completed the entire experiment. Of the total initial number of interested participants (40) nine were non-schematics as regards punctuality. In the end, five of these nine completed the experiment and were included in the analysis.

Sample Description. Average age for the sample was 36 years, with the youngest participant being 23 and the oldest 72 years of age. The oldest participant was notably older than the rest, but the participant was an experienced iPhone user, had no characteristics in choice of daily tasks or otherwise that stood out from the rest of the sample and so the participant was not considered an outlier. Nine participants out of the 13 were female, but the analysis does not consider gender a critical factor within the scope of the experiment. A clear majority (11) had used in iPhone for more than six months, making them familiar with the test device itself. As regards punctuality schematicism, the sample includes more schematics than non-schematics, meaning that the majority of the participants identify themselves as people who value punctuality and timeliness.

4.2 Data Analysis

The collected data was analyzed for variance both for task success (Tsucc) and task satisfaction (Tsat). These scores were also checked for correlation with Perceived Unobtrusiveness (PU). The PU scores were also analyzed for variance between the test groups.

Analysis of variance showed no significant effect of time of measurement in the Task success scores (time of measurement here referring to each of the five days of the experiment). The daily score used in the analysis is an averaged score from the three

---

[2] NASA TLX: Task Load Index. http://humansystems.arc.nasa.gov/groups/tlx/.

[3] System Usability Scale (SUS). http://www.usability.gov/how-to-and-tools/methods/system-usability-scale.html.

tasks participants reported each day in order to show a more consolidated day-by-day view of the development over time. The RT group's task scores were measured at different times of the day, depending upon what time their set tasks took place, while the UT group reported all three scores at one self-set time. The extended delay between completing a task and reporting it in retrospect was part of the timing strategy difference between the conditions.

The collected means in Fig. 2 show the development of means for each variable and factor over the five days. The interesting movements in the chart (Fig. 2) concern the beginning and the end of the period. At the beginning User-defined timing group scores drop after the first day before they gradually climb back up to the starting levels and even beyond. The Random timing group is seen to climb up to the same levels at the end as the user-defined timing group, but task satisfaction in particular appears to climb up in a steady and even manner.

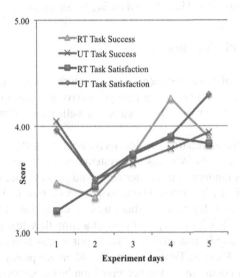

Fig. 2. Self-evaluation scores: means for each group per day.

UT group participants' Tsucc and Tsat scores compared with PU scores pointed to a very small linear relationship (r = −31 for Tsucc, r = −.20 for Tsat). In the RT group the correlation coefficients indicated a stronger positive linear relationship, with r = .62 for Tsucc and r = .56 for Tsat. These indications of strength in the linear relationship are extremely interesting considering that the PU score is given on negative statements: the higher the score, the stronger the agreement with statements that indicate obtrusiveness. In other words, participants in Group A (Random Timing) tended to rate the system more obtrusive as their Task Success and Task Satisfaction increased. In the UT group, on the other hand, the system was rated less obtrusive as the Task Success and Task Satisfaction increased.

One of the initial hypotheses was that Random Timing of persuasive messaging may be experienced as being more obtrusive than timing set by the system user. We do not have exact information as to the reasons why participants dropped out from the experiment, as it was their right to do so without explanation, but it is worth noting that of the 31 initial participants assigned to test groups 17 were assigned to Random Timing and 15 to User-defined Timing groups. For these groups, the completion rate was only 5 participants (approx. 30 %) in the RT group and 8 (approx. 50 %) in the UT group. One possible avenue of thought for explaining the difference in the drop-out rate could be the difference in the obtrusiveness between the two experiment conditions.

A one-way ANOVA of the PU scores does not show statistical significance variance between the groups either, but as predicted, it is the RT group whose scores point towards a more pronounced experience of obtrusiveness. Therefore, while performance related scores improved over the experiment period, the participants in the RT group perceived the system to be more obtrusive than the participants in the UT group. In this questionnaire a higher score (the 'agree' end of the scale) indicated agreement on negative statements. In other words, here, too, there is some slight indication that Random timing might be experienced as more obtrusive than User-defined timing of persuasive messaging.

5   Discussion and Conclusion

The primary purpose of the experiment was to explore the problem field around the concept of unobtrusive user experience with persuasive systems so that a more robust exploration could then be carried out by means of a well-informed model of influencing factors.

The difference in the correlation coefficients between the test groups is a particularly interesting avenue of analysis. When using a system that sends messages, reminders and evaluation requests at random times, better perceived performance (Tsucc) and higher satisfaction in one's own achievement (Tsat) do not seem to translate into an unobtrusive experience of the system. By contrast, there was an indication of the opposite effect when system users dealt with the system only at a time they had chosen themselves. Admittedly, the linearity in this case was weak, but it was observably in a different direction than with the Random Timing group. The difference prompts various questions as regards the role of cognitive load in perceived unobtrusiveness. *How strongly does the awareness and sense of being disturbed, interrupted or otherwise reminded of an on-going task at random moments result in negative affect towards the system?* In this small sample and over this short period of time performance and satisfaction did not differ significantly, and neither did the final experience scores; but does the correlation result suggest potential problems in terms of perceived unobtrusiveness in a longer time frame? Or does this suggest that it might be possible to achieve acceptable behavior change results even when minimizing interruption-based cognitive load?

As it was, statistically we ended up with an inconclusive set of results: the differences between the groups in terms of Task Success and Task Satisfaction ratings are not significant, and while there is an observable difference between the Perceived Unobtrusiveness rating between the conditions, the difference is not statistically significant. The significance of the drop-out rate difference between the two groups calls for further exploration in order to determine if the perceived unobtrusiveness was even more pronounced in the Random Timing group than presently reported. As it was, the freedom to drop out of the experiment does not allow for more than speculative conclusions based on the fact that more participants dropped out from the Random Timing group than from the User-defined Timing group.

Further research is certainly required, but the findings from this study can be used in identifying meaningful factors that are at play in defining appropriate timing strategies. One way of looking at the relationship between 'timing strategies' and an 'opportune moment' is to regard 'opportune moment' as one end of a continuum and an abysmally inappropriate moment as the other. Where a persuasive system falls on that continuum can depend on the timing strategies, whether random vs. set, sensor-based or context-based, etc. The ideal is to hit upon the kairos moment and achieve behavior change with minimal cognitive load, but such rarities apart, we must search for ways of providing an unobtrusive user experience without compromising the behavior change target.

References

1. Kuonanoja, L., Lanqrial, S., Lappalainen, R., Lappalainen, P., Oinas-Kukkonen, H.: Treating depression with a behavior change support system without face-to-face therapy. AIS Trans. Hum. Comput. Interact. **7**(3), 192–210 (2015)
2. Lappalainen, P., Langrial, S., Oinas-Kukkonen, H., Tolvanen, A., Lappalainen, R.: Web-based acceptance and commitment therapy for depressive symptoms with minimal support: treatment efficacy and participants' experiences: a randomized controlled trial. Behav. Modif. **39**(6), 805–834 (2015)
3. NovoNordisk. Cornerstones4Care Diabetes Healthcoach, 30 July 2015. https://www.cornerstones4care.com
4. Oinas-Kukkonen, H.: Prerequisites for successful measuring of ambient persuasive technology, pp. 491–494 (2010)
5. Oinas-Kukkonen, H.: A foundation for the study of behavior change support systems. Pers. Ubiquit. Comput. **17**(6), 1223–1235 (2013)
6. Fogg, B.J.: Persuasive Technology: Using Computers to Change What We Think and Do. Morgan Kaufmann Publishers, San Francisco (2003)
7. Räisänen, T., Oinas-Kukkonen, H., Pahnila, S.: Finding kairos in quitting smoking: smokers' perceptions of warning pictures. In: Oinas-Kukkonen, H., Hasle, P., Harjumaa, M., Segerståhl, K., Øhrstrøm, P. (eds.) PERSUASIVE 2008. LNCS, vol. 5033, pp. 254–257. Springer, Heidelberg (2008)
8. Bailey, B.P., Iqbal, S.T.: Understanding changes in mental workload during execution of goal-directed tasks and its application for interruption management. ACM Trans. Comput. Hum. Interact. **14**(4), 1–28 (2008)
9. Bailey, B.P., Konstan, J.A.: On the need for attention-aware systems: measuring effects of interruption on task performance, error rate, and affective state. Comput. Hum. Behav. **22**(4), 685–708 (2006)
10. Miyata, Y., Norman, D.A.: The control of multiple activities. In: Norman, D.A., Draper, S.W. (eds.) User-Centered System Design: New Perspectives on Human-Computer Interaction. Lawrence Erlbaum Associates, Hillsdale (1986)
11. Paas, F., Renkl, A., Sweller, J.: Cognitive load theory: instructional implications of the interaction between information structures and cognitive architecture. Instru. Sci. **32**(1/2), 1–8 (2004)
12. Sweller, J.: Cognitive load during problem solving. Cogn. Sci. **12**, 257–285 (1988)

13. Vohs, K.D., Baumeister, R.F., Schmeichel, B.J., Twenge, J.M., Nelson, N.M., Tice, D.M.: Making choices impairs subsequent self-control: a limited-resource account of decision making, self-regulation, and active initiative. J. Pers. Soc. Psychol. **94**(5), 883–898 (2008)
14. Kahneman, D.: Attention and Effort. Prentice-Hall Inc., Englewood Cliffs (1973)
15. Czerwinski, M., Cutrell, E., Horvitz, E.: Instant messaging: effects of relevance and timing. In: People and Computers XIV: Proceedings of HCI, British Computer Society, pp. 71–76 (2000)
16. Frein, S.F., Jones, S.L., Gerow, J.E.: When it comes to Facebook there may be more to bad memory than just multitasking. Comput. Hum. Behav. **29**(6), 2179–2182 (2013)
17. Kinneavy, J.L.: Kairos: a neglected concept in classical rhetoric. In: Moss, J.D. (ed.) Rhetoric and Praxis: the Contribution of Classical Rhetoric to Practical Reasoning, pp. 79–105. The Catholic University of America Press, Washington (1986)
18. Drozd, F., Lehto, T., Oinas-Kukkonen, H.: Exploring perceived persuasiveness of a behavior change support system: a structural model. In: Bang, M., Ragnemalm, E.L. (eds.) PERSUASIVE 2012. LNCS, vol. 7284, pp. 157–168. Springer, Heidelberg (2012)
19. Lehto, T., Oinas-Kukkonen, H., Drozd, F.: Factors affecting perceived persuasiveness of a behavior change support system. In: ICIS 2012 Proceedings of Human Behavior in IT Adoption and Use: Paper 18 (2013)
20. Oinas-kukkonen, H., Harjumaa, M.: Persuasive systems design: key issues, process model, and system features. Commun. Assoc Inf. Syst. **24**(1), 28 (2009)
21. Ploderer, B., Reitberger, W., Oinas-Kukkonen, H., van Gemert-Pijnen, J.: Social interaction and reflection for behaviour change. Pers. Ubiquit. Comput. **18**(7), 1667–1676 (2014). doi: 10.1007/s00779-014-0779-y
22. Anhalt, J., Smailagic, A., Siewiorek, D.P., Gemperle, F., Salber, D., Weber, S. Jennings, J.: Toward context-aware computing: experiences and lessons. IEEE Intell. Syst. **16**(3), 38–46 (2001)
23. Beeftink, F., van Eerde, W., Rutte, C.G.: The effect of interruptions and breaks on insight and impasses: do you need a break right now? Creativity Res. J. **20**(4), 358–364 (2008)
24. Markus, H.: Self-schemata and processing information about the self. J. Pers. Soc. Psychol. **35**(2), 63–78 (1977)
25. Sheeran, P., Orbell, S.: Self-schemas and the theory of planned behaviour. Eur. J. Soc. Psychol. **30**, 533–550 (2000)
26. Cacioppo, J.T., Petty, R.E., Sidera, J.A.: The effects of a salient self-schema on the evaluation of proattitudinal editorials: top-down versus bottom-up message processing. J. Exp. Soc. Psychol. **18**, 324–338 (1982)
27. Wheeler, C.S., Petty, R.E., Bizer, G.Y.: Self-schema matching and attitude change: situational and dispositional determinants of message elaboration. J. Consum. Res. **31**, 787–797 (2005)
28. Faul, F., Erdfelder, E., Lang, A.-E., Buchner, A.: G*Power 3: a flexible statistical power analysis program for the social, behavioral, and biomedical sciences. Behav. Res. Methods **39**(2), 175–191 (2007)
29. DeLonzor, D.: Never Be Late Again, 7 Cures for the Punctually Challenged. Post Madison Publishing, San Francisco (2003)
30. Kendzierski, D.: Self-schemata and exercise. Basic Appl. Soc. Psychol. **9**(1), 45–59 (1988). http://doi.org/10.1207/s15324834basp0901_4
31. Lehto, T. Oinas-Kukkonen, H.: Explaining and predicting perceived effectiveness and use continuance intention of a behaviour change support system for weight loss. Behav. Inf. Technol. **34**(2), 176–189 (2015). http://dx.doi.org/10.1080/0144929X.2013.866162
32. Baddeley, A.D.: Working memory. Science **225**, 556–559 (1992)
33. Rubinstein, J., Meyer, D., Evans, J.: Executive control of cognitive processes in task switching. J. Exp. Psychol. Hum. Percept. Perform. **27**(4), 763–797 (2001)

Persuasive Information Security: Techniques to Help Employees Protect Organizational Information Security

Marc Busch[1]([✉]), Sameer Patil[2,3], Georg Regal[1], Christina Hochleitner[1], and Manfred Tscheligi[1]

[1] AIT Austrian Institute of Technology GmbH, Giefinggasse 2,
1210 Vienna, Austria
{March.Busch,Georg.Regal,Christina.Hochleitner,
Manfred.Tscheligi}@ait.ac.at
[2] Department of Computer Science and Engineering, New York University,
Brooklyn, NY 11201, USA
sameer.patil@nyu.edu
[3] Helsinki Institute for Information Technology HIIT / Aalto University,
P.O. Box 15600, 00076 Aalto, Finland

Abstract. Digital information is an important corporate asset. Organizations typically devise policies and guidelines to help employees protect the security of such information. Complying with these rules can often be confusing and difficult and may obstruct the task at hand, leading employees to circumvent or ignore policies. Commercial technology and training programs to mitigate this issue suffer from various shortcomings. To address these shortcomings, we designed six persuasive features: Security Points, Security Quiz, Challenges, Statistics, Personalization, and Risk Communication. A design probe that implemented the features sheds light on how *persuasive security* features could influence intentions to follow secure work practices. We apply the findings to offer suggestions for further enhancing the six persuasive features.

Keywords: Usable security · Persuasive design · Information security policy · Security compliance · Organizational information systems

1 Introduction

Breaches in organizational information security can lead to the loss or theft of sensitive digital information, potentially costing significant financial amounts and damaging the organization's reputation. Studies show that a sizable proportion of information security breaches are caused inadvertently in the course of routine work of employees, despite absence of malicious intent. A recent study

This research was conducted when Dr. Patil was a researcher at the Helsinki Institute for Information Technology HIIT / Aalto University, Finland.

© Springer International Publishing Switzerland 2016
A. Meschtscherjakov et al. (Eds.): PERSUASIVE 2016, LNCS 9638, pp. 339–351, 2016.
DOI: 10.1007/978-3-319-31510-2_29

that included more than 1400 employees of 277 companies in 9 countries found that 35 percent of data breaches were caused by such "human factors" [5].

One of the mechanisms organizations use for the protection of information is an information security policy, i.e., the rules and guidelines defining permitted and forbidden actions related to information assets. Naturally, organizations expect employees to adhere to the policy. However, employees often find it challenging to comply. Factors underlying these difficulties include individual attitudes toward the policy, beliefs about organizational norms, and efficacy to comply [1].

Solutions to ensure compliance with information security policies may be technology- or human-centric. Enforcement via technical means (e.g., denying access when the network connection is insecure) takes away employee autonomy and may lead to potentially insecure workarounds, thus undermining, rather than enhancing, security. Moreover, automated technological enforcement affects only the corresponding work practices, not employee *attitudes*. In contrast, human-centric approaches (such as training and awareness programs [12,17]) aim to influence attitudes and motivate employees to follow secure information practices. However, such approaches are expensive and time consuming and need repetition. The effectiveness of security education programs is further limited because they are typically decontextualized from work practices and decoupled from the situations under consideration (viz., actual policy breaches).

We believe that a key to enhancing the effectiveness of such tools and methods is *educating* employees regarding the risks and rationale that form the basis of the policy and *engaging* them by incentivizing secure information practices. Toward this end, we designed six features aimed at increasing employee awareness and knowledge of the organizational information security policy and changing attitudes and behavioral intention toward compliance. Our goal was to identify the effectiveness and promise of the features for raising employee awareness of the organization's information security policy and increasing policy compliance. Specifically, we explored the following research question: *Which persuasive features are likely to effect a change in attitudes and behavior intention regarding organizational information security?*

To tackle the above question, we carried out a user study in which we evaluated the perceived persuasiveness of these features via an interface implementation in the form of a design probe. We found that persuasive strategies could indeed be beneficial for promoting secure work practices, albeit to varying extents. We apply our findings to offer suggestions for further exploration of the design space of persuasive security features.

Our contribution lies in the application of persuasive strategies for organizational security. Persuasive technology has not been systematically explored for usable security in general and organizational security in particular. By extending persuasive design to this domain, we promote an approach to security policy compliance that engages with and educates the human in the loop.

2 Related Work

Technological approaches to improve organizational information security policy compliance include commercial applications that manage endpoint security. Such applications monitor company-owned devices and networks and enforce access controls for information assets. For instance, the application could forbid access via a non-trusted and insecure network. The user interfaces of these applications are typically geared toward information security managers and system administrators, rather than end-users of the devices. Further, the systems often enforce information security policies without helping end users understand the importance of the rules and the consequences of violations. To mitigate this shortcoming, approaches such as training [12] and security awareness campaigns [10] have been suggested to educate employees regarding the importance, threats, risks, and compliance procedures associated with security rules. Research shows that training and awareness programs can be useful and effective [12,17], especially when personalized [11]. However, this utility incurs high financial and time costs, and the program may need periodic repetition. Moreover, these programs provide generic prescriptive guidance and, unlike our approach, do not include incentives for incorporating the advice in work practice [15].

So far, only a few studies have applied persuasive technology for usable security. Forget et al. [7–9] utilized persuasive technology to raise the strength of user-chosen text passwords, while Chiasson et al. [3,4] achieved similar success in helping users choose strong graphical passwords. Other researchers have used persuasive technology to implement games targeting security related behavior. Yeo et al. [19] demonstrated the effectiveness of a Web based multiple-choice quiz to improve password management and virus protection, and Sheng et al. [14] found that an anti-phishing game was effective in educating users about secure Internet behavior. However, all of these studies utilized relatively small student samples, not knowledge workers. Additionally, these explorations were limited to specific actions, such as choosing passwords, rather than considering *all* work practices that impact the security of an organization's information resources. We tackle this broader challenge and explore the effectiveness of several individual persuasive strategies and their combinations.

3 Design Probe of Persuasive Features

To explore persuasive technology for organizational information security, we built a Web based design probe in the form of an interactive front-end interface based on several persuasive strategies. We treated compliance with the organizational security policy as the target behavior; the security policy defines permissible actions, thus setting the desired direction for a change in security-related behavior.

We selected 8 persuasive strategies from the collection of 28 described by Oinas-Kukkonen and Harjumaa [13]. Our selection was based on a combination of factors, viz., applicability to organizational information security, application in past usable security studies, amenability to implementation as a concrete and distinct interface mechanism, and the necessity to limit strategies to a reasonable number. Specifically, the probe covered the following eight persuasive strategies:

- Rewards: Rewarding the target behavior (with Security Points and Badges).
- Tailoring: Personalizing to one's interests and personality (via a questionnaire to determine features of potential interest to the employee).
- Competition: Promoting competition with others (through Challenges).
- Simulation: Providing a means for understanding the connection between behavior and its consequences (by communicating potential risks).
- Social comparison: Comparing one's performance with others (using Statistics of past security behavior).
- Suggestions: Recommending appropriate behavior at opportune moments (by suggesting interesting features determined using questionnaire responses).
- (Social) learning: Facilitating learning about target behavior (in the form of a Security Quiz with questions about the information security policy).
- Self monitoring: Providing a means to track one's performance and status (using Statistics of past security behavior).

We term an operational system *implementation* of one or more persuasive strategies as a persuasive *feature*. Our probe incorporated the above eight persuasive strategies in the form of six persuasive features, viz., Security Points, Security Quiz, Challenges, Statistics, Personalization, and Risk Communication. The feature design followed Oinas-Kukkonen and Harjumaa's [13] suggested process model for designing persuasive technologies. Table 1 shows the mapping between the strategies and the features. With the exception of Security Points, each feature operationalized a primary and a secondary strategy. We summarize each of these features below. Busch et al. [2] provide further details.

Table 1. Mapping between probe features and persuasive strategies.

Probe feature	Primary strategy	Secondary strategy
Security points	Rewards	–
Security quiz	(Social) learning	Rewards
Challenges	Competition	Rewards
Statistics	Self monitoring	Social comparison
Personalization	Tailoring	Suggestion
Risk communication	Simulation	Rewards

Security Points: Users could collect virtual *rewards* in the form of Security Points (see Fig. 1a). Security Points could be earned by taking a Security Quiz, completing Challenges, or answering the Personalization questionnaire. Users were awarded Badges corresponding to the progressive accumulation of Security Points, viz., Beginner, Intermediate, Expert, Professional, and Master. Security

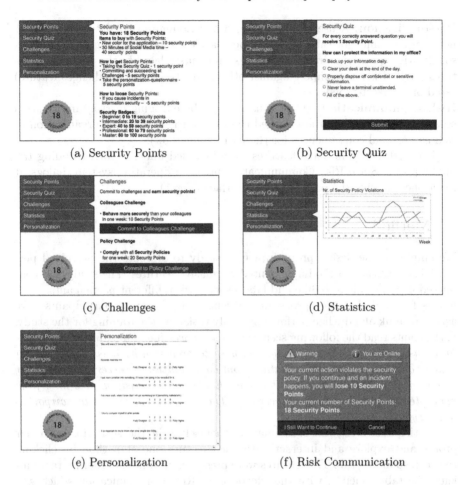

(a) Security Points

(b) Security Quiz

(c) Challenges

(d) Statistics

(e) Personalization

(f) Risk Communication

Fig. 1. Screenshots of the six persuasive features implemented in the probe.

Points could be used to 'buy' perks, such as time to use social media and colors to change the look-and-feel of the interface. Points were deducted if the user's actions were deemed insecure.

Security Quiz. In order to facilitate *learning*, users were presented with quizzes on work scenarios related to the information security policy (see Fig. 1b).

Challenges. This feature provided motivation in the form of *competition* among employees (see Fig. 1c). Users could accept Challenges that were either group based (e.g., "Behave more securely than your colleagues for one week.") or individual (e.g., "Comply fully with the security policy for one week.").

Statistics. The probe showed Statistics of security-related behavior, e.g., the number of policy violations committed by the user per week as well as the average number of violations for all employees across the organization (see Fig. 1d).

Personalization. A user could answer a questionnaire that determined his or her persuadability for each of the six persuasive features (see Fig. 1e). The Personalization questionnaire consisted of statements related to the persuasive features (e.g., "I like to compete against others" related to the Challenges feature) rated on a Likert-type scale.

Risk Communication. When a user might be engaging in risky information security practices, the probe warned the user of the risk for the organization as well as personal consequences for the user (*simulation*).

The first five persuasive features were included under a corresponding tab in the probe. Since Risk Communication involved operating system dialogs, it functioned outside the probe's main interface (Fig. 1).

4   Method

We employed the design probe in a user study to evaluate the perceived persuasiveness of each of the implemented persuasive features. The study was conducted in two modes – online and laboratory – with different participants. Both modes followed the *same* procedure, except that laboratory participants were asked to think aloud when performing study tasks. As the framing for the study, participants read the following scenario: *You are waiting at the airport to embark on a business trip. While waiting, you wish to prepare a business document for which you need sensitive information from your company's servers. The security policy of your employer states that you should access sensitive files only from encrypted (secure) network connections. The wireless Internet at the airport is unencrypted.*

Participants were asked to imagine themselves in the scenario, open our probe, and explore and interact with each feature one at a time by clicking the corresponding tab. The features were presented in random order by randomizing the tab sequence, with the exception of Risk Communication which was excluded from randomization because it operated outside the probe interface; it was always the final task. To evaluate Risk Communication, participants were asked to open another application called 'File Explorer.' Within this application, participants were instructed to (try to) open 'Low-Sensitive Document.pdf,' 'Medium-Sensitive Document.pdf,' and 'High-Sensitive Document.pdf.' Clicking on the 'Low-Sensitive Document.pdf' brought up a warning regarding a security policy violation (see Fig. 1f). Given the low sensitivity of the file, the warning allowed the user to proceed if he or she desired. The warning popup for the other two files blocked opening the file with no user override.

4.1   Influence of Persuasive Features

After encountering each persuasive feature, participants rated it using the following items in random order on a 7-point Likert-type scale from Strongly disagree (1) to Strongly agree (7):

– Usefulness: *I find this feature useful.*

- Enjoyment: *I enjoy using this feature.*
- Increase in Awareness: *This feature would make me more aware of organizational information security.*
- Attitude Change: *This feature would have a positive influence on my attitude toward organizational information security.*
- Behavior Change: *This feature would lead me to comply with organizational information security.*

The items measured the perceived persuasiveness of each feature and were adapted from Drozd et al. [6] and Venkatesh and Bala [18]. We further allowed participants to provide open-ended opinions regarding the feature.

Recruiting and Sample. Participants were recruited from a database of research volunteers from Austria. We screened potential online participants to include only those who were employed full- or part-time. For the laboratory mode, we selected participants on the basis of the relevance of information security policies for their jobs and recruited them by telephone. Nearly all participants worked in professions such as consulting, management, administration, programming, marketing, etc., requiring the handling of digital information, As participation incentive, online participants were entered into a raffle for 20 gift certificates of €30 for Amazon.com, while each laboratory participant received a gift certificate of €30 redeemable at a variety of brick-and-mortar stores.

5   Findings

Of the 81 online participants, we retained the responses of the 64 who met our screening criterion of the presence of explicit information security policies in their organizations. Of these, 48 (75 %) were employed full-time and 16 (25 %) part-time (33 females / 31 males) with ages ranging from 21 to 60 (median = 32).[1] A further 15 participants completed the study in the laboratory (12 employed full-time and 3 part-time; 8 females and 7 males) ranging in age from 27 to 43 (median = 36).

The lowest value of Cronbach's alpha for the set of items for rating each feature (see Sect. 4) was 0.94, indicating excellent internal consistency. Therefore, we combined the ratings into a persuasiveness score by averaging the five individual ratings. Figure 2 shows notched box plots of the persuasiveness scores for each feature (higher values indicate greater persuasiveness). The notches in the boxes indicate the 95 percent confidence interval of the median. The line at 4 on the y-axis marks the neutral mid-point of the 7-point Likert-type scale. We found that Risk Communication, Statistics, and Security Quiz were rated more persuasive compared to Security Points, Challenges, and Personalization.

We consulted the open-ended answers of the online and laboratory participants to the question "What is your opinion about this feature?" The first author

---

[1] Four participants declined to provide their age.

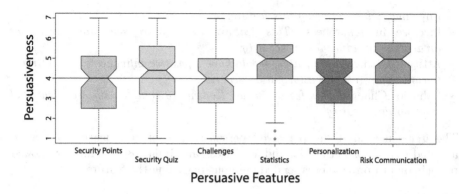

Fig. 2. Persuasiveness rating for each feature (1 = Strongly Disagree to 7 = Strongly Agree).

and a researcher not connected with the study independently read all responses and used open coding [16] to generate potential descriptors. Upon comparison and discussion, the two independent sets of descriptors were consolidated into a single set of 14 characteristics describing the features: *instructive, easy to understand, useful, playful, motivating, informative, innovative, efficient, pleasing, context appropriate, appealing, competition inducing, privacy protecting,* and *detailed.*

The coding further indicated whether the answer expressed positive or negative views regarding the particular characteristic since this was identified as an important dimension during open coding. For almost every feature, opinions were split. For example, playfulness was seen positively (*enjoyable*) or negatively (*childish*). Statistics received the greatest proportion of positive remarks (64.8 %) and Security Points the most negative (65.1 %). For a nuanced understanding, we examined salient comments. On the positive side, many participants found each feature to be understandable and useful. Several participants expressed positive opinions about the ability of the Security Quiz, Statistics, and Risk Communication features to raise security awareness and promote learning. On the negative side, a roughly equivalent number of participants deemed the features useless, unhelpful, or confusing. Several commented that the playfulness of features like Security Points was childish and unprofessional. (*"This is like a game. This will not be appropriate in my company. Employees should do important stuff."*). Participants found Risk Communication disruptive to the ongoing task. Further, several expressed displeasure that they were allowed to dismiss the warning. (*"It is weird that I can open a 'Low sensitive' document although it's against the security policy."*). Instead, some preferred being denied access altogether. (*"If I am not allowed to open it, it should not open."*). Further, participants felt that the competition introduced by Challenges could have a negative effect on relationships with colleagues. (*"To be better than others means showing that someone else is worse."*). Other negative responses were an artifact of the prototype nature of the probe. For instance, participants complained that the Statistics were not sufficiently detailed and nuanced and the purpose, and subsequent use, of the Personalization questionnaire was unclear.

Verbalized thoughts of the laboratory participants while interacting with the probe confirmed that the various annoyances and shortcomings arose chiefly due to the missing detail and polish of the probe, rather than the underlying persuasive strategies. For instance, laboratory participants expressed desires for more practical benefits for Security Points, such as meals, breaks, vacation, etc. (*"Not an incentive for me. Better: new tablet, free meals in the cafeteria."*). Similar to typed open-ended responses, the verbalized thoughts included demand for more detail. For instance, participants wished that the Statistics included not only the number but also the severity of security breaches. They also alluded to various opportunities for pertinent system feedback, such as the extent of correctness of each option in the Security Quiz and the secure way to deal with the Risk Communication warning.

6   Discussion and Implications

It was beneficial to conduct the study in two modes. Although the number of laboratory participants was small, having access to their thinking as they interacted with the probe was valuable for understanding the reactions to the features and illuminating the underlying reasons. It also helped confirm that participants understood the scenario and were immersed in it.

Security is secondary to the task at hand, often obstructing the ongoing activity. Users are inclined to view security requirements with frustration rather than enjoyment. While the neutral ratings for some of our persuasive features are reflective of this fact, the overall comments referring to user experience and adoption illustrate the general positive reception for the persuasive features, suggesting that the underlying strategies could contribute to reducing the annoyance of an otherwise unenjoyable task. Our results thus indicate the promise of *persuasive security* for helping employees understand and follow work practices compliant with the organizational security policy.

At the same time, results also show that individuals could react to a particular feature in opposite ways. It might be impossible to resolve certain fundamental divergences, such as whether one views playfulness as enjoyable or unprofessional. Ensuring coverage across a diversity of views may require combining several features and strategies, instead of relying on a single approach. Appropriate personalization could also mitigate the impact of differences by tailoring system operation to individual preferences.

The probe merely served as the means to achieving our goal of evaluating the individual persuasive features. Rather than implementation as a separate system, such as our probe, we envision and advocate that the features be appropriately integrated within existing security applications (e.g., virus scanners, password change systems, access control mechanisms, etc.) and integrated across all systems that comprise the organizational security infrastructure. In this regard, our findings point to specific design implications for each of the persuasive features we evaluated:

Security Points. It is important to take into account whether playful and game-like elements such as Security Points and Badges are suitable in an organizational context where they might run counter to expected professionalism and seriousness. Moreover, rewards like Security Points should be designed to provide tangible value. The utility of such features could be significantly increased if users could convert them from a *virtual* state to a personally meaningful incentive, such as meals, gift certificates, etc.

Security Quiz. We found that it is essential not only to reveal the correct answer to the quiz but also to explain the rationale behind how it was obtained. In the case of multiple possible answers, the quiz ought to support and explain relative rankings of the choices. Toward this end, it might be helpful to administer quizzes at regular intervals (e.g., 'Quiz of the Day') as well as at contextually appropriate times (e.g., when the user engages in an insecure action).

Challenges. While competition caters to the inner human desire for rivalry and accomplishment, it might have a negative impact on work dynamics and collegiality among colleagues. Some participants in our study suggested including Challenges based on cooperation. Cooperative security tasks could help employees learn from each other and foster a positive group dynamic and team spirit.

Statistics. The Statistics feature was well-liked. We believe that the appeal stemmed from the usefulness of the information for comparing one's practices with the larger picture as well as the visual presentation that made it easy to comprehend. At the same time, findings indicated that the feature needs to incorporate a large range of possible factors to visualize and to support modifying the visualizations to reveal important nuance. The former could be implemented by incorporating a diversity of aspects covered by the information security policy, such as security updates, VPN, etc. To add nuance, the interface ought to facilitate examination of relative as well as absolute measures. It can be beneficial to allow additional sensemaking operations such as classifying, grouping, sorting, and filtering the visualized information based on relevant aspects, such as importance, severity, recency, etc.

Personalization. Participants found it difficult to understand the Personalization feature and its connection with information security. These difficulties appeared to be driven largely by the one-time nature of the study and the nonfunctioning nature of this feature in the probe. Nonetheless, we obtained useful insight from participant complaints regarding the length of the questionnaire and the lack of clarity regarding how the answers were used. For instance, a personalization questionnaire in a deployed system could be administered one question at a time and completed over a longer period. Interaction data regarding employee use of devices and information resources could further augment the quality and the nature of personalization.

Risk Communication. While participants appreciated the contextual nature of Risk Communication, they complained about disruption and obtrusiveness.

Moreover, they were frustrated that it did not offer guidance on achieving the task securely. These findings illustrate that effective Risk Communication needs to balance a variety of tensions, such as whether to allow a policy violation to avoid interrupting the task and blocking user action. Regardless of the approach, whenever Risk Communication is necessary, it is an opportunity for contextual security training via effective information presentation.

7   Limitations

There were interdependencies among the persuasive features. For instance, Security Points were incorporated in the Security Quiz, Challenges, Personalization, and Risk Communication features. These interdependencies might have led to overlapping effects. Additionally, randomization to avoid order effects may have resulted in somewhat unnatural sequencing, thus hampering full understanding of a feature. Risk Communication may have been affected by an order effect because it was encountered at the end. We examined a single usage instance using an interface probe lacking back-end functionality. Moreover, participants had no prior exposure to the probe. A longitudinal study of user behavior within a functioning system is needed to verify that our self-reported intentions extend to actual user practices and to examine how they are affected by usage experience and learning. Given our self-selected and geographically-restricted sample, replication is needed to verify generalizability.

8   Conclusion

Our goal was to investigate if persuasive features could raise employee awareness of their organization's information security policy and promote policy compliant behavior. To achieve this objective, we applied eight persuasive strategies to implement six persuasive features in a design probe. Online and laboratory evaluation suggests that the features hold promise but could be enhanced by additional feedback and concretely beneficial incentives. A functioning real-life deployment is needed to study the longitudinal impact of the persuasive features on contextual behavior. We hope that these findings spur explorations to investigate how persuasive strategies could be employed to develop additional persuasive security features.

Acknowledgments. We thank the study participants. We acknowledge Elke Mattheiss for help in coding open-ended responses. This work was partially funded by the European Union Seventh Framework Programme (FP7/2007-2013) under grant agreement 318508 (MUSES: Multiplatform USable Endpoint Security). Dr. Patil's participation in the research was funded by the Helsinki Institute of Information Technology (HIIT) Visitor Programme.

References

1. Bulgurcu, B., Cavusoglu, H., Benbasat, I.: Information security policy compliance: An empirical study of rationality-based beliefs and information security awareness. MIS Q. **34**(3), 523–548 (2010)
2. Busch, M., Wolkerstorfer, P., Hochleitner, C., Regal, G., Tscheligi, M.: Designing a persuasive application to improve organizational information security policy awareness, attitudes and behavior. In: Poster Abstract, 10th Symposium on Usable Privacy and Security, SOUPS 2014 (2014)
3. Chiasson, S., Forget, A., Biddle, R., van Oorschot, P.C.: Influencing users towards better passwords: Persuasive cued click-points. In: Proceedings of the 22nd British HCI Group Annual Conference, BCS-HCI 2008, pp. 121–130, British Computer Society, Swinton, UK (2008)
4. Chiasson, S., Stobert, E., Forget, A., Biddle, R., Van Oorschot, P.: Persuasive cued click-points: Design, implementation, and evaluation of a knowledge-based authentication mechanism. IEEE Trans. Dependable Secur. Comput. **9**(2), 222–235 (2012)
5. Department for Business, Innovation & Skills: Information security breaches survey (2013). http://www.pwc.co.uk/assets/pdf/cyber-security-2013-exec-summary.pdf
6. Drozd, F., Lehto, T., Oinas-Kukkonen, H.: Exploring perceived persuasiveness of a behavior change support system: a structural model. In: Bang, M., Ragnemalm, E.L. (eds.) PERSUASIVE 2012. LNCS, vol. 7284, pp. 157–168. Springer, Heidelberg (2012)
7. Forget, A., Chiasson, S., Biddle, R.: Persuasion as education for computer security. In: Bastiaens, T., Carliner, S. (eds.) Proceedings of World Conference on E-Learning in Corporate, Government, Healthcare, and Higher Education 2007, pp. 822–829. AACE, Quebec City, Canada, October 2007
8. Forget, A., Chiasson, S., Biddle, R.: Lessons from brain age on persuasion for computer security. In: CHI 2009 Extended Abstracts on Human Factors in Computing Systems, CHI EA 2009, pp. 4435–4440. ACM, NY, USA, New York (2009)
9. Forget, A., Chiasson, S., van Oorschot, P.C., Biddle, R.: Persuasion for stronger passwords: Motivation and pilot study. In: Oinas-Kukkonen, H., Hasle, P., Harjumaa, M., Segerståhl, K., Øhrstrøm, P. (eds.) PERSUASIVE 2008. LNCS, vol. 5033, pp. 140–150. Springer, Heidelberg (2008)
10. Khan, B., Alghathbar, K.S., Khan, M.K.: Information security awareness campaign: An alternate approach. In: Kim, T., Adeli, H., Robles, R.J., Balitanas, M. (eds.) ISA 2011. CCIS, vol. 200, pp. 1–10. Springer, Heidelberg (2011)
11. Mangold, L.V.: Using ontologies for adaptive information security training. In: Proceedings of the 2012 Seventh International Conference on Availability, Reliability and Security, ARES 2012, pp. 522–524. IEEE Computer Society (2012)
12. Merhi, M.I., Midha, V.: The impact of training and social norms on information security compliance: A pilot study. In: International Conference on Information Systems: Research in Progress, ICIS 2012 (2012)
13. Oinas-Kukkonen, H., Harjumaa, M.: A systematic framework for designing and evaluating persuasive systems. In: Oinas-Kukkonen, H., Hasle, P., Harjumaa, M., Segerståhl, K., Øhrstrøm, P. (eds.) PERSUASIVE 2008. LNCS, vol. 5033, pp. 164–176. Springer, Heidelberg (2008)
14. Sheng, S., Magnien, B., Kumaraguru, P., Acquisti, A., Cranor, L.F., Hong, J., Nunge, E.: Anti-phishing Phil: The design and evaluation of a game that teaches people not to fall for phish. In: Proceedings of the 3rd Symposium on Usable Privacy and Security, SOUPS 2007, pp. 88–99. ACM, NY, USA, New York (2007)

15. Siponen, M.T.: A conceptual foundation for organizational information security awareness. Inf. Manage. Comput. Secur. **8**(1), 31–41 (2000)
16. Strauss, A., Corbin, J.: Open coding. Basics Qual. Res.: Grounded Theor. Proc. Tech. **2**, 101–121 (1990)
17. Thomson, M.E., von Solms, R.: Information security awareness: Educating your users effectively. Inf. Manage. Comput. Secur. **6**(4), 167–173 (1998)
18. Venkatesh, V., Bala, H.: Technology acceptance model 3 and a research agenda on interventions. Decis. Sci. **39**(2), 273–315 (2008)
19. Yeo, A.C., Rahim, M.M., Ren, Y.Y.: Use of persuasive technology to change end users' IT security aware behavior: a pilot study. Int. J. Psychol. Behav. Sci. **1**(1), 48–54 (2009)

Lock Up the Lighter: Experience Prototyping of a Lively Reflective Design for Smoking Habit Control

Kenny K.N. Chow[✉]

School of Design, The Hong Kong Polytechnic University,
Hung Hom, Hong Kong
sdknchow@polyu.edu.hk

Abstract. Mobile apps have been employed in assisting people to control various addictive habits including smoking. These apps track users' behavior mainly via self-reporting, which demands users' patience in making explicit input. This paper presents Lock Up, which requires users to lock their lighters in a smart case connected to an app. It heuristically estimates the continuous time of a user without smoking and metaphorically overshadows the lighter by foregrounding the smoking consequence due to the accessibility of the lighter. After reviewing major behavior models, we extend the notion of lively interactive systems grounded in cognitive science and phenomenology, and introduce a design framework promoting behavior control via provoking imagination and reflection. An experience prototype of Lock Up has been built for participants to use in the laboratory environment. The evaluation is exploratory and generative, providing qualitative data to enrich the proposed user experiences and informing orientation toward the next iteration.

Keywords: Reflective design · Liveliness · Embodied interaction · Conceptual blending · Imagination · Behavior change

1 Introduction

When searching Apple's App Store or Google Play with the keyword 'smoking', one would find many mobile apps aiming to assist users to control their smoking behavior or even to quit smoking. These apps usually track how much time has passed since their users smoked last time, or how many cigarettes their users has smoked each day, by requiring one to self-report. Users have to remember to launch the apps and input whenever they smoke. This is demanding even to self-motivated users. Although these apps usually provide the users' progress statistics (e.g., how much money saved, how many days of life regained based on scientific estimation, etc.) as a hopeful encouragement, the factual data needs sparks for highlighting the immediate pleasure or pain and the contingent hope or fear. We believe incorporating reflective design [1] and the liveliness framework [2] can create those sparks.

Lock Up is a reflective, lively interactive system aiming to assist users in controlling their smoking habit via provoking imagination, emotion, and so reflection in them. The initial idea originated from a design student (Ms. Lui Yan Yan, School of

A. Meschtscherjakov et al. (Eds.): PERSUASIVE 2016, LNCS 9638, pp. 352–364, 2016.
DOI: 10.1007/978-3-319-31510-2_30

Design, The Hong Kong Polytechnic University)'s graduation project, which we have further developed into an experience prototype based on the design framework of liveliness. Grounded in cognitive semantics in cognitive science, the psychology of emotion, and phenomenological approaches to interaction design, the notion of liveliness suggests drawing on analogies with everyday life experience in designing interactive systems in order to provoke user imagination and emotion at multiple cognitive levels. Users immediately understand how to operate the systems at initial moments of use, and then make metaphorical, reflective meaning during the later contingent moments. The two levels of meaning construction enabled by liveliness can be employed to create sparks for highlighting the motivators for behavior change.

Lock Up requires users to put their lighters in a smart case and lock it up. This is a heuristic way to estimate how much time a user has passed without smoking. After closing the hinged cover tightly, the user sees the LED (light-emitting diode) lights on the case moving fast back and forth (Fig. 1). The mobile app then shows a wireless connection set up with the case. To create a spark for highlighting the immediate pain as a motivator, the user is required to blow at the smartphone for a lung capacity test (Fig. 2). The app responds with a default result: a skeleton graphic and a message saying that the user has been seriously infected (Fig. 3a). The skeleton, together with the fast moving lights on the case, seems to signal emergency and call for action. After spending some time on sports activities, the user gets improvement in the lung capacity test, from the skeleton, to a zombie (Fig. 3b), then a half-zombie-half-human (Fig. 3c), a healthy human (Fig. 3d), and so on. An immediate understanding comes about in the user's mind that locking up the lighter and doing workout make progress, which also project a hopeful future.

Yet, the future is contingent. The user is given a leeway to get around the strict smoking control. One can unwrap the case and take out the lighter anytime, but the lung capacity test result then quickly drops back to the skeleton, even though the user keeps doing sports. During these contingent moments, the unexpected change in health status makes the user wonder. The user may invoke different interpretive frames, for instance the infection frame, to make sense of the contingency. The lighter is the source of infection. This metaphorical, reflective meaning is another spark that highlights the

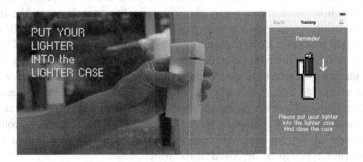

Fig. 1. Lock Up requires the user to put the lighter into the case, and the lights on the case start moving.

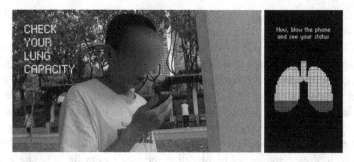

Fig. 2. Lock Up allows the user to blow at the smartphone for the lung capacity test.

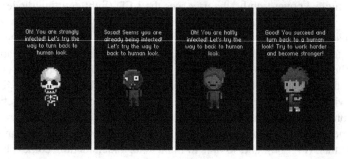

Fig. 3. a-d. The default result of the first test is the skeleton, followed by the zombie, the half-zombie-half-human, the healthy human, and so on.

contingent fear (or hope) in the future. The user may see the lighter in a very different way and want to lock it up again.

The design of Lock Up demonstrates an application of the liveliness framework in reflective design for behavior control. During initial moments of use, the system's sensory feedback is a spark highlighting the immediate pain or pleasure, resulting in immediate understanding of the action. During later contingent moments, the system's unexpected changes are another spark foregrounding the contingent fear or hope in the future of which the user makes a metaphorical, reflective meaning that 'the lighter is evil'. An experience prototype has been built for participants to use in the laboratory. This evaluation process is more exploratory and generative than validating. The design framework provides guidelines for designers and researchers to propose possible, intended meaning in terms of user imagination, emotion, and reflection, while the evaluation assists in finding real and particular instances in order to support and enrich the user experience narratives predicted via the framework. This paper first articulates the theoretical framework, followed by the research design, experience prototyping, and discussion of the findings. The conclusion is the design implication for next iteration of prototypes to be deployed in the wild.

2 Theoretical Framework

2.1 Behavior Models

Fogg Behavior Model (FBM). The design of Lock Up refers to a few influential models of human behavior. B. J. Fogg [3] introduces a behavior model for designing persuasive systems. The three determinants for a person to perform a behavior include motivation, ability, and triggers. Motivation includes immediate results (i.e., pleasure vs. pain), foreseeable outcomes (i.e., hope vs. fear), and social conforming. Ability is related to perceived probability of success, which can be improved through empowering the users. With sufficient motivation and ability, people become determined but still need triggers for taking action. Fogg introduces three types of triggers that are applicable to the design of Lock Up. Spark is used to foreground the relevant motivators to the user (e.g., using iconic representation to show immediate status and assist in projecting foreseeable development). Facilitator is to make the behavior easier or harder to do (e.g., locking up the lighter). Signal is to provide timely and relevant reminder.

While motivation and ability are dependent on many internal and external factors that are less controllable to designers, triggers have become more accessible means to designers with today's ubiquitous technologies. FBM's triggers are an important consideration in designing persuasive systems, especially when different stages of behavior change are concerned.

Five Stages of Change. James O. Prochaska and his colleagues [4] summarize research on self-initiated and professionally assisted change of addictive behaviors in five stages. At the pre-contemplation stage, the individual does not see the problem and so has no intention to change. At the contemplation stage, the individual is aware of the problem and starts seriously thinking of overcoming it, without taking any action yet. At the preparation stage, one is about to take action. At the action stage, the modification is visible and even recognized by others. Finally the maintenance stage is about whether the change can endure for more than six months without relapse, which is generally regarded as a successful indicator. Based on this model, designing for behavior change needs overview of the whole journey but also identification of a focusing stage. The pre-contemplation stage requires persuasively informing people of the problem. Spark can be added to bring hope or fear to the people (e.g., showing exaggerated graphic images of current status). The contemplation and preparation stages have to enable and even empower the people. Using facilitators to make the behavior easier or harder to do is an effective intervention (e.g., hiding the lighter from one's sight). At the action and maintenance stages, the design has to provide reminder or progress report (e.g., showing incremental changes of the status).

In summary, Lock Up has the following features based on the above models:

- Focusing on the contemplation and preparation stages, Lock Up helps the user temporarily forget smoking by hiding the lighter from the user's sight. It makes the key to smoking less accessible.

- To foreground the relevant motivators, Lock Up shows the user's lung capacity in terms of iconic images like skeleton and zombie. Subsequent images assist the user in projecting foreseeable improvement, or conversely bring fear to those still in the pre-contemplation stage.
- Lock Up shows incremental signs of successful performance from skeleton to healthy human and even superhero to strengthen the user's determination. It is important for those in the action and maintenance stages.

2.2   Lively Interactive Artifacts for Behavior Control

Lock Up demonstrates how lively interactive artifacts can be used for promoting behavior change via provoking reflection in users. Designing lively artifacts [5] usually draws on embodied interaction [6] and conceptual metaphors [7, 8], making the interactions reminiscent of users' past experiences in everyday life and stimulating meaning construction at multiple cognitive levels during different moments of use.

During initial moments of use, the user acts upon the artifact and perceive quick feedback. The interaction between the user and the lively artifact, represented by two arrows in Don Norman's conceptual model diagram [9], is so instantaneous that turns into a loop, resulting in immediate understanding of the operation with a sense of control (Fig. 4a). The operation is similar, but not exactly, to a common experience, triggering an immediate blend of the current experience and the past. Blending, a theory introduced by Gilles Fauconnier and Mark Turner [10], is a pervasive cognitive operation that integrates concepts and outputs new one. At this immediate level, the output is an embodied imagination between familiar (past experience) and unfamiliar (new experience).

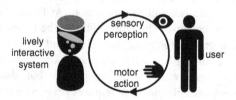

Fig. 4a. A sensorimotor feedback loop between a user and a lively interactive system during initial moments of use, giving the user a sense of control.

During later contingent moments of use, the lively artifact shows unexpected changes, bringing the user a sense of wonder (Fig. 4b). The user then invokes an interpretive frame [11] to make sense of and account for the changes. The frame comes with a past scenario in the user's memory. The user analogically maps the current experience of the changes with the past scenario, and elaborates a metaphorical blend, resulting in an imaginative scenario with reflective meaning.

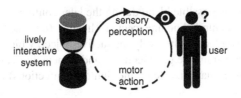

Fig. 4b. Unexpected changes seemingly unrelated to user input during contingent moments, bringing the user a sense of wonder.

We illustrate the above cognitive processes based on Fauconnier and Turner's integration diagrams [10]. An integration diagram consists of circles representing mental spaces, each of which contains conceptual elements of a scenario, such as actors, objects, actions, or relations. The two horizontal spaces are input for the blend, while the one below is the output. The horizontal solid lines between the two input spaces are links connecting the counterparts respectively. These outer-space links are compressed into inner-space relations inside the blend. Other elements are only selectively projected from either input to the blend. Figure 5a shows a possible immediate blend. What we add to the integration diagram includes the sensorimotor feedback loop, which envelops motor action (e.g., blow at the phone, lock the lighter up, etc.) and sensory perception (e.g., see the skeleton and the warning, see fast moving lights, etc.) in the mental space. The left input is the current experience enabled by a lively interactive object featuring a loop mobilized by one's impulsive desire and automatic emotional appraisal, which is analogical to a past experience (e.g., walk to security check with a buzz) denoted by the right input. The result is an immediate blend (e.g., "I'm forced to put it away").

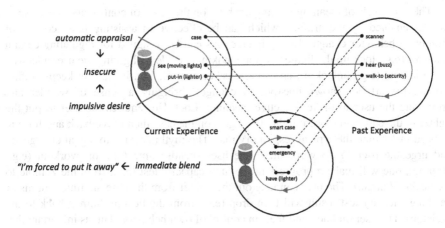

Fig. 5a. A possible immediate blend triggered by Lock Up at initial moments

Figure 5b illustrates a possible blend during the later contingent moments. The loop is fading in the user's mind, but unexpected changes (e.g., see the skeleton again despite exercising) take place in the lively interactive object, which prompts the user to invoke an interpretation frame (e.g., infection), and a metaphorical blend results. This gives rise to an imagined narrative (e.g., the lighter is infectious) and elicits emotions (e.g., fear).

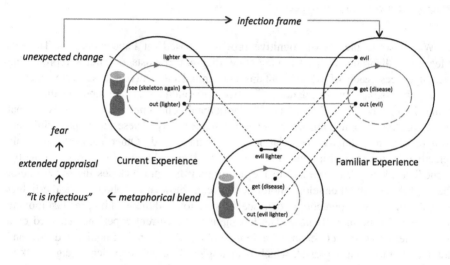

Fig. 5b. A possible metaphorical blend taking place at Lock Up's contingent moments

The two levels of meaning making are built on the sense of control and the sense of wonder enabled by the artifact, which can be effective in assisting habit control or promoting behavior change. Lively interactions can be designed for regulating certain behavior (e.g., lock up the lighter to stop smoking), while still giving the user a leeway to get around (e.g., unlock it), and so a sense of control. Yet, if the user keeps getting around, the artifact shows unexpected changes, bringing a sense of wonder and prompting the user to make reflective meaning. Lock Up requires the user to put the lighter in the case and close it tight. The lights on the case then move back and forth at a speed faster than the typical respiratory rate. The rhythm seems to signal emergency and urge the user to do workout. If the user spends some time on workout (e.g., running), one will make a progress in the lung capacity test (e.g., from the zombie to the healthy human). The user can take out the lighter from the case anytime, but his or her lung capacity test result will then drop (e.g., from the healthy human back to the skeleton). The user on one hand feels in control of own behavior. This is important that one would not feel being tightly regulated. On the other hand, the user wonders what makes the health status reverted. After knowing the culprit is the lighter, one may invoke the infection frame and want to stay away from the lighter.

3 Experience Prototyping

Aligning the design framework of liveliness with major behavior models allows us to predict the possible user experiences of Lock Up in terms of conceptual integration diagrams. To substantiate the proposed blends in Figs. 5a and 5b (i.e., for those in italic in the figures), experience prototyping has been conducted to generate real and particular instances. Experience prototyping conveys an experience, from the sensory to the cognitive, with a design to designers or target users [12]. It can be in any kind of representation or medium. In this project, we have built both physical and digital artifacts and let participants experience in a simulated environment in the laboratory.

The experience prototype of Lock Up includes the lighter case with a hinged cover and a series of LED lights on its side, together with the mobile app. When the case is closed with something in it, the lights start to move in a line back and forth. When the case is open, the lights move only toward the hinged cover direction for a while and then go off. The mobile app allows the user to blow at the smartphone's built-in microphone for the lung capacity test, and then responds with results according to the script of the experience test. The app can also forge a sign of wireless connection with the closed case.

The study was conducted in our usability study room with one participant (having smoking habit) a time, including activities and semi-structured interviews. The activities started with launching the app and asking the participant to blow at the smartphone. The result was scripted to be the skeleton. The participant was then asked to put his or her lighter into the case and close the hinged cover tight by wrapping it with medical tape. The lights on the case started to move back and forth. The participant was led to a treadmill and ran for three minutes, followed by the second lung capacity test. The result was scripted to be the zombie. This time the participant was tempted whether he or she would like to take the lighter out. Another three-minute run and then the third blow followed. If the lighter had already been taken out, the result reverted to the skeleton; otherwise, the half-zombie-half-human was shown. This concluded the activity session.

The in-depth semi-structured interview was divided into two sessions. The outline roughly matched the timeline of the predicted user experience based on the liveliness framework. The first session is about the initial moments, questioning about immediate blends, impulsive desires, and automatic appraisals. After the first session, the participant was asked to do the lung capacity test again. The result was scripted to be the skeleton again, because the lighter was not in the case. The second session then follows, questioning about the later contingent moments related to unexpected changes, metaphorical blends, and extended appraisals. Table 1 summarizes the questions.

Six participants, all males, have taken the test. One of them (DJ) is at the age between 18 and 25 years. The other participants are at the age between 25 and above and having smoking habit for more than three years. Three of them (XX, LL, and DJ) have background in Design or related disciplines, and three (CL, XR, and ZB) in Land Surveying. The questionnaire results informed that all of them smoked at least four or five times a day, with XR being the most frequent smoker (about 10 times a day). XX was at the preparation stage (was focusing on sports activities to reduce smoking frequency). Others were at the contemplation stage, being fully aware of the health problems associated with smoking. Half of them (DJ, CL, XR) were more motivated to discontinue smoking.

Table 1. Questions asked during interviews refer to the theoretical framework

About immediate blends	• *When you blew the first time, what did you see?* • *When you put the lighter into the case, what did you see? What did it mean to you? Could you recall any slice of life like this?* • *When you blew after the first run, what did you see? What about after the second run? What did it mean to you?* • *Could you recall anything similar in your life?*
About impulsive desires and automatic appraisals	• *How did you feel after seeing zombie?* • *How did you feel after seeing half-zombie?* • *How did you feel when seeing the flash right after putting lighter in?*
About unexpected changes, interpretive frames, and metaphorical blends	• *Do you notice any changes? Is it what you expected? What do you think? (If don't know why, show the app reminder)* • *Could you recall any similar scenarios from your past experience?* • *How would you see the relationship between smoking and the lighter?* • *How would you like the lighter? How would you describe it?* • *What do you want to do now? What else (other than exercising) in your mind?* • *From skeleton to zombie, how would you project your goal?*
Extended appraisals	• *What do you think now? What did you feel about it overall?*

3.1 Qualitative Findings

The findings include qualitative data such as participants' quotes during the interviews, which reveal their thoughts and feelings. This paper only highlights (Table 2) some of those used to fill in Figs. 5a and 5b.

Table 2. Significant responses from the 6 participants

About immediate blends	To DJ, the flashing rate of the lights seemed like charging or downloading. XX, CL, and XR recalled the moments they could not have the lighter with them (e.g., forgot to bring, during swimming, being on plane, etc.).
About impulsive desires and automatic appraisals	Putting the lighter into the case, most participants (XX, CL, and XR) felt insecure, anxious. CL said, "do not want to tape the lighter", but then conversely "felt negatively after removing the tape."

(Continued)

Table 2. (*Continued*)

About unexpected changes, interpretive frames, and metaphorical blends	All participants said the reverted status was unexpected. Most of them tried to interpret with logic or science, like "I smoked too much before this test" (ZB), or "maybe exercise generates some chemicals in my body and after some time when there is no chemical, I feel like having a cigarette again" (XX).
	Only DJ remembered that putting the lighter in the case was one condition.
	Being reminded of the lighter, participants invoked different interpretive frames to predict the next move.
	The infection frame:
	"As it told me I was infected so maybe the lighter is the infection, and when you put it in the box, you may not get the infection." (DJ)
	"It doesn't seem like my lighter anymore ... it causes me some disease, made me lose all my effort." (XR)
	The partnership frame:
	"Key and lock, the lighter is like a key to light a cigarette." (ZB)
	The devil frame:
	"Lighters and exercise may be like devil and angel." (LL)
Extended appraisals	*Satisfied:*
	"Overall satisfied, also realized if I don't put lighter inside, I am a skeleton, not living a healthy life." (DJ)
	"If putting the lighter back, would like to try doing something to stay away from smoking." (CL)
	Uneasy:
	"Overall experience is like going to swimming pool and putting things like money and cards in a box. We can't use it..." (ZB)

4   Discussion

4.1   The Immediate Level

The lights on the case are designed to move back and forth at a speed faster than the respiratory rate to create an illusion that the lighter is resisting inside the case. This is to anthropomorphize the lighter. Yet, this metaphor was not obvious to the participants, who unconsciously assumed the case was a device and the lighter was a tool, and so the light movement seemed like charging or downloading (DJ). On the other hand, half of the participants felt tense after putting the lighter in the case. They closed the hinged cover tightly and wrapped it by tape. Meanwhile, they saw the lights moving fast. The frequency seemed to suggest alertness. The sensorimotor feedback loop evoked a slice of life in them. At least two participants (XX, XR) mentioned the moments of having no access to lighters on plane. Lighters are classified as dangerous goods and cannot be carried. The immediate blend between putting the lighter into the case and the experience of boarding resulted in a message that the dangerous lighter should be put away (Fig. 5a). To facilitate this blend, the lights should be made to flash faster.

After exercising and making progress in the app, all participants became increasingly happy or satisfied. Participant CL even had a negative feeling when taking back the lighter, because this made smoking possible to him again.

4.2   The Reflective Level

All participants felt shock when they saw the test results reverting back to the skeleton in the middle of the interviews. Nearly all of them, except Participant DJ, attributed the downgrade to the hiatus of exercising. They invoked different frames based on logic or science to account for the unexpected change. For example, Participant ZB thought it was because of heavy smoking just before coming to the test; Participant XX even imagined the "good" chemicals generated from exercising had been fading away.

Only Participant DJ remembered the lighter was in the case during the workout, and so figured out that was the reason for the skeleton result. He could even point out the system knew how long the lighter was in the case and gave the scores. Other than running, walking or watching movies would also do. The text messages of the app evoked the infection frame in his mind. The lighter was the source of infection, and putting it in the case could save him. This metaphorical blend is shown in Fig. 5b.

Other participants who were unaware of the lighter were then shown with the instructional screen of the app they have seen earlier. They immediately realized the key role played by the lighter. They invoked different interpretive frames. Participant XR, initially thought the lung capacity tests were not serious, turned to see the lighter with the infection frame and feared of it. Three participants (XX, CL, ZB) invoked the partnership frame to see the coupling of lighters and cigarettes. They worked together like the key-and-lock relationship. They could do harm, yet either one did not (cf. Fig. 5b). Participant ZB explicitly said lighters might remind him of smoking. Hiding the lighter could be a good strategy for him to control the habit.

Participant LL was skeptical of the singularity of the lighter. He argued the system could not know if he smoked by using another lighter. Yet, he still saw lighters in general like the devil. In summary, the system has successfully cast a shadow on lighters, from dangerous goods, infection, to evil partners. To facilitate these metaphorical blends, the system should highlight whether the lighter is locked or not.

5 Conclusion and Future Work

Designing systems assisting people to control or even change their addictive habits is a major yet challenging mission. Behavior models, including FBM and Five Stages of Change, inform important factors for predicting and anticipating behavior change. Together with our design framework of liveliness, we have developed Lock Up, a reflective lively system, which assists users to reduce or stop smoking via provoking imagination, emotion, and reflection in them. The theoretical framework helps delineate the intended and possible user perceptions, actions, and cognitive processes in terms of conceptual integration diagrams. Experience prototyping generates real and particular samples to substantiate the proposed narratives in terms of blends, emotions, and interpretive frames.

Although the current empirical study consists of only six participants, useful findings include many nuances in the perceptions of different participants. For instance, the moving lights are supposed to arouse the sense of alertness or emergency, but not all participants could recall similar moments in their past experiences. This suggests stronger color (e.g., red) and higher frequency of the moving lights. Most participants focused too much on the workout and forgot the relevance of the lighter during the interviews. This suggests more reminders of the lighter in the mobile app. These insights generated from the tests will be used to further develop Lock Up into the next iteration of prototyping and testing not only in the laboratory but also in the field.

Acknowledgments. The grant GRF from Hong Kong Research Grants Council (PolyU 5412/13H).

References

1. Sengers, P., Boehner, K., David, S., Kaye, J.J.: Reflective design. In: Proceedings of 4th Decennial Conference on Critical Computing, pp. 49–58, Aarhus, Denmark (2005)
2. Chow, K.K.N.: Animation, Embodiment, and Digital Media Human Experience of Technological Liveliness. Palgrave Macmillan, Basingstoke (2013)
3. Fogg, B.J.: A behavior model for persuasive design. In: Persuasive 2009, Claremont, California, USA (2009)
4. Prochaska, J.O., DiClemente, C.C., Norcross, J.C.: In search of how people change: applications to addictive behaviors. Am. Psychol. **47**, 1102–1114 (1992)
5. Chow, K.K.N., Harrell, D.F., Yan, W.K.: Designing and analyzing swing compass: a lively interactive system provoking imagination and affect for persuasion. In: MacTavish, T., Basapur, S. (eds.) PERSUASIVE 2015. LNCS, vol. 9072, pp. 107–120. Springer, Heidelberg (2015)
6. Dourish, P.: Where the Action Is: the Foundations of Embedded Interaction. MIT Press, Cambridge (2001)
7. Lakoff, G., Johnson, M.: Metaphors We Live By. University of Chicago Press, Chicago (2003)
8. Lakoff, G., Turner, M.: More than Cool Reason: a Field Guide to Poetic Metaphor. University of Chicago Press, Chicago (1989)

9. Norman, D.A.: The Design of Everyday Things. Basic Books Inc., New York (2002)
10. Fauconnier, G., Turner, M.: The Way We Think: Conceptual Blending and the Mind's Hidden Complexities. Basic Books, New York (2002)
11. Fillmore, C.J.: Frames and the semantics of understanding. Quaderni di Semantica **6**, 222–254 (1985)
12. Buchenau, M., Suri, J.F.: Experience prototyping. In: DIS 2000 Proceedings of the 3rd Conference on Designing Interactive Systems, pp. 424–433, Brooklyn, New York (2000)

Author Index

Printed in the United States
By Bookmasters